The New Complete
MEDICAL
and HEALTH
ENCYCLOPEDIA

The New Complete
MEDICAL
and HEALTH
ENCYCLOPEDIA

EDITED BY
Richard J. Wagman, M.D., F.A.C.P.

Assistant Clinical Professor of Medicine
Downstate Medical Center
New York, New York

AND BY
the J. G. Ferguson Editorial Staff

Volume Three

J. G. FERGUSON PUBLISHING COMPANY/CHICAGO

Editor

Richard J. Wagman, M.D., F.A.C.P.
Assistant Clinical Professor of
    Medicine
Downstate Medical Center
New York, New York

Contributors to The New Complete Medical and Health Encyclopedia

Consultant in Surgery

N. Henry Moss, M.D., F.A.C.S.
Associate Clinical Professor of
  Surgery
Temple University Health Sciences
  Center and Albert Einstein
  Medical Center;
Past President, American Medical
  Writers Association;
Past President, New York Academy
  of Sciences

Consultant in Gynecology

Douglass S. Thompson, M.D.
Clinical Professor of Obstetrics and
  Gynecology and Clinical Associate
  Professor of Community Medicine
University of Pittsburgh School of
  Medicine

Consultant in Pediatrics

Charles H. Bauer, M.D.
Clinical Associate Professor of
  Pediatrics and Chief of Pediatric
  Gastroenterology
The New York Hospital-Cornell
  Medical Center
New York, New York

Consultants in Psychiatry

Julian J. Clark, M.D.
Assistant Professor of Psychiatry
              and
Rita W. Clark, M.D.
Clinical Assistant Professor of
  Psychiatry
Downstate Medical Center

Consulting Editor

Kenneth N. Anderson
Formerly Editor
Today's Health

Bruce O. Berg, M.D.
Associate Professor
Departments of Neurology and
  Pediatrics
Director, Child Neurology
University of California
San Francisco, California

D. Jeanne Collins
Assistant Professor
College of Allied Health Professions
University of Kentucky
Lexington, Kentucky

Anthony A. Davis
Vice President and Education
    Consultant
Metropolitan X-Ray and Medical
    Sales, Inc.
Olney, Maryland

Peter A. Dickinson
Editor Emeritus
Harvest Years/Retirement Living

Gordon K. Farley, M.D.
Associate Professor of Child
    Psychiatry
Director, Day Care Center
University of Colorado Medical
    Center

Arthur Fisher
Group Editor
Science and Engineering
Popular Science

Edmund H. Harvey, Jr.
Editor
Science World

Helene MacLean
Medical writer

Ben Patrusky
Science writer

Stanley E. Weiss, M.D.
Assistant Attending Physician, Renal
    Service
Beth Israel Hospital and Medical
    Center, New York

Jeffrey S. Willner, M.D.
Attending Radiologist
Southampton Hospital
Southampton, New York

Contents

Volume III

21

Skin and Hair

Not many people have perfectly proportioned faces and bodies, but practically anyone, at any age, can present an attractive appearance if skin is healthy-looking and glowing and hair is clean and shining. Healthy skin and hair can be achieved through good health habits, cleanliness, and personal grooming. Expensive skin-and-hair products may boost self-confidence, but they are a poor substitute for proper diet, exercise, enough sleep, and soap and water or cleansing creams.

The condition of skin and hair reflects a person's physical and emotional health. Of course, general appearance is determined not only by what is going on inside the body but also by outward circumstances, such as extremes of temperature or the use of harsh soaps. Appearance can also be altered temporarily by cosmetics and permanently by surgery.

The Skin

The skin is one of the most important organs of the body. It serves as protection against infection by germs and shields delicate underlying tissue against injury. Approximately one-third of the bloodstream flows through the skin, and as the blood vessels contract or relax in response to heat and cold, the skin acts as a thermostat that helps control body temperature. The two million sweat glands in the skin also regulate body temperature through the evaporation of perspiration. The many delicate nerve endings in the skin make it a sense organ responsive not only to heat and cold but also to pleasure, pain, and pressure.

Certain cells in the skin produce a protective pigmentation that determines its color and guards against overexposure to the ultraviolet rays of the sun. By absorption and elimination, the skin helps regulate the body's chemical and fluid balance. One of the miracles of the skin is that it constantly renews itself.

Structure of the Skin

The skin is made up of two layers. The outer layer, or *epidermis,* has a surface of horny, nonliving cells that form the body's protective envelope. These cells are constantly being shed and replaced by new ones, which are made in the lower or inner layer of the epidermis.

Underneath the epidermis is the *dermis,* the thicker part of the skin. It contains blood vessels, nerves, and connective tissue. The sweat glands are located in the dermis, and they collect fluid containing water, salt, and waste products from the blood. This fluid is sent through tiny canals that end in pores on the skin's surface.

The oil, or *sebaceous,* glands that secrete the oil that lubricates the surface of the skin and hair are also located in the dermis. They are most often associated with hair *follicles.*

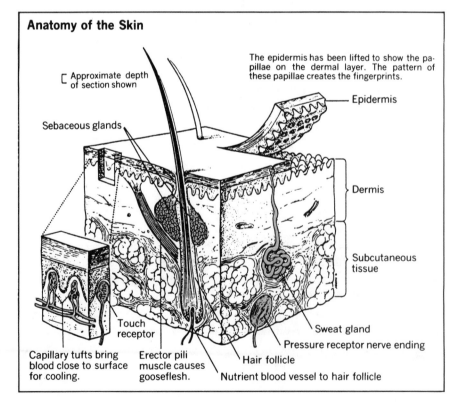

Anatomy of the Skin

The epidermis has been lifted to show the papillae on the dermal layer. The pattern of these papillae creates the fingerprints.

⌈ Approximate depth of section shown

Epidermis

Sebaceous glands

Dermis

Subcutaneous tissue

Touch receptor

Sweat gland

Pressure receptor nerve ending

Capillary tufts bring blood close to surface for cooling.

Erector pili muscle causes gooseflesh.

Hair follicle

Nutrient blood vessel to hair follicle

Hair follicles and oil glands are found over most of the body, with the exception of the palms of the hands and the soles of the feet.

The layer of fatty tissue below the dermis, called *subcutaneous* tissue, acts as an insulator against heat and cold and as a shock absorber against injury.

Skin Color

The basic skin color of each person is determined at birth, and is a part of his heritage that cannot be changed.

Melanin

There are four pigments in the normal skin that affect its color: melanin, oxygenated hemoglobin, reduced hemoglobin, and various carotenes. Of these, *melanin* is the most powerful. The cells that produce it are the same in all races, but there is wide variation in the amount produced, and wide variation in its color, which ranges from black to light tan. Every adult has about 60,000 melanin-producing cells in each square inch of skin.

Melanin cells also affect eye color. When the cells are deep in the eye, the color produced is blue or green. When they are close to the surface, the eye is brown. An *albino,* a person with no melanin, has eyes that appear pink, because the stronger pigment that ordinarily masks the blood vessels is lacking.

Hemoglobin

The pigment that gives blood its color, called *hemoglobin,* has the next greatest effect on skin color. When it is combined with oxygen, a bright red is the result, and this in turn produces the rosy complexion associated with good health in light-skinned people. When such people suffer from reduced hemoglobin because of anemia, they appear to be excessively pale. A concentration of reduced hemoglobin gives the skin a bluish appearance. Because hemoglobin has a weaker coloring effect than the melanin that determines basic skin color, these variations are more visible in lighter-skinned individuals.

Carotenes

The weakest pigments in the skin are the *carotenes*. These produce a yellowish tone that is increased by eating excessive amounts of carrots and oranges. In people with black or brown skin, excess carotene is usually masked by the melanin pigment.

Aging Skin

Skin appearance is affected by both internal and external factors. A baby's skin has a silken quality because it has not yet begun to show the effects of continued exposure to sun and wind. The skin problems associated with adolescence reflect the many glandular changes that occur during the transition to adulthood. As the years pass, the skin becomes the most obvious indicator of aging.

Heredity, general health, and exposure to the elements are some of the factors that contribute to aging skin. Because people with darker skin have built-in protection against the ravages of the sun, their skin usually has a younger appearance than that of lighter-skinned people of comparable age.

In general, the skin of an older person is characterized by wrinkles and shininess. It feels thinner when pinched because it has lost its elasticity and part of the underlying fat that gives firmness to a younger skin.

Constant exposure to sunlight is now thought to play a more important role in the visible aging of skin than the aging process itself. Such exposure also appears to be directly related to the greater frequency of skin cancer among farmers, sailors, and others who spend most of their working hours out of doors.

Care of the Skin

Healthy, normal skin should be washed regularly with mild soap and warm water to remove grease, perspiration, and accumulated dirt. For those with a limited water supply or inadequate bath and shower facilities, sponge baths are a good substitute if the sponge or washcloth is thoroughly rinsed as various parts of the body are washed. Many people feel that a shower is a much more efficient way of getting clean than a bath, since the bath water becomes the receptacle for the dirt washed from the body, instead of its being rinsed away.

No matter what method is used, all soap should be thoroughly rinsed off the skin after washing. Unless specifically prescribed by a physician, medicated or germicidal soaps should not be used, since they may be an irritant. Skin should be dried with a fluffy towel, and bath towels should never be shared. Hands should be washed several times a day, and fingernails kept clean.

Facial skin requires special care because of its constant exposure. The face should be cleaned in the morning and before bedtime. Some people may prefer to use a cleansing cream rather than soap and water. Everyone should avoid massaging soap into the skin, because this may cause drying.

Dry and Oily Skin

Both heredity and environment account for the wide variation in the amount of oil and perspiration secreted by the glands of different people. Also, the same person's skin may be oily in one part of the body and dry in another. Skin on the nose and chin tends to be the oiliest.

Dry Skin

This condition is the result of loss of water from the outer surface of the epidermis and its insufficient replacement from the tissues below. Some causes of the moisture loss are too frequent use of soap and detergents, and constant exposure to dry air. Anyone spending a great deal of time in air-conditioned surroundings in which the humidity has been greatly lowered is likely to suffer from dry skin.

To correct the condition, the use of soap and water should be kept to a minimum for those parts of the body where the skin is dry. Cleansing creams or lotions containing lanolin should be used on the face, hands, elbows, and wherever else necessary. If tub baths are taken, a bath oil can be used in the water or applied to the skin after drying. Baby oil is just as effective and much cheaper than glamorously packaged and overadvertised products. Baby oil or a protective lotion should also be used on any parts of the body exposed to direct sunlight for any extended length of time. Applying oil to the skin will not, however, prevent wrinkles.

Oily Skin

The amount of oil that comes to the surface of the skin through the sebaceous glands is the result not only of heredity but also of temperature and emotional state. In warm weather, when the skin perspires more freely, the oil spreads like a film on the surface moisture. Nonoily foundation lotions can be helpful in keeping the oil spread to a minimum, and so can frequent washing with soap and water. When washing is inconvenient during the day, cleansing pads packaged to fit in pocket or purse are a quick and efficient solution for both men and women.

Too much friction from complexion brushes, rough washcloths, or harsh soaps may irritate rather than improve an oily skin condition.

Deodorants and Antiperspirants

Sweat glands are present almost everywhere in the skin except for the lips and a few other areas. Most of them give off the extremely dilute salt water known as sweat, or perspiration. Their purpose is to cool the body by evaporation of water. Body odors are not produced by perspiration itself but by the bacterial activity that takes place in the perspiration. The activity is most intense in warm, moist parts of the body from which perspiration cannot evaporate quickly, such as the underarm area.

Deodorants

The basic means of keeping this type of bacterial growth under control is through personal cleanliness of both skin and clothing. Deodorant soaps containing antiseptic chemicals are now available. Though they do not kill bacteria, they do reduce the speed with which they multiply.

Underarm deodorants also help to eliminate the odor. They are not meant to stop the flow of perspiration but rather to slow down bacterial growth and mask body odors with their own scent. Such deodorants should be applied immediately after bathing. They are usually more effective if the underarm area is shaved, since the hair in this unexposed area collects perspiration and encourages bacterial growth.

Antiperspirants

Antiperspirants differ from deodorants in that they not only affect the rate of bacterial growth but also reduce the amount of perspiration that reaches the skin surface. Because the action of the chemical salts they contain is cumulative, they seem to be more effective with repeated use. Antiperspirants come under the category of drugs, and their contents must be printed on the container. Deodorants are considered cosmetics, and may or may not name their contents on the package.

No matter what the nature of the advertising claim, neither type of product completely stops the flow of perspiration, nor would it be desirable to do so. Effectiveness of the various brands differs from one person to another. Some may produce a mild allergic reaction; others might be too weak to do a good job. It is practical to experiment with a few different brands, using them under similar conditions, to find the type that works best for you.

Creams and Cosmetics

The bewildering number of creams and cosmetics on the market and the exaggerated claims of some of their advertising can be reduced to a few simple facts. Beauty preparations should be judged by the user on their merits rather than on their claims.

Cold Creams and Cleansing Creams

These two products are essentially the same. They are designed to remove accumulated skin secretions, dirt, and grime, and should be promptly removed from the skin with a soft towel or tissue.

Lubricating Creams and Lotions

Also called night creams, moisturizing creams, and conditioning creams, these products are supposed to prevent the loss of moisture from the skin and promote its smoothness. They are usually left on overnight or for an extended length of time. Anyone with dry skin will find it helpful to apply a moisturizer under foundation cream. This will help keep the skin from drying out even further, and protect it against the effects of air-conditioning.

Vanishing Creams and Foundation Creams

These products also serve the purpose of providing the skin with moisture, but are meant to be applied immediately before putting on makeup.

Rejuvenating Creams

There is no scientific proof that any of the "royal jelly," "secret formula," or "hormone" creams produce a marked improvement on aging skin. They cannot eliminate wrinkles, nor can they regenerate skin tissue.

Medicated Creams and Lotions

These products should not be used except on the advice of a physician, since they may cause or aggravate skin disorders of various kinds.

Lipsticks

Lipsticks contain lanolin, a mixture of oil and wax, a coloring dye, and pigment, as well as perfume. Any of these substances can cause an allergic reaction in individual cases, but such reactions are uncommon. Sometimes the reaction is caused by the staining dye, in which case a "nonpermanent" lipstick should be used.

Cosmetics and the Sensitive Skin

Anyone with a cosmetic problem resulting from sensitive skin should consult a *dermatologist,* a physician specializing in the skin and its diseases. Cosmetic companies will inform a physician of the ingredients in their products, and he or she can then recommend a brand that will agree with the patient's specific skin problems. The physician may also recommend a special nonallergenic preparation.

Eye Makeup

Eye-liner and mascara brushes and pencils—and lipsticks, for that matter—can carry infection and should never be borrowed or lent. *Hypoallergenic* makeup, which is specially made for those who get allergic reactions to regular eye makeup, is available.

Suntanning Creams and Lotions

Growing awareness that exposure to the sun may cause skin cancer (see "Skin Cancer" in Ch. 18, *Cancer*) has led to a demand for a variety of skin creams and lotions. The preparations protect the skin or speed the tanning process. Many of the "sunblocks" and "sunscreens" keep the ultraviolet radiation in sunlight from reaching the skin. They are adapted to six basic skin types, ranging from type 1, which burns easily and never tans, to types 5 and 6, which never burn and usually tan well.

Skin lotions and creams are rated according to a "sun protection factor" (SPF). Among the basic ratings are SPF 4, providing "moderate protection;" SPF 8, a "maximal" sunscreen; and SPF 15, with "ultra" protection. Other ratings range up to SPF 50. Some medical authorities question the need for sunscreens rated higher than 15 or 20. Food and Drug Administration ratings go only to SPF 15. Many newer sunscreens are greaseless, hypoallergenic, waterproof, or PABA-free. PABA, or para-aminobenzoic acid, is a sunscreen chemical that can irritate skin and stain clothing.

Sunscreen ratings indicate, in theory, how long the user can stay in the sun without burning. A lotion or cream with a rating of SPF 2 should allow users to remain exposed twice as long as they could with no protection at all. The Skin Cancer Foundation believes that persons who burn in the sun should uniformly wear an SPF 15 protective preparation.

Persons who want suntans have many products from which to choose. "Tanning accelerators" in lotion form speed up the tanning process. A pocket-sized "sun exposure meter" operated electronically alerts the user when overexposure may be taking place. The meter is programmed with the individual's skin type and SPF.

Tanning Pills

Case-studies have proven that tanning pills can cause serious medical problems, possibly resulting in death. Ailments include aplastic anemia (a decrease in the production of red blood cells), orange skin, headaches, weight loss, easy bruising, and increased fatigue. Treatment involves blood transfusion therapy. Physicians believe that the ingredient canthaxanthin is responsible for the disorders.

This drug is not approved as a prescription or an over-the-counter preparation by the Federal Drug Administration. Ultimately, this product serves no purpose, and it is best to avoid using it.

Hair

Hair originates in tiny sacs or follicles deep in the dermis layer of skin tissue. The part of the hair below the skin surface is the root; the part above is the shaft. Hair follicles are closely connected to the sebaceous glands, which secrete oil to the scalp and give hair its natural sheen. Hair grows from the root outward, pushing the shaft farther from the scalp.

Texture

Each individual hair is made up of nonliving cells that contain a tough protein called *keratin*. Hair texture differs from one part of the body to another. It also differs between the sexes, among individuals, and among the different races.

If an individual hair is oval in cross-section, it is curly along its length. If the cross-section is round, the hair is straight. Thick, wiry hair is usually triangular or kidney-shaped. The fineness or coarseness of hair texture is related to its natural color.

Curling

Anyone using a home permanent preparation should follow the instructions with great care: improper mixing, application, or exposure time could result in serious damage to the hair.

Electric curling irons are not safe, because they may cause pinpoint burns in the scalp that are hardly noticeable at the time but may lead to permanent small areas of baldness. The danger can be minimized, however, if instructions for use are followed exactly. It is especially important that the iron not be hot enough to singe the hair. Setting lotions used with rollers or clips have a tendency to dull the hair unless they are completely brushed out.

Straightening

The least harmful as well as the least effective way of straightening the hair temporarily is the use of pomades. They are usually considered unsatisfactory by women because they are too greasy, but are often used by men with short, unruly hair. Heat-pressing the hair with a metal comb is longer-lasting but can cause substantial damage by burning the scalp. The practice of ironing the hair should be discouraged, since it causes dryness and brittleness, with resultant breakage. Chemical straighteners should be used with great care, since they may cause serious burns. Special efforts must be made to protect the eyes from contact with these products.

Hair Color

In the same way that melanin colors the skin, it also determines hair color. The less melanin, the lighter the hair. As each hair loses its melanin pigment, it gradually turns gray, then white. It is assumed that the age at which hair begins to gray is an inherited characteristic and therefore can't be postponed or prevented by eating special foods, by taking vitamins, or by the external application of creams. The only way to recolor gray hair is by the use of a chemical dye.

Dyes and Tints

Anyone wishing to make a radical change in hair color should consult a trained and reliable hairdresser. Trying to turn black hair bright red or dark red hair to blond with a home preparation can sometimes end up with unwanted purplish or greenish results. When tints or dyes are used at home to lighten or darken the hair color by one or two shades, instructions accompanying the product must be followed carefully. Anyone with a tendency to contract contact dermatitis should make a patch test on the skin to check on possible allergic reactions. Hair should be tinted or dyed no more often than once a month.

Dye Stripping

The only safe way to get rid of an unwanted dye color that has been used on the hair is to let it grow out. The technique known as stripping takes all color from the hair and reduces it to a dangerously weak mass. It is then redyed its natural color. Such a procedure should never be undertaken by anyone except a trained beautician, if at all.

Bleaching

Hydrogen peroxide is mixed with a hair lightener to prebleach hair before applying blond tints. Bleaching with peroxide alone can cause more damage to the hair than dyeing or tinting it with a reliable commercial preparation, because it causes dryness, brittleness, and breakage.

General Hair Care

Properly cared for hair usually looks clean, shiny, and alive. Unfortunately, too many people mask the natural good looks of their hair with unnecessary sprays and "beauty" preparations.

Washing the Hair

Hair should be washed about once a week—more often if it tends to be oily. The claims made by shampoo manufacturers need not always be taken too seriously, since most shampoos contain nothing more than soap or detergent and a perfuming agent. No shampoo can restore the natural oils to the hair at the same time that it washes it. A castile shampoo is good for dry hair, and one containing tincture of green soap is good for oily hair.

Thorough rinsing is essential to eliminate any soap deposit. If the local water is hard, a detergent shampoo can be rinsed off more easily than one containing soap.

Drying the Hair

Drying the hair in sunlight or under a heat-controlled dryer is more satisfactory than trying to rub it dry with a towel. Gentle brushing during drying reactivates the natural oils that give hair its shine. Brushing in general is excellent for the appearance of the hair. Be sure to wash both brush and comb as often as the hair is washed.

Hair pomades should be avoided or used sparingly, since they are sometimes so heavy that they clog the pores of the scalp. A little bit of olive oil or baby oil can be rubbed into dry hair after shampooing. This is also good for babies' hair.

There is no scientific evidence that creme rinses, protein rinses, or beer rinses accomplish anything for the hair other than making it somewhat more manageable if it is naturally fine and flyaway.

Dandruff

Simple dandruff is a condition in which the scalp begins to itch and flake a few days after the hair has been washed. There is no evidence that the problem is related to germ infection.

Oiliness and persistent dandruff may appear not only on the scalp but also on the sides of the nose or the chest. In such cases, a dermatologist should be consulted. Both light and serious cases often respond well to prescription medicines containing tars. These preparations control the dandruff, but there is no known cure for it.

Nits

Head lice sometimes infect adults as well as children. These tiny parasites usually live on the part of the scalp near the nape of the neck, and when they bite, they cause itching. They attach their eggs, which are called *nits,* to the shaft of the hair, and when they are plentiful, they can be seen by a trained eye as tiny, silvery-white ovals. This condition is highly contagious and can be passed from one head to another by way of combs, brushes, hats, head scarfs, and towels. A physician can be consulted for information on effective ways of eliminating nits—usually by the application of chemicals and the use of a fine-tooth comb.

Baldness

Under the normal circumstances of combing, brushing, and shampooing, a person loses anywhere from 25 to 100 hairs a day. Because new hairs start growing each day, the loss and replacement usually balance each other. When the loss rate is greater than the replacement rate, thinning and baldness are the result.

Alopecia

The medical name for baldness is *alopecia,* the most common form of which is *male pattern baldness.* Dr. Eugene Van Scott, Professor of Dermatology of Temple University's Health Sciences Center, sums up the opinion of medical authorities on the three factors responsible for this type of baldness: sex, age, and heredity. Unfortunately, these are three factors over which medical science has no control.

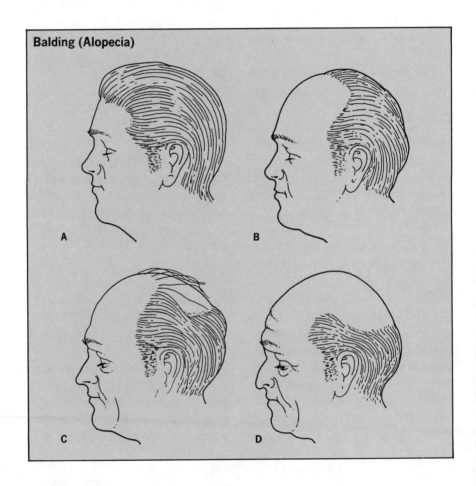

Balding (Alopecia)

Other Causes of Baldness

Other forms of baldness may be the result of bacterial or fungal infections, allergic reactions to particular medicines, radiation, or continual friction. It has also been suggested that constant stress from hair curlers or tightly pulled ponytails can cause loss of hair. These forms of baldness usually disappear when the cause is eliminated.

Although diet has very little to do with baldness, poor nutrition can result in hair that is dry, dull, and brittle enough to break easily. Any serious illness can lead to hair loss as well. It is thought that vitamin A taken in grossly excessive amounts can contribute to hair loss.

Women ordinarily lose some of their hair at the end of pregnancy, after delivery, and during the menopause, but regrowth can be expected in a few months.

It is now possible for anyone suffering from temporary baldness or from male pattern baldness to choose from a wide variety of attractively styled wigs and hairpieces.

A surgical procedure for treating male pattern baldness and baldness in women is called hair transplantation; it is discussed in Ch. 20, *Surgery.*

Hair Removal

Over the centuries and around the world, fashions in whiskers and beards come and go, but the average American male still subjects at least part of his face to daily shaving. Although feminine shaving practices are a more recent phenomenon, most American women now consider it part of good grooming to remove under-arm and leg hair with a razor as often as twice a week. Shaving removes not only the dead skin cells that make up the protective layer of the body's surface but also some of the living skin underneath. Instead of being harmful, this appears to stimulate rather than damage new skin growth.

Male Shaving

The average beard grows about two-tenths of an inch a day. However, the density of male face hair varies a great deal depending on skin and hair color. In all races, the concentration is usually greatest on the chin and in the area between the nose and upper lip.

There is no proof that an electric razor is safer or better for all types of skin than a safety razor. Both types result in nicks and cuts of the living skin tissue, depending on the closeness of the shave.

Twice as many men prefer wet shaving to dry because the use of soap and hot water softens the hair stubble and makes it easier to remove. Shaving authorities point out that thorough soaking is one of the essentials of easy and safe shaving. Leaving the shaving lather on the face for at least two minutes will also soften whiskers a good deal.

The razor should be moistened with hot water throughout the process, and the chin and upper lip left for last so that the heavier hair concentration in these areas has the longest contact with moisture and lather.

Oily Skin

Men with oily skin should use an aerosol shaving preparation or a lather-type applied with a brush. These are really soaps and are more effective in eliminating the oils that coat the face hair, thus making it easier to shave.

Dry Skin

A brushless cream is advisable for dry skin, since it lubricates the skin rather than further deprives it of oil.

Ingrown Hairs

One of the chief problems connected with shaving is that it often causes ingrown hairs, which can lead to pore-clogging and infection. Hair is more likely to turn back into the skin if it is shaved against the grain, or if the cutting edge of the blade is dull and rough rather than smooth. Men with coarse, wiry, curly, rather than fine, hair may find that whisker ends are more likely to become ingrown than men with fine hair. The problem is best handled by shaving with the grain, using a sharp blade, and avoiding too close a shave, particularly in the area around the neck.

Shaving and Skin Problems

For men with acne or a tendency to skin problems, the following advice is offered by Dr. Howard T. Behrman, Director of Dermatological Research, New York Medical College:

- Shave as seldom as possible, perhaps only once or twice a week, and always with the grain.
- If wet shaving is preferred, use a new blade each time, and shave as lightly as possible to avoid nicking pimples.
- Wash face carefully with plenty of hot water to make the beard easy to manage, and after shaving, rinse with hot water followed by cold.
- Use an antiseptic astringent face lotion.
- Instead of plucking out ingrown hairs, loosen them gently so that the ends do not grow back into the skin.
- Although some people with skin problems find an electric shaver less irritating, in most cases, a wet shave seems best.

Female Shaving

Millions of American women regularly shave underarm and leg hair, and most of them do so with a blade razor. In recent years, various types of shavers have been designed with blade exposure more suited to women's needs than the standard type used by men. To make shaving easier and safer, the following procedures are recommended.

- Since wet hair is much easier to cut, the most effective time to shave is during or immediately following a bath or shower.

- Shaving cream or soap lather keeps the water from evaporating, and is preferred to dry shaving.

- Underarm shaving is easier with a contoured razor designed for this purpose. If a deodorant or antiperspirant causes stinging or irritation after shaving, allow a short time to elapse before applying it.

- Light bleeding from nicks or scrapes can be stopped by applying pressure to a sterile pad placed on the injured area.

Unwanted Hair

The technical word for excess or unwanted hair on the face, chest, arms, and legs is *hirsutism*. The condition varies greatly among different ethnic strains, and so does the attitude toward it. Women of southern European ancestry are generally hairier than those with Nordic or Anglo-Saxon ancestors. Caucasoid peoples are hairier than Negroid peoples. The sparsest amount of body hair is found among the Mongolian races and American Indians. Although heredity is the chief factor of hirsutism, hormones also influence hair growth. If there is a sudden appearance of coarse hair on the body of a young boy or girl or a woman with no such former tendency, a glandular disturbance should be suspected and investigated by a physician.

A normal amount of unwanted hair on the legs and under the arms is usually removed by shaving. When the problem involves the arms, face, chest, and abdomen, other methods of removal are available.

Temporary Methods of Hair Removal

Bleaching

Unwanted dark fuzz on the upper lip and arms can be lightened almost to invisibility with a commercially prepared bleach or with a homemade paste consisting of baking soda, hydrogen peroxide (bleaching strength), and a few drops of ammonia. Soap chips can be used instead of baking soda. The paste should be left on the skin for a few minutes and then washed off. It is harmless to the skin, and if applied repeatedly, the hair will tend to break off as a result of constant bleaching.

Chemical Depilatories

These products contain alkaline agents that cause the hair to detach easily at the skin surface. They can be used on and under the arms, and on the legs and chest. However, they should not be used on the face unless the label says it is safe to do so. Timing instructions should be followed carefully. If skin irritation results, this type of depilatory should be discontinued in favor of some other method.

Abrasives

Devices that remove hair from the skin surface by rubbing are cheap but time-consuming. However, if an abrasive such as pumice is used regularly, the offending hairs will be shorter with each application. A cream or lotion should be applied to the skin after using an abrasive.

Waxing

The technique of applying melted wax to the skin for removal of excess facial hair is best handled by an experienced cosmetician. The process involves pouring hot wax onto the skin and allowing it to cool. The hairs become embedded in the wax, and are plucked out from below the skin surface when the wax is stripped off. Because this method is painful and often causes irritation, it is not very popular, although the results are comparatively long-lasting.

Plucking

The use of tweezers for removing scattered hairs from the eyebrows, face, and chest is slightly painful but otherwise harmless. It is not a practical method for getting rid of dense hair growth, however, because it takes too much time.

Permanent Hair Removal by Electrolysis

The only permanent and safe method of removing unwanted hair is by *electrolysis*. This technique destroys each individual hair root by transmitting electric current through fine wire needles into the opening of the hair follicle. The hair thus loosened is then plucked out with a tweezer. The older type of electrolysis machine uses galvanic current. The newer type, sometimes called an *electrocoagulation machine*, uses modified high-frequency current. In either case, the efficiency and safety of the technique depends less on the machine than on the care and skill of the operator.

Because the process of treating each hair root is expensive, time-consuming, and uncomfortable, it is not recommended for areas of dense hair growth, such as the arms or legs. Before undertaking electrolysis either at a beauty salon or at home, it would be wise to consult a dermatologist about individual skin reaction.

Nails

Fingernails and toenails are an extension of the epidermis, or outer layer of the skin. They are made of elastic tissue formed from keratin, the substance that gives hair its strength and flexibility.

Some of the problems associated with fingernails are the result of too much manicuring. White spots, for example, are often caused by too much pressure at the base of the nail when trying to expose the "moon"— the white portion that contains tissue not yet as tough as the rest of the nail.

To ensure the health of toenails, feet should be bathed once a day and the nails cleaned with a brush dipped in soapy water. Shoes should fit properly so that the toenails are not subjected to pressure and distortion. To avoid ingrown toenails, trimming should be done straight across rather than by rounding or tapering the corners.

Splitting

Infection or injury of the tissue at the base of a fingernail may cause its surface to be rigid or split. Inflammation of the finger joints connected with arthritis will also cause nail deformity. For ordinary problems of splitting and

Nail Anatomy

Dead cells
Germinal layer
Bone
Cuticle
Nail root

peeling, the nails should be kept short enough so that they don't catch and tear easily. For practical purposes, the top of the nail should not be visible when the palm is held about six inches from the eye. As the nails grow stronger, they can be grown longer without splitting.

Brittleness

This condition seems to be caused by such external factors as the chemicals in polish removers, soaps, and detergents. It is also a natural consequence of aging. Commercial nail-hardening preparations that contain formaldehyde are not recommended, because they are known to cause discoloration, loosening, or even loss of nails in some cases.

Nail damage can be reduced by wearing rubber gloves while doing household chores. Hand cream massaged into the skin around the nails will counteract dryness and lessen the possibility of hangnails. Although nail polish provides a shield against damage, it should not be worn all the time, particularly if the nail is polished right down to the base; this prevents live tissue from "breathing."

Disorders of the Skin

The skin is subject to a large number of disorders, most of which are not serious even though they may be temporarily uncomfortable. A disorder may be caused by one or another type of allergy; by excessive heat or cold; or by infection from fungi, bacteria, viruses, or parasites. Many skin ailments are caused or aggravated by emotional disturbances.

The symptoms and treatment of the more common disorders are discussed in the following pages. Any persistent change in skin condition should be brought to the attention of a physician.

Allergies and Itching

Itching and inflammation of the skin may be caused by an allergic reaction, by exposure to poisonous plants, or by a generalized infection.

Dermatitis

Dermatitis is the term used for an inflammation of the skin. The term for allergic reactions of the skin resulting from surface contact with outside agents is *contact dermatitis*. This condition is characterized by a rash and may be brought out by sensitivity to cosmetics, plants, cleaning materials, metal, wool, and so on. Other forms of dermatitis can be caused by excesses of heat or cold, by friction, or by sensitivity to various medicines. Dermatitis is usually accompanied by itching at the site of the rash.

Poison Ivy

This common plant, unknown in Europe but widespread everywhere in the United States except in California and Nevada, produces an allergic reaction on the skin accompanied by a painful rash and blisters. Some people are so sensitive to it that they are affected by contact not only with the plant itself but with animal fur or clothing that might have picked up the sap weeks before.

A mild attack of poison ivy produces a rash and small, watery blisters that get progressively larger. The affected area of the skin becomes crusty and dry, and after a few weeks, all symptoms vanish. If the exposed area is thoroughly washed with laundry soap immediately after contact, the poison may not penetrate the skin.

If the symptoms do develop, they can be relieved with Burow's solution—one part solution to fifteen parts of cool water—or with the application of calamine lotion. If the symptoms are severe, and especially if the area around the eyes is involved, a physician should be consulted. He may prescribe an application or an injection of cortisone.

The best way to avoid the unpleasantness of a poison ivy attack is to learn to recognize the plant and stay away from it. Children especially should be warned against putting the leaves and berries in their mouths.

Poison oak and poison sumac produce somewhat the same symptoms and should also be avoided.

Under no circumstances should these plants be burned to eliminate them, because the inhaling of the contaminated smoke even from a distance can cause a serious case of poisoning. The application of special sprays, if the instructions are followed carefully, will get rid of the plants without affecting people or the neighborhood greenery.

Hives

These are large, irregularly shaped swellings on the skin that burn and itch. The cause is unknown, but allergic reactions to certain foods and medicine or to insect bites have been suggested as possible causes. The swellings of hives usually disappear within a day or so, but they can be very uncomfortable while they last. The itching and burning can often be relieved by applying cold water and a calamine solution. However, some people are sensitive to cold and develop wheals when subjected to intense cold. Commercial preparations containing surface anesthetics are seldom effective and may cause allergic reactions.

If the outbreak of hives can be traced to a specific food, such as shellfish or strawberries, the food should be eliminated from the diet. If a medicine such as penicillin or a sulfa drug is the cause, a physician should be told about the reaction.

Eczema

This condition is an allergic reaction that produces itching, swelling, blistering, oozing, and scaling of the skin. It is more common among children than among adults and may sometimes cover the entire body, although the rash is usually limited to the face, neck, and folds of the knees and elbows. Unlike contact dermatitis, it is likely to be caused by an allergy to a food or a pollen or dust. Advertised cures for eczema cannot control the cause and sometimes make the condition worse. A physician should be consulted if the symptoms are severe, particularly if the patient is an infant or very young child.

Itching

The technical name for the localized or general sensation on the skin that can be relieved by scratching is *pruritus*. Itching may be caused by many skin disorders, by infections, by serious diseases such as nephritis or leukemia, by medicines, or by psychological factors such as tension. A physician should always be consulted to find the cause of persistent itching, because it may be the symptom of a basic disorder. Repeated scratching may provide some relief, but it can also lead to infection.

Anal Pruritus

If itching in the anal area is so severe that only painful scratching will relieve it, the condition is probably *anal pruritus*. It is often accompanied by excessive rectal mucus that keeps the skin irritated and moist. This disorder is most commonly associated with hemorrhoids, but many other conditions, such as reactions to drugs, can cause it. Anxiety or tension can also contribute to it. Sitz baths with warm water are usually recommended. Every effort should be made to reduce scratching and to keep the anal skin clean and dry. Cortisone cream may be prescribed in persistent cases.

Skin Irritations and Weather

Extremes of weather produce local inflammations and other skin problems for many people.

Chapping

In cold weather, the sebaceous glands slow down the secretions that lubricate the skin, causing it to become dry. When dry skin is exposed to wintry weather, it becomes irritated and is likely to crack, particularly around the lips. Chapped skin is especially sensitive to harsh soaps. During such periods of exposure, the skin can be protected with a mild cream or lotion. A lubricating ointment should be used on the lips to prevent them from

cracking. Children who lick their lips continually no matter what the weather can benefit from this extra protection. Chapped hands caused by daily use of strong soaps and detergents can be helped by the use of a lubricating cream and rubber gloves during housework.

Frostbite

Exposure to extreme cold for a prolonged period may cause freezing of the nose, fingers, toes, or ears, thus cutting off the circulation to the affected areas. Frostbitten areas are of a paler color than normal and are

numb. They should not be rubbed with snow or exposed to intense heat. Areas should be thawed gradually, and a physician should be consulted for aftercare in extreme cases.

Chilblain

A localized inflammation of the skin called *chilblain* is common among people who are particularly sensitive to cold because of poor circulation. Chilblain may occur in the ears, hands, feet, and face, causing itching, swelling, and discoloration of the skin. Anyone prone to chilblain should dress protectively during the cold

weather and use an electric pad or blanket at night. Affected parts should not be rubbed or massaged, nor should ice or extreme heat be applied directly, since these measures may cause additional damage. Persistent or extreme attacks of chilblain should be discussed with a physician.

Chafing

This condition is an inflammation of two opposing skin surfaces caused by the warmth, moisture, and friction of their rubbing together. Diabetics, overweight people, and those who perspire heavily are particularly prone to chafing. Chafing is accompanied by itching and burning, and sometimes infection can set in if the superficial skin is broken. Parts of the body subject to chafing are the inner surfaces of the thighs, the anal region, the area

under the breasts, and the inner surfaces between fingers and toes.

To reduce the possibility of chafing, lightweight clothing should be worn and strenuous exercise avoided during hot weather. Vaseline or a vitamin A and D ointment may be applied to reduce friction. In general, the treatment is the same as that for diaper rash in infants. If the condition becomes acute, a physician can prescribe more effective remedies.

Prickly Heat

This skin rash is usually accompanied by itching and burning. It is caused by an obstruction of the sweat ducts such that perspiration does not reach the surface of the skin but backs up and causes pimples the size of a pinhead. If the obstruction is superficial, the pimples are white; if it is deeper, they are red. The condition can be brought on by other minor skin irritations, by continued exposure to moist heat, such as a compress, or by exercise in humid weather. Infants and people who are overweight are especially prone to prickly heat.

The discomfort can be eased by wearing lightweight, loose-fitting clothing, especially at night, and keeping room temperature low. Alcoholic beverages, which tend to dehydrate the body, should be avoided. Tepid baths and the application of cornstarch to the affected skin areas will usually relieve itching. If the rash remains for several days, a physician should be consulted to make sure it does not arise from some other cause.

Calluses and Corns

As a result of continued friction or pressure in a particular area, the skin forms a tough, hard, self-protecting layer known as a *callus*. Calluses are common on the soles of the feet, the palms of the hands, and, among guitarists and string players, on the tips of the fingers. A heavy callus that presses against a bone in the foot because of poorly fitted shoes can be very painful. The hard surface can be reduced somewhat by the use of pumice, or by gently paring it with a razor blade that has been washed in alcohol.

Corns are a form of callus that appear on or between the toes. They usually have a hard inner core that causes pain when pressed against underlying tissue by badly fitted shoes.

A hard corn that appears on the surface of the little toe can be removed by soaking for about ten minutes and applying a few drops of ten percent salicylic acid in collodion. The surface should be covered with a corn pad to reduce pressure, and the corn lifted off when it is loose enough to be released from the skin. Anyone suffering from a circulatory disease and particularly from diabetes should avoid home treatment of foot disturbances. Those with a tendency to callus and corn formations should be especially careful about the proper fit of shoes and hose. A *chiropodist* or *podiatrist* is a trained specialist in foot care who can be visited on a regular basis to provide greater foot comfort.

Fungus Infections

Fungi are plantlike parasitic growths found in the air, in water, and in the soil. They comprise a large family that includes mushrooms, and are responsible for mildew and mold. Only a small number cause disease.

Ringworm

This condition is caused not by a worm but by a group of fungi that live on the body's dead skin cells in those areas that are warm and damp because of accumulated perspiration. One form of ringworm attacks the scalp, arms, and legs, especially of children, and is often spread by similarly affected pets. It appears as reddish patches that scale and blister and frequently feel sore and itchy. Ringworm is highly contagious and can be passed from person to person by contaminated objects such as combs and towels. It should therefore be treated promptly by a physician. Ringworm can best be prevented by strict attention to personal cleanliness.

Athlete's Foot

Another form of ringworm, *athlete's foot,* usually attacks the skin between the toes and under the toenails. If not treated promptly, it can cause an itching rash on other parts of the body. Athlete's foot causes the skin to itch, blister, and crack, and as a result, leaves it vulnerable to more serious infection from other organisms. The disorder can be treated at home by gently removing the damaged skin, and, after soaking the feet, thoroughly drying and dusting between the toes with a medicated foot powder. Some of the powder should be sprinkled into shoes. If the condition continues, a fungicidal ointment can be applied in the morning and at night. Persistent cases require the attention of a physician.

Scabies

An insectlike parasite causes the skin irritation called *scabies,* otherwise known as "the itch." The female itch mite burrows a hole in the skin, usually in the groin or between the fingers or toes, and stays hidden long enough to build a tunnel in which to deposit her eggs. The newly hatched mites then work their way to the skin surface and begin the cycle all over again. There is little discomfort in the early period of infestation, but in about a week, a rash appears, accompanied by extreme itching, which is usually most severe at night. Constant scratching during sleep can lead to skin lesions that invite bacterial infection.

Scabies is very contagious and can spread rapidly through a family or through a community, such as a summer camp or army barracks. It can also be communicated by sexual contact.

Treatment by a physician involves the identification of the characteristic tunnels from which sample mites can be removed for examination. Hot baths and thorough scrubbing will expose the burrows, and medical applications as directed by the physician usually clear up the condition in about a week.

Bacterial Infections

The skin is susceptible to infection from a variety of bacteria. Poor diet and careless hygiene can lower the body's resistance to these infectious agents.

Boils

These abscesses of the skin are caused by bacterial infection of a hair follicle or a sebaceous gland. The pus that accumulates in a boil is the result of the encounter between the bacteria and the white blood cells that fight them. Sometimes a boil subsides by itself and disappears. Sometimes the pressure of pus against the skin surface may bring the boil to a head; it will then break, drain, and heal if washed with an antiseptic and covered with a sterile pad. Warm-water compresses can be applied for ten minutes every hour to relieve the pain and to encourage the boil to break and drain. A fresh, dry pad should be applied after each period of soaking.

Anyone with a serious or chronic illness who develops a boil should consult a physician. Since the bacteria can enter the bloodstream and cause a general infection with fever, a physician should also be consulted for a boil on the nose, scalp, upper lip, or in the ear, groin, or armpit.

Carbuncles

This infection is a group of connected boils and is likely to be more painful and less responsive to home treatment. Carbuncles may occur as the result of poor skin care. They tend to occur in the back of the neck where the skin is thick, and the abscess tends to burrow into deeper tissues. A physician usually lances and drains a deep-seated carbuncle, or he may prescribe an antibiotic remedy.

Impetigo

This skin infection is caused by staphylococcal or streptococcal bacteria, and is characterized by blisters that break and form yellow crusted areas. It is spread from one person to another and from one part of the body to another by the discharge from the sores. Impetigo occurs most frequently on the scalp, face, and arms and legs. The infection often is picked up in barber shops, swimming pools, or from body contact with infected people or household pets.

Special care must be taken, especially with children, to control the spread of the infection by keeping the fingers away from infected parts. Bed linens should be changed daily, and disposable paper towels, as well as paper plates and cups, should be used during treatment. A physician should be consulted for proper medication and procedures to deal with the infection.

Barber's Itch

Sycosis, commonly called *barber's itch,* is a bacterial infection of the hair follicles of the beard, accompanied by inflammation, itching, and the formation of pus-filled pimples. People with stiff, curly hair are prone to this type of chronic infection, because their hair is more likely to curve back and reenter the skin. The infection should be treated promptly to prevent scarring and the destruction of the hair root.

In some cases, physicians recommend antibiotics. If these are not effective, it may be necessary to drain the abscesses and remove the hairs from the inflamed follicles. During treatment, it is best to avoid shaving, if possible. If one must shave, the sterilization of all shaving equipment and the use of a brushless shaving cream are recommended.

Erysipelas

An acute streptococcal infection of the skin, *erysipelas* can be fatal, particularly to the very young or very old, if not treated promptly. One of its symptoms is the bright redness of the affected areas of the skin. These red patches enlarge and spread, making the skin tender and painful. Blisters may appear nearby. The patient usually has a headache, fever, chills, and nausea. Erysipelas responds well to promptly administered antibiotics, particularly penicillin. The patient is usually advised to drink large amounts of fluid and to eat a nourishing, easily digested diet.

Viral Infections

The most common skin conditions caused by viruses are cold sores, shingles, and warts, discussed below.

Cold Sores

Also called fever blisters, *cold sores* are technically known as *herpes simplex.* They are small blisters that appear most frequently in the corners of the mouth, and sometimes around the eyes and on the genitals. The presumed cause is a virus that lies dormant in the skin until it is activated by infection or by excessive exposure to sun or wind. There is no specific cure for cold sores, but the irritation can be eased by applying drying or cooling agents such as camphor ice or cold-water compresses. Recurrent cold sores, especially in infants, should be called to a physician's attention.

Recent studies have shown that a variety of the herpes simplex virus called HSV-II (for herpes simplex virus-Type II) can be a serious danger to the fetus of a pregnant woman. For a discussion of this condition, see Ch. 25, *Women's Health.* The variety that causes cold sores is called Type I.

Shingles

The virus infection of a sensory nerve, accompanied by small, painful blisters that appear on the skin along the path of the nerve—usually on one side of the chest or abdomen—is called *shingles.* The medical name for the disorder, which is caused by the chicken pox virus, is *herpes zoster,* Latin for "girdle of blisters." When a cranial nerve is involved, the blisters appear on the face near the eye. The preliminary symptom is neuritis with severe pain and, sometimes, fever. The blisters may take from two to four weeks to dry up and disappear. Although there is no specific cure, the pain can be alleviated by aspirin. In severe cases, or if the area near the eye is involved, a physician should be seen.

Warts

These growths are caused by a virus infection of the epidermis. They never become cancerous, but can be painful when found on the soles of the feet. In this location, they are known as *plantar warts,* and they cause discomfort because constant pressure makes them grow inward. Plantar warts are most likely to be picked up by children because they are barefooted so much of the time, and by adults when their feet are moist and they are walking around in showers, near swimming pools, and in locker rooms. Warts can be spread by scratching, by shaving, and by brushing the hair. They are often transmitted from one member of the family to another. Because warts can spread to painful areas, such as the area around or under the fingernails, and because they may become disfiguring, it is best to consult a physician whenever they appear.

In many ways, warts behave rather mysteriously. About half of them go away without any treatment at all. Sometimes, when warts on one part of the body are being treated, those in another area will disappear. The folklore about "witching" and "charming" warts away has its foundation in fact, because apparently having faith in the cure, no matter how ridiculous it sounds, sometimes brings success. This form of suggestion therapy is especially successful with children.

There are several more conventional ways of treating warts. Depending on their size and the area involved, electric current, dry ice, or various chemicals may be employed. A physician should be consulted promptly when warts develop in the area of the beard or on the scalp, because they spread quickly in these parts of the body and thus become more difficult to eliminate.

Sebaceous Cysts

When a sebaceous gland duct is blocked, the oil that the gland secretes cannot get to the surface of the skin. Instead, it accumulates into a hard, round, movable mass contained in a sac. This mass is known as a *sebaceous cyst.* Such cysts may appear on the face, back, ears, or in the genital area. A sebaceous cyst that forms on the scalp is called a *wen,* and may become as large as a billiard ball. The skin in this area will become bald, because the cyst interferes with the blood supply to the hair roots.

Some sebaceous cysts just disappear without treatment. However, those that do not are a likely focus for secondary infection by bacteria, and they may become abscessed and inflamed. It is therefore advisable to have cysts examined by a physician for possible removal. If such a cyst is superficial, it can be punctured and drained. One that is deeper is usually removed by simple surgical procedure in the physician's office.

Acne

About 80 percent of all teenagers suffer from the skin disturbance called *acne.* It is also fairly common among women in their twenties. Acne is a condition in which the skin of the face, and often of the neck, shoulders, chest, and back, is covered to a greater or lesser extent with pimples, blackheads, whiteheads, and boils.

The typical onset of acne in adolescence is related to the increased activity of the glands, including the sebaceous glands. Most of the oil that they secrete gets to the surface of the skin through ducts that lead into the pores. When the surface pores are clogged with sebaceous gland secretions and keratin, or when so much extra oil is being secreted that it backs up into the ducts, the result is the formation of the skin blemishes characteristic of acne. Dirt or makeup does not cause acne.

The blackheads are dark not because they are dirty but because the fatty material in the clogged pore is oxidized and discolored by the air that reaches it. When this substance is infected by bacteria, it turns into a pimple. Under no circumstances should such pimples be picked at or squeezed, because the pressure can rupture the surrounding membrane and spread the infection further.

Although a mild case of acne usually clears up by itself, it is often helpful to get the advice of a physician so that it does not get any worse.

Cleanliness

Although surface dirt does not cause acne, it can contribute to its spread. Therefore, the affected areas should be cleansed with a medicated soap and hot water twice a day. Hair should be shampooed frequently and brushed away from the face. Boys who are shaving should soften the beard with soap and hot water. The blade should be sharp and should skim the skin as lightly as possible to avoid nicking pimples.

Creams and Cosmetics

Nonprescription medicated creams and lotions may be effective in reducing some blemishes, but if used too often, they make the skin dry. They should be applied according to the manufacturer's instructions and should be discontinued if they cause additional irritation. If makeup is used, it should have a nonoily base and be completely removed before going to bed.

Forbidden Foods

Although acne is not caused by any particular food, it can be made worse by a diet overloaded with candy, rich pastries, and fats. Chocolate and cola drinks must be eliminated entirely in some cases.

Professional Treatment

A serious case of acne, or even a mild one that is causing serious emotional problems, should receive the attention of a physician. He or she may prescribe antibiotics, usually considered the most effective treatment, or recommend sunlamp treatments. A physician can also be helpful in dealing with the psychological aspects of acne that are so disturbing to teenagers.

Psoriasis

Psoriasis is a noncontagious chronic condition in which the skin on various parts of the body is marked by bright red patches covered with silvery scales. The areas most often affected are the knees, elbows, scalp, and trunk, and less frequently, the areas under the arms and around the genitals.

The specific cause of psoriasis has not yet been discovered, but it is thought to be an inherited abnormality in which the formation of new skin cells is too rapid and disorderly. In its mild form, psoriasis responds well to a variety of long-term treatments. When it is acute, the entire skin surface may be painfully red, and large sections of it may scale off. In such cases, prompt hospitalization and intensive care are recommended.

Conditions That Can Bring On an Outbreak

The onset or aggravation of psoriasis can be triggered by some of the following factors:

- bruises, burns, scratches, and overexposure to the sun

- sudden drops in temperature—a mild, stable climate is most beneficial
- sudden illness from another source, or unusual physical or emotional stress

- infections of the upper respiratory tract, especially bacterial throat in- fections and the medicines used to cure them

Treatment

Although there is no specific cure for psoriasis, these are some of the recommended treatments:

- controlled exposure to sunlight or an ultraviolet lamp

- creams or lotions of crude coal tar or tar distillates, used alone or in combination with ultraviolet light

- psoralen and ultraviolet light (PUVA), a combined systemic-external therapy in which a psoralen drug is taken orally before exposure to ultraviolet light

- systemic drugs, such as methotrexate, which can be taken orally

- steroid hormone medications applied to the skin surface under dressings

Pigment Disorders and Birthmarks

The mechanism that controls skin coloration is described above under "Skin Color." Abnormalities in the creation and distribution of melanin result in the following disorders, some of which are negligible.

Freckles

These are small spots of brown pigment that frequently occur when fair-skinned people are exposed to the sun or to ultraviolet light. For those whose skin gets red rather than tan during such exposure, freckles are a protective device. In most cases, they recede in cold weather. A heavy freckle formation that is permanent can be covered somewhat by cosmetic preparations. No attempt should be made to remove freckles with commercial creams or solutions unless supervised by a physician.

Liver Spots

Flat, smooth, irregularly placed markings on the skin, called *liver spots,* often appear among older people, and result from an increase in pigmentation. They have nothing to do with the liver and are completely harmless. Brownish markings of similar appearance sometimes show up during pregnancy or as a result of irritation or infection. They usually disappear when the underlying cause is eliminated.

Liver spots are permanent, and the principal cause is not aging but the accumulated years of exposure to sun and wind. They can be disguised and treated in the same way as freckles. A liver spot that becomes hard and thick should be called to a physician's attention.

Moles

Clusters of melanin cells, called *moles,* may appear singly or in groups at any place on the body. They range in color from light tan to dark brown; they may be raised and hairy or flat and smooth. Many moles are present at birth, and most make their appearance before the age of 20. They rarely turn into malignancies, and require medical attention only if they become painful, if they itch, or if they suddenly change in size, shape, or color.

There are several ways of removing moles if they are annoying or particularly unattractive. They can be destroyed by the application of an electric needle, by cauterizing, and by surgery. A mole that has been removed is not likely to reappear. The hairs sometimes found in moles can be clipped close to the surface of the skin, or they can be permanently removed. Hair removal often causes the mole to get smaller.

Vitiligo

Vitiligo is an autoimmune disease in which the body's white cells attack its pigment cells, causing a loss of pigment in the skin. About 1 percent of the U.S. population suffers from this condition, which can appear any time up to middle age and is believed to be inherited. Vitiligo can occur anywhere on the body, from small spots to large patches, but the nose, hands, feet, and genital area are the most common areas affected.

There is no cure for vitiligo, but it can be treated with drugs and exposure to ultraviolet A radiation. The condition itself is not physically painful, but many vitiligo sufferers, particularly dark-skinned persons, experience emotional pain and embarrassment.

Birthmarks

About one-third of all infants are born with the type of birthmark called a *hemangioma,* also known as a vascular birthmark. These are caused by a clustering of small blood vessels near the surface of the skin. The mark, which is flat, irregularly shaped, and either pink, red, or purplish, is usually referred to as "port wine stain." There is no known way to remove it, but with cosmetic covering creams, it can usually be successfully masked.

The type of hemangioma that is raised and bright red—called a strawberry mark—spontaneously disappears with no treatment in most cases during early childhood. If a strawberry mark begins to grow rather than fade, or if it begins to ulcerate, a physician should be promptly consulted.

See Ch. 18, *Cancer,* for a discussion of skin cancer; see Ch. 3, *The Teens,* for a discussion of adolescent skin problems; see Ch. 23, *Aches, Pains, Nuisances, Worries,* for further discussion of minor skin problems.

22

The Teeth and Gums

Although a human baby is born without teeth, a complete set of 20 *deciduous,* or baby, teeth (also called *primary teeth*) already has formed within the gums of the offspring while it still is within the mother's womb. The buds of the permanent or secondary teeth are developing even before the first baby tooth appears at around the age of six months. The baby teeth obviously are formed from foods eaten by the mother. Generally, if the mother follows a good diet during pregnancy, no special food items are required to ensure an adequate set of deciduous teeth in the baby.

It takes about two years for the full set of deciduous teeth to appear in the baby's mouth. The first, usually a central incisor at the front of the lower jaw, may erupt any time between the ages of three and nine months. The last probably will be a second molar at the back of the upper jaw. As with walking, talking, and other characteristics of infants, there is no set timetable for the eruption of baby teeth. One child may get his first tooth at three months while another must wait until nine months, but both would be considered within a normal range of tooth development.

The permanent teeth are never far behind the deciduous set. The first permanent tooth usually appears around the age of six years, about four years after the last of the baby teeth has erupted. But the last of the permanent molars, the third molars or *wisdom teeth,* may not break through the gum line until the offspring is an adult.

Types of Teeth

The permanent teeth number 32. In advancing from deciduous to permanent teeth, the human gains six teeth in the lower jaw, or *mandible,* and six in the upper jaw, or *maxilla,* of the mouth. The primary set of teeth includes the following:

UPPER JAW	LOWER JAW
2 central incisors	2 central incisors
2 lateral incisors	2 lateral incisors
2 cuspids	2 cuspids
2 first molars	2 first molars
2 second molars	2 second molars

The permanent set of teeth has an equivalent combination of incisors, cuspids, and first and second molars. But it also includes:

2 first bicuspids	2 first bicuspids
2 second bicuspids	2 second bicuspids
2 third molars	2 third molars

An *incisor* is designed to cut off particles of food, which is then pushed by muscles of the tongue and cheeks to teeth farther back in the mouth for grinding. The front teeth, one on each side, upper and lower, are central incisors. Next to each central incisor is a lateral incisor.

A *cuspid* is so named because it has a spear-shaped crown, or *cusp.* It is

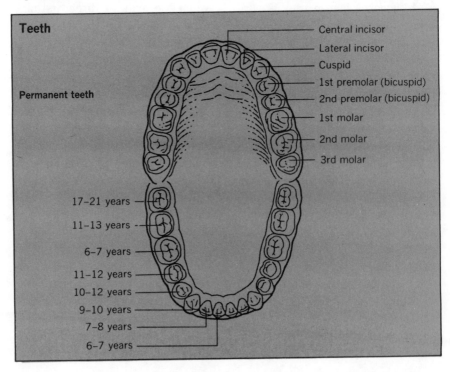

Teeth

Permanent teeth

Central incisor
Lateral incisor
Cuspid
1st premolar (bicuspid)
2nd premolar (bicuspid)
1st molar
2nd molar
3rd molar

17–21 years
11–13 years
6–7 years
11–12 years
10–12 years
9–10 years
7–8 years
6–7 years

designed for tearing as well as cutting. Cuspids sometimes are called *canine teeth* or *eyeteeth; canine teeth* owe their name to the use of these teeth by carnivorous animals, such as dogs, for tearing pieces of meat. There are four cuspids in the mouth, one on the outer side of each lateral incisor in the upper and lower jaws.

Bicuspids sometimes are identified as *premolars*. The term "bicuspid" suggests two cusps, but a bicuspid may in fact have three cusps. The function of the bicuspids is to crush food passed back from the incisors and cuspids. The permanent set of teeth includes a total of eight bicuspids.

The *molars,* which also number eight and are the last teeth at the back of the mouth, are the largest and strongest teeth, with the job of grinding food. The third molars, or wisdom teeth, are smaller, weaker, and less functional than the first and second molars.

Structure of the Tooth

The variety of shapes of teeth make them specialized for the various functions in preparing food for digestion— biting, chewing, and grinding. All varieties, however, have the same basic structure.

Enamel

The outer covering of the part of the tooth that is exposed above the gum line is *enamel,* the hardest substance in the human body. Enamel is about 97 percent mineral and is as tough as some gemstones. It varies in thickness, with the greatest thickness on the surfaces that are likely to get the most wear and tear.

Enamel begins to form on the first tooth buds of an embryo at the age of about 15 weeks, depending upon substances in the food eaten by the mother for proper development.

Structure of Tooth

Lymphatic system
Gingiva
Alveolar bone of jaw
Periodontal ligament

Enamel
Dentin
Nerve supply
Vascular supply
Pulp
Cement

Once the tooth has formed and erupted through the gum line, there is nothing further that can be done by natural means to improve the condition of the enamel. The enamel has no blood supply, and any changes in the tooth surface will be the result of wearing, decay, or injury.

While the health and diet of the mother can affect the development of tooth enamel in the deciduous teeth, certain health factors in the early life of a child can result in defective enamel formation of teeth that have not yet erupted. Some infectious or metabolic disorders, for example, may result in enamel pitting.

Dentin

Beneath the enamel surface of a tooth is a layer of hard material—though not as hard as enamel—called *dentin,* which forms the bulk of a tooth. The dentin forms at the same time that enamel is laid down on the surface of a developing tooth, and the portion beneath the crown of the tooth probably is completed at the same time as the enamel. However, the dentin, which is composed of calcified material, is not as dense as the enamel; it is formed as myriad tubules that extend downward into the pulp at the center of the tooth. There is some evidence that dentin formation may continue slowly during the life of the tooth.

Cementum

The *cementum* is a bonelike substance that covers the root of the tooth. Though harder than regular bone, it is softer than dentin. It contains attachments for fibers of a periodontal ligament that holds the tooth in its socket. The periodontal ligament serves as a kind of hammock of fibers that surround and support the tooth at the cementum surface, radiating outward to the jawbone. This arrangement allows the tooth to move a little while still attached to the jaw. For example, when the teeth of the upper and lower jaws are brought together in chewing, the periodontal ligament allows the teeth to sink into their sockets. When the teeth of the two jaws are separated, the hammocklike ligament permits the teeth to float outward again.

Pulp

The cavity within the dentin contains the *pulp.* There is a wide pulp chamber under the crown of the tooth and a pulp canal that extends from the chamber down through the root or roots. Some teeth, such as the molars, may contain as many as three roots, and each of the roots contains a pulp canal.

The pulp of a tooth contains the blood vessels supplying the tooth and the lymphatic system. Although the blood supply arrangement is not the same for every tooth, a typical pattern includes a dental artery entering through each passageway, or *foramen*, leading into the root of a tooth. The artery branches into numerous capillaries within the root canal. A similar system of veins drains the blood from the tooth through each foramen. A lymphatic network and nerve system also enter the tooth through a foramen and spread through the pulp, as branches from a central distribution link within the jawbone. The nerve fibers have free endings in the tooth, making them sensitive to pain stimuli.

Supporting Structures

The soft, pink gum tissue that surrounds the tooth is called the *gingiva*, and the bone of the jaw that forms the tooth socket is known as *alveolar bone*. The gingiva, alveolar bone, and periodontal ligaments sometimes are grouped into a structural category identified as the *periodontium*. Thus, when a dentist speaks of periodontal disease, he is referring to a disorder of these supporting tissues of the teeth. The ailment known as *gingivitis* is an inflammation of the gingiva, or gum tissue around the teeth.

Care of the Teeth and Gums

Years ago, loss of teeth really was unavoidable. Today, thanks to modern practices of preventive dentistry, it is possible for nearly everyone to enjoy the benefits of natural teeth for a lifetime. But natural teeth can be preserved only by daily oral-hygiene habits and regular dental checkups.

The Dental Examination

During the teen years, careful supervision by the dentist and cooperation from the teenager are especially necessary. The poor eating habits of many youngsters are reflected in high cavity rates, which may be greater during adolescence than in later life. Neglect of proper dental care also occurs in the middle years when an often used excuse is that eventual loss of teeth is inevitable. After the permanent teeth are established, the dentist should be visited every six months, or at whatever intervals he recommends for an individual patient who may need more or less care than the typical patient.

The dentist, like the family physician, usually maintains a general health history of each patient, in addition to a dental health history. He examines each tooth, the gums and other oral tissues, and the *occlusion*, or bite. A complete set of X-ray pictures may be taken on the first visit and again at intervals of perhaps five to seven years. During routine visits, the dentist may take only a couple of X-ray pictures of teeth on either side of the mouth; a complete set of X rays may result in a file of 18 or 20 pictures covering every tooth in the mouth.

X-rays constitute a vital part of the dental examination. Without them the dentist cannot examine the surfaces between the teeth or the portion of the tooth beneath the gum, a part that represents about 60 percent of the total length of the tooth. The X-rays will reveal the condition of the enamel, dentin, and pulp, as well as any impacted wisdom teeth and the alveolar bone, or tooth sockets. Caps, fillings, abscessed roots, and bone loss resulting from gum disease also are clearly visible on a set of X-rays.

Other diagnostic tests may be made, such as a test of nerve response. Sometimes the dentist will make an impression of the teeth, an accurate and detailed reverse reproduction, in plaster of paris, plastic impression compound, or other material. Models made from these impressions are used to study the way the teeth meet. Such knowledge is often crucial in deciding the selection of treatment and materials.

After the examination, the dentist will present and explain any proposed treatment. After oral restoration is completed, he will ask the patient to return at regular intervals for a checkup and *prophylaxis,* which includes cleaning and polishing the teeth. Regular checkups and prophylaxis help prevent periodontal diseases affecting the gum tissue and underlying bone. Professional cleaning removes hard deposits that trap bacteria, especially at the gum line, and polishing removes stains and soft deposits.

Dental Care in Middle Age

Although periodontal (gum) disease and cavities—called *dental caries* by dentists—continue to threaten oral health, two other problems may assume prominence for people of middle age: replacing worn-out restorations, or fillings, and replacing missing teeth. No filling material will last forever. The whitish restorations in front teeth eventually wear away. Silver restorations tend to crack and chip with age because they contract and expand slightly when cold or hot food and drinks come in contact with them. Even gold restorations, the most permanent kind, are subject to decay around the edges, and the decay may spread underneath.

If a needed restoration is not made or a worn-out restoration is not replaced, a deep cavity may result. When the decay reaches the inner layer of the tooth—the dentin—temporary warning twinges of pain may occur. If the tooth still is not restored, the decay will spread into the pulp that fills the inner chamber of the tooth. A toothache can result from inflammation of the pulp, and although the pain may eventually subside, the pulp tissue dies and an abscess can form at the root of the tooth.

Dental Care During Pregnancy

It may be advisable for a pregnant woman to arrange for extra dental checkups. Many changes take place during pregnancy, among them increased hormone production. Some pregnant women develop gingivitis (inflammation of the gums) as an indirect consequence of hormonal changes. A checkup by the dentist during the first three months of pregnancy is needed to assess the oral effects of such changes, and to make sure all dental problems are examined and corrected. Pregnant women should take special care to brush and floss their teeth to minimize these problems.

Infection

To avoid the problem of toxic substances or poisons circulating in the mother's bloodstream, all sources of infection must be removed. Some of these sources can be in the mouth. An abscessed tooth, for example, may not be severe enough to signal its presence with pain, but because it is directly connected to the bloodstream it can send toxic substances and bacteria through the mother's body with possible harmful effects to the embryo.

It is during pregnancy that tooth buds for both the deciduous and permanent teeth begin to form in the unborn child. If the mother neglects her diet or general health care during this period, the effects may be seen in the teeth of her child.

Maintaining Good Oral Hygiene

Fluoridation

Among general rules to follow between dental checkups are using fluorides, maintaining a proper diet, and removing debris from the teeth by brushing and by the use of dental floss. Fluorides are particularly important for strengthening the enamel of teeth in persons under the age of 15. Many communities add fluorides to the water supply, but if the substance is not available in the drinking water, the dentist can advise the patient about other ways of adding fluoride to water or other fluids consumed each day. Studies show that children who drink fluoridated water from birth have up to 65 percent fewer cavities than those who do not drink fluoridated water. However, using excessive amounts of fluoride in the drinking water can result in mottled enamel.

Diet

Although a good diet for total health should provide all of the elements needed for dental health, several precautions on sugars and starches should be added. Hard or sticky sweets should be avoided. Such highly refined sweets as soft drinks, candies, cakes, cookies, pies, syrups, jams, jellies, and pastries should be limited, especially between meals.

One's intake of starchy foods, such as bread, potatoes, and pastas, should also be controlled. Natural sugars contained in fresh fruits can provide sweet flavors with less risk of contributing to decay if the teeth are brushed regularly after eating such foods. Regular chewing gum may help remove food particles after eating, but it deposits sugar; if you chew gum, use sugarless gum.

Because decay is promoted each time sugars and other refined carbohydrates are eaten, between-meals snacks of sweets should be curtailed to lessen the chances of new or additional caries. Snack foods can be raw vegetables, such as carrots or celery, apples, cheese, peanuts, or other items that are not likely to introduce refined carbohydrates into the mouth between meals.

Brushing

Brushing the teeth is an essential of personal oral hygiene. Such brushing rids the mouth of most of the food debris that encourages bacterial growth, which is most intense 20 minutes after eating. Therefore, the teeth should be cleaned as soon as possible after a meal.

There is no one kind of toothbrush that is best for every person. Most dentists, however, recommend a soft toothbrush with a straight handle and flat brushing surface that can clean the gums without irritating them. As for claims about whether toothbrushes should have bristles with square corners or rounded shapes, a dentist may point out that there are both curved and straight surfaces in the mouth, so what one design offers in advantages may be offset by equivalent disadvantages. There also are special brushes for reaching surfaces of crooked teeth or cleaning missing-tooth areas of the mouth.

Although several different methods may be used effectively, the following is the technique most often recommended. Brush the biting surfaces, or tops, of the back upper and lower teeth. The lines and grooves on these surfaces make them prone to decay. They should be brushed first, before moisture has softened the brush. The cheek and tongue surfaces of the lower teeth are brushed next. Hold the brush parallel to the teeth with the bristle edges angled against and touching the gums. Using short strokes, move the brush back and forth several times before proceeding to the next one or two teeth. Use the same technique on all the inner surfaces of your teeth as well. For the hard-to-brush inner surfaces of the front teeth, hold the handle of the brush out in front of the mouth and apply the tip in an up-and-down motion. For all brushing, a scrubbing motion—but without too much pressure—should be used.

Some people prefer electric toothbrushes, which require less effort to use than ordinary toothbrushes. These are available with two basic motions—up and down and back and forth. Your dentist may advise which kind best serves an individual's needs

Brushing

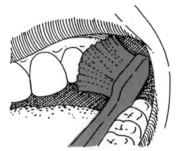

Begin by brushing the tops of the upper and lower molars, using a scrubbing motion without much pressure. A soft toothbrush with a straight handle is most recommended.

Next, keeping the brush parallel to the teeth, angle the bristles against the lower gums and brush back and forth with short strokes against both sides of every tooth. Use the same technique for the upper teeth.

Apply the tip of the brush to the backs of upper and lower front teeth. Scrub in an up-and-down motion holding the brush handle directly out in front.

and proper use of equipment. Some dentists point out that back-and-forth brushing applied with too much pressure can have an abrasive effect on tooth enamel because it works against the grain of the mineral deposits. The American Dental Association also evaluates electric toothbrushes and issues reports on the safety and effectiveness of various types.

Removing Debris with Dental Floss

Brushing often does not clean debris from between the teeth. But plaque and food particles that stick between the teeth usually can be removed with dental floss. A generous length of floss, about 18 inches, is needed to do an effective job. The ends can be wrapped several times around the first joint of the middle finger of each hand. Using the thumbs or index fingers, the floss is inserted between the teeth with a gentle, sawing, back-and-forth motion. Then it is slid gently around part of a tooth in the space at the gum line and gently pulled out; snapping the floss in and out may irritate the gums. After brushing and flossing, the mouth should be rinsed with water. A mouthwash is unnecessary, but it may be used for the good taste it leaves in the mouth.

The dentist may recommend the use of an oral irrigating device as part of dental home care. These units produce a pulsating stream of water that flushes food debris from between teeth. They are particularly useful for patients wearing orthodontic braces or for those who have had recession of the gums, creating larger spaces between the teeth.

The person who wants to see the areas of plaque on his teeth can chew a *disclosing tablet,* available at most pharmacies, which leaves a harmless temporary stain on plaque surfaces. Some dentists recommend the use of disclosing tablets about once a week so that patients can check on the effectiveness of their tooth-cleaning techniques.

Flossing

(1) Wrap floss several times around middle fingers and pull center section taut between thumbs or index fingers. (2) Insert floss between teeth and gently slide back and forth against every tooth. Work floss into the space between tooth and gumline. (3) To remove, pull floss gently downward along the angle of the tooth. Snapping it in and out may cause gum irritation.

Tooth Decay

In addition to wear, tear, and injury, the major threat to the health of a tooth is bacteria. Bacteria can cause tooth decay, and the human mouth is a tremendous reservoir of bacteria because the mouth is warm, dark, moist, and usually contains tiny particles of food that help nourish the organisms. The bacteria found in the mouth are of two kinds, *aerobic* and *anaerobic.* Aerobic bacteria need oxygen to survive; anaerobic bacteria do not. Anaerobic bacteria can find their way through cracks and crevices into areas of the mouth or teeth where there is little or no oxygen and continue their *cariogenic,* or decay, activity.

Saliva

Saliva offers some protection against the decay germs, for reasons not well understood, but there are crevices and deep pockets around the teeth and gums where saliva does not penetrate. Paradoxically, saliva itself contains millions of different bacterial organisms. Dental scientists have calculated that one ounce of saliva may contain as many as 22 billion bacteria. Even a presumably healthy mouth may contain more than ten varieties of bacteria, plus protozoa and yeast cells. The yeast cells and at least three of the different kinds of bacteria are capable of producing acids that erode the tough enamel surface of a tooth.

Bacterial Acids and Plaque

The acids produced by decay bacteria actually are waste products of the organisms' digestive processes; bacteria, like other living creatures, eventually excrete waste products after a meal. As unpleasant as the thought may be, tooth decay can be the result of feeding a colony of germs in the mouth. Bacterial growth—hence the production of harmful acids—is encouraged by the consumption of too many foods composed of refined sugars. The sugars of candies, cakes, soft drinks, and the like are easier for the bacteria to eat and digest than those of fruits, vegetables, and other less thoroughly processed foods. Even a tiny bit of food remaining in the mouth after a meal may be enough to support many millions of bacteria for 24 hours or more.

An additional contributing factor to tooth decay is *plaque* formation. Plaque is a sticky, transparent substance that forms a film over the surface of the teeth. Plaque forms every day, which is the reason that the teeth must be brushed every day. Plaque frequently begins with deposits of soft food debris along the gum line after a meal; it consists mainly of bacteria and its products. When mixed with mucus, molds, tissue cells from the membranes lining the mouth, and mineral salts, it takes the form of a white, cheesy substance called *materia alba*. If not removed regularly by brushing and the use of dental floss, this substance becomes a thick, sticky mass that has been compared to epoxy cement. Then it becomes a rough-surfaced hard substance with the texture of stone, otherwise known as *dental calculus,* or *tartar.*

Other Causes of Decay

Bacterial acid is not the only way in which the tooth enamel may be damaged to permit the entry of decay bacteria. Certain high-acid foods and improper dental care can erode the molecules of enamel. Temperature extremes also can produce cracks and other damage to the enamel; some dental scientists have suggested that repeated exposure to rapid temperature fluctuations of 50° F., as in eating alternately hot and cold foods or beverages, can cause the enamel to develop cracks.

Complications of Tooth Decay

Once decay activity breaks through the hard enamel surface, the bacteria can attack the dentin. Because the dentin is about 30 percent organic material, compared to 5 percent in the enamel layer, the decay process can advance more rapidly there. If the tooth decay is not stopped at the dentin layer, the disease organisms can enter the pulp chamber, where they will multiply quickly, producing an acute inflammation and, if unchecked, spread through the blood vessels to other parts of the body. Osteomyelitis, an infection of the membrane covering the skeletal bones, and endocarditis, an extremely dangerous heart ailment, are among diseases in other parts of the body that can begin with untreated tooth decay.

Periodontal disease, described below, is another possible complication of tooth decay.

Treatment of Tooth Decay

The portion of a tooth invaded by decay is called a *cavity;* it may be compared to an ulcer that develops because of disease in soft tissues. In treating the decay process, the dentist tries to prevent further destruction of the tooth tissue. The dentist also tries to restore as much as possible the original shape and function of the diseased tooth. The procedure used depends on many factors, including the surfaces affected (enamel, dentin, etc.) and the tooth face and angle involved, as well as whether the cavity is on a smooth area or in a pit or fissure of the tooth surface.

The decayed portions of the tooth are removed with various kinds of carbide burrs and other drill tips, as well as with hand instruments. The dentist may also use a caries removal system that reduces or eliminates drilling. In this system two solutions are combined in one liquid and squirted in a pulsating stream onto the decayed area. The stream does not harm gums or healthy teeth; rather, it softens the caries so that it can easily be scraped away. Used, generally, in conjunction with rotary

Tooth Restoration

The portion of the tooth affected by decay is known as a *cavity.* After removal of this diseased area (2), using drill, hand instrument, or other method, the dentist fills the cleaned cavity with a base or liner material (3). Finally, the tooth is filled with a restorative substance such as an amalgam, inlay, or ceramic material.

or hand instruments, the "squirt" system may make anesthesia unnecessary.

In other cases an anesthetic may be injected for the comfort of the patient. The dentist usually asks whether the patient prefers to have an anesthetic before work commences. In the cleaning process, an effort is made to remove all traces of diseased enamel or dentin, but no more of the tooth material than is necessary.

The cleaned cavity is generally filled in a layering procedure. The layers of liners and bases used before insertion of the filling are determined by the depth of the cavity and other factors. If pulp is exposed, special materials may be applied to help the pulp recover from the irritation of the procedure and to form a firm base for the amalgam, inlay, or other restorative substance that becomes the filling.

In the 1980s, new ceramic materials came into use for fillings. Many dentists believed that ceramics could provide more natural-looking restorations. With ceramics, also, teeth would be less sensitive to changes of temperature—a problem with some more traditional materials.

Tooth Extraction

When it becomes necessary to remove a diseased, damaged, or malpositioned tooth, the procedure is handled as a form of minor surgery, usually with administration of a local anesthetic to the nerves supplying the tooth area. However, there is no standard routine for extraction of a tooth, because of the numerous individual variations associated with each case. The dentist usually has a medical history of the patient available, showing such information as allergies to drugs, and medications used by the patient that might react with those employed in oral surgery. Because the mouth contains many millions of bacteria, all possible precautions are taken to prevent entry of the germs into the tooth socket.

The condition of the patient is checked during and immediately after tooth extraction, in the event that some complication develops. The patient is provided with analgesic (pain-killing) and other needed medications, along with instructions regarding control of any postoperative pain or bleeding. The dentist also may offer special diet information with suggested meals for the recovery period, which usually is quite brief.

Dry Socket

Severe pain may develop several days after a tooth has been extracted if a blood clot that forms in the socket becomes dislodged. The condition, commonly called *dry socket*, can involve infection of the alveolar bone that normally surrounds the roots of the tooth; loss of the clot can expose the bone tissue to the environment and organisms that produce *osteitis*, or inflammation of the bone tissue. Dry socket may be treated by irrigating the socket with warm salt water and packing it with strips of medicated gauze. The patient also is given analgesics, sedatives, and other medications as needed to control the pain and infection.

General anesthetics are sometimes necessary for complicated oral surgery. In such cases, there are available dental offices or clinics that are as well equipped and staffed as hospital operating rooms.

Endodontic Therapy

Tooth extraction because of caries is less common today than in previous years, although an estimated 25 million Americans have had all of their teeth removed. Modern preventive dentistry techniques of *endodontics* now make it possible to save many teeth that would have been extracted in past decades after the spread of decay into the pulp canal. The procedures include *root canal therapy, pulp capping,* and *pulpotomy.*

Root Canal Therapy

Once the tooth has fully developed in the jaw, the nerve is not needed, so if the pulp is infected the nerve as well as the pulp can be removed. Only minor effects are noticeable in the tooth structure after the pulp is removed, and the dentist compensates for these in filling the tooth after root canal therapy.

Briefly, the procedure of root canal work begins by examination and testing of the pulp viability. The pulp may be tested by heat, cold, or an electrical device called a *vitalometer,* which measure the degree of sensation the patient feels in a tooth. If the

Root Canal Therapy

(1) The first step of root canal, or removal of the nerve of a tooth, begins with examining the infected pulp to determine its vitality. (2) The depth of the root is measured by X ray and, after administering local anesthetic, the dentist extracts the pulp with drill or hand instrument marked to indicate when the end of the root has been reached. (3) When the entire pulp and nerve have been removed the canal is sterilized to prevent infection. (4) After filling the tooth with silver or a tough plastic substance known as *gutta-percha,* or sometimes a combination of both, the dentist then caps the tooth.

pulp is dead, the patient will feel no sensation, even at the highest output of current.

After the degree of vitality in the pulp has been determined, a local anesthetic is injected and the dentist begins removing the pulp, using rotary drills and hand instruments. By means of X-ray pictures, the dentist measures the length of the root, which may be about one and a half times the length of the crown. Stops or other markers are placed on the root excavation tools to show the dentist when the instrument has reached the end of the root. The canal is then sterilized and filled with gutta-percha—a tough plastic substance—silver, or a combination of the two, and a cap is added.

Pulp Capping

Pulp capping consists of building a cap over the exposed pulp with layers of calcium hydroxide paste, which is covered by zinc oxide and topped with a firm cement.

Pulpotomy

A pulpotomy procedure involves removal of the pulp in the pulp chamber within the crown of the tooth, while leaving the root canal pulp in place. The amputated pulp ends are treated and a pulp-capping procedure is used to restore the crown of the tooth.

Periodontal Disease

It is important in the middle years of life and later to continue good oral-hygiene habits and the practice of having regular dental checkups. Studies have found that after the age of 50 more than half the people in America have periodontal disease. At the age of 65, nearly everybody has this disease.

The Course of the Disease

The combination of bacterial action described above and the roughness of the resulting calculus injures the surrounding gum tissue and makes it susceptible to infection and recession. The irritation causes swelling, inflammation, and bleeding into the crevices between the teeth and gums, which is one of the early signs of impaired tissue health.

The inflammation of the gums, known as *gingivitis,* can spread to the roots of the teeth if not treated. The gums separate from the teeth, forming pockets that fill up with more food particles and colonies of bacteria. As

Periodontal Disease

1   2   3   4

(1) If allowed to build up at the gumline, deposits of plaque and calculus result in damage to the gum tissues (periodontal disease). (2) As gums become increasingly irritated and inflamed, they may bleed easily and begin to recede from the tooth itself. (3) Untreated, the inflammation spreads to the roots of the teeth. Bacteria and particles of food lodge in the pockets between tooth and gums, aggravating the condition. (4) A tooth held by the diseased gum loses most of its bony support structure, causing it to loosen and move out of position. Eventually, such teeth may need to be extracted.

the disease progresses, the bone support for the teeth is weakened and the affected teeth begin to loosen and drift from their normal position. Finally, unless the disease is treated in time, the teeth may be lost.

Periodontal disease is sometimes called *pyorrhea,* a Greek word meaning a discharge of pus. But "pyorrhea" is a somewhat misleading term, because it identifies only one manifestation of the disease, an abscess that usually forms along the side of an affected tooth. In some cases, a membrane forms around the abscess, creating a pus-filled cyst in the tooth socket.

Other Signs and Complications

Another manifestation of periodontal disease is periodontal atrophy, or recession of the gingiva, or gum tissue, and the underlying bone away from the outer layer of the tooth that joins it to its socket. Recession tends to expose the dentin below the gum line, which is not protected by a layer of enamel. The exposed dentin may be hypersensitive to hot or cold foods or beverages, air, and sweet or sour food flavors.

Inflammation of the gingival tissue in periodontal disease may be increased in intensity by toxic chemicals from tobacco smoke, bacterial infections, vitamin deficiencies, and defective dental restorations. The normal pink color of the gingival tissue may be altered by periodontal disease to a bright red or a darker coloration ranging to bluish purple.

The inflamed gingival tissue may lead to a complication called *periodontitis* in which the bone under the gum tissue is gradually destroyed, widening the crevice between the tooth and surrounding tissues. Pregnant women seem particularly vulnerable to periodontitis and gingivitis if they have been experiencing periodontal disorders, because the temporary hormonal imbalance of the pregnancy tends to exaggerate the effects of this condition.

One kind of gingivitis that involves projections of gum tissue between the teeth is sometimes referred to as *trench mouth,* because it was not an uncommon form of periodontal disease affecting soldiers during World War I. The infection is associated with poor oral hygiene, along with nutritional deficiencies and general depressed condition of health.

Causes

At one time it was assumed that periodontal diseases were associated with the life styles of persons living in more technologically advanced societies, where soft, rich foods are eaten regularly, providing materials toward the formation of plaque and support of bacteria in the plaque. But recent investigations show that people living in the less developed nations, who are relatively free of tooth decay, eventually develop periodontal disease. However, this does not alter the fact that the accumulation of plaque and harmful bacteria are the chief causes of periodontal disease, as well as of tooth decay.

Although periodontal disease generally becomes troublesome in middle age, there is some evidence that early symptoms of gingival disorders occur during childhood or adolescence. Also, because more people live longer today, periodontal disease has become more common than in the past.

Bruxism

Bruxism—the nervous habit, often unconsciously done, of clenching and grinding the teeth—can contribute to the development of periodontal disease. Bruxism frequently occurs during sleep.

Malocclusion

Another contributing cause to periodontal disease is repeated shock or undue pressure on a tooth because of *malocclusion,* or an improper bite. This effect accelerates damage to the tooth and gum structure during such simple activities as biting and chewing.

Treatment

Periodontal treatment may include a variety of techniques ranging from plaque removal to oral surgery to form new contours on the alveolar bone surrounding the tooth. If treatment is not begun until periodontal disease is well advanced, it may be difficult to fit replacement teeth, or *dentures,* as substitutes for lost teeth. Dentures fit over the ridges of the jaws, and if the top edge of the ridge has been destroyed by periodontal disease, the procedure for holding the denture firmly in place will be complicated.

Dentures

I f it becomes necessary to have some teeth removed, they should be replaced as soon as possible with a *bridge*—a mounting for false teeth anchored to natural teeth on either side—or a partial or full denture.

Why Missing Teeth Must Be Replaced

Chewing ability and clarity of speech may be impaired if missing teeth are not replaced. Also, each tooth functions to hold the teeth on either side and opposite it in place. If a tooth is lost, the tooth opposite may erupt further and the teeth on either side shift in their positions because there is no counterforce to keep them in place. Food particles lodge in the spaces created by the shifting teeth, plaque forms, and periodontal disease develops, causing the loss of additional teeth. This loss may take years if the movement of intact teeth is slow, but if they tilt and shift rapidly into the empty spaces, the remaining teeth may be lost in a much shorter time.

The loss of a few teeth can also alter a person's appearance. The cheeks may become puckered and the lips drawn together, making the individual look older.

Fitting of Dentures

Modern techniques and materials of construction and the skill of modern dentists should assure well-fitting, natural-looking dentures. The dentist selects the tooth shade and shape that are best for an individual's face size, contours, and coloring. No one, however, has perfectly arranged, perfectly white natural teeth. Tooth coloring depends upon genetic factors and changes as one grows older. These factors must be considered in designing dentures.

Partial Denture
Anchoring teeth
Denture
Upper palate

Bridges and Partial Dentures

Several different types of dental appliances may be constructed to fill empty spaces. Some, such as dental bridges, may be attached to the remaining natural teeth by cementing them. Others, such as complete sets of dentures, are removable.

A bridge may be made entirely of gold, a combination of gold and porcelain, or combinations of gold and porcelain and other materials. If there is a sound natural tooth on either side of the space, a *pontic*, or suitable substitute for the missing tooth, may be fused to the metal bridge. The crown retainer on either side of the pontic may then be cemented to the crowns of the neighboring natural teeth.

If there are no natural teeth near the space created by an extracted tooth, a partial denture may be constructed to replace the missing teeth. This appliance usually fastens by a clasp onto the last tooth on each side of the space. A bar on the inside of the front teeth provides stability for the partial denture.

A "Maryland bridge," a fixed partial denture developed by the University of Maryland's Baltimore College of Dental Surgery, eliminates the need for crowns to anchor false teeth. With the Maryland bridge, hidden metal "wings" are used to anchor the partial denture. The wings are bonded to the backs of neighboring teeth. Because it eliminates the need for drilling, the Maryland bridge saves healthy teeth, makes anesthesia unnecessary, and reduces costs considerably.

New materials have brought bonding into more common use as an alternative to crowning and for cosmetically restoring chipped, malformed, stained, or widely spaced teeth. In the bonding process the dentist isolates a tooth with a rubber dam, cleans and dries the tooth, and applies a phosphoric acid solution that produces microscopic pores in the enamel. The etched area is then filled in with a liquid plastic. To that base the dentist applies thin layers of tooth-colored plastics known as composite resins. The layers can be sculpted, hardened with a beam of light or by some other method, contoured, and polished.

A removable partial denture should be taken out and cleaned whenever the natural teeth are brushed. A special brush, usually cone-shaped to fit into the clasp, is available as a cleaning tool. The pontic, or tooth substitute of a bridge, remains in place permanently and is brushed like a natural tooth.

A bridge or partial denture helps prevent further deterioration of the mouth if it is kept clean and in good condition. But a dentist should check bridges and partial dentures periodically to make sure they have not become loosened. A loose clasp of a partial denture can rock the teeth to which the device is attached, causing damage and possible loss.

Complete Dentures

Before a full set of removable dentures is constructed, the dentist will take X rays to determine whether there are any abnormalities in the gum ridges, such as cysts or tooth root tips that may have to be removed. If the gums are in poor condition, treatments may be needed to improve the surfaces of the ridges on which the dentures will be fitted. The dentist may also have to reconstruct the bone underlying the gums—the alveolar ridge. Human bone "harvested" from another part of the patient's body has for decades been used in such reconstruction, but is today giving way to ceramic materials.

Two ceramic materials used in such surgery are hydroxylapatite and beta tricalcium phosphate. Oral surgeons have reported good results with both. The new materials are said to be safer and simpler to use and less expensive than human bone. They also eliminate the need for preliminary surgery to obtain transplants of the patient's bone.

With preliminary work done, the dentist makes an impression of the patient's mouth. Tooth and shade choices are discussed. Several other appointments may be arranged before the new dentures are delivered to the patient. Appointments may be needed for "try-ins" of dentures as they are being constructed and for adjustments after completion of the set.

Although dentures do not change with age, the mouth does. Therefore, it is necessary for the denture-wearer to have occasional dental checkups. At denture checkup appointments, the dentist examines oral tissues for irritation and determines how the dentures fit with respect to possible changing conditions of the mouth. If the dentures no longer fit properly, a replacement may be recommended. The dentist also seeks to correct any irritations of the oral tissues of the mouth and polishes the dentures, making them smooth and easier to keep clean between checkups. If any of the teeth in the dentures has become damaged, the dentist can repair or replace the denture tooth.

Care of Dentures

Dentures should be cleaned daily with a denture brush and toothpaste; once a week they should be soaked for seven or eight hours in a denture cleaner. To avoid breaking them during the brushing process, fill a wash basin with water and place it under the dentures while they are being cleaned; if they are dropped, the dentures will be cushioned by the water. A harsh abrasive that could scratch the denture surface should not be used. Scratches allow stains to penetrate the surface of the dentures, creating permanent discoloration.

The use of adhesives and powders is only a temporary solution to ill-fitting dentures. In time, the dentist may rebuild the gum side of the denture to conform with the shape of the patient's gum ridge. The patient should never try to make his own changes in the fit of dentures. Rebuilding the gum side of the dentures, or *relining,* as it is called, usually begins with a soft temporary material if the patient's gums are in poor condition, and requires several appointments over a period of two or three weeks while the gum tissues are being restored to good health.

Most patients show some concern over the replacement of natural teeth with dentures, even when a set of complete dentures is needed to replace an earlier set. Some people associate the loss of teeth with old age in the same way that others resist the advice that they should wear eyeglasses or a hearing aid. The fact is that many millions of persons of all ages have found they can improve their eating, speaking, and physical appearance by obtaining attractive and well-fitted dentures.

Orthodontics

*O*rthodontics is a term derived from the Greek words for straight, or normal, teeth. Straight teeth are easier to keep clean and they make chewing food more efficient. There also is a cosmetic benefit in being able to display a smile with a set of straight teeth, although many dentists consider the cosmetic aspect of orthodontics as secondary to achieving proper occlusion, or bite.

Causes of Improper Bite

Orthodontic problems can be caused by hereditary factors, by an infectious or other kind of disease, by the premature loss of primary teeth, by the medications used in treatment, or by individual factors such as injury or loss of permanent teeth. A person may have congenitally missing teeth resulting in spaces that permit drifting of neighboring teeth or collapse of the dental arch. Or he may develop extra (supernumerary) teeth resulting from an inherited factor. The supernumerary teeth may develop during the early years of life while the deciduous teeth are in use. A supernumerary tooth may force permanent teeth into unnatural positions.

Nutritional disorders can also affect the development of jaws and teeth, while certain medications can cause abnormal growth of gingival, or gum, tissues, resulting in increased spaces between the teeth.

Teeth that erupt too early or too late, primary teeth that are too late in falling out when permanent teeth have developed, and habits such as grinding of the teeth, thumb-sucking, or pushing the tongue against the

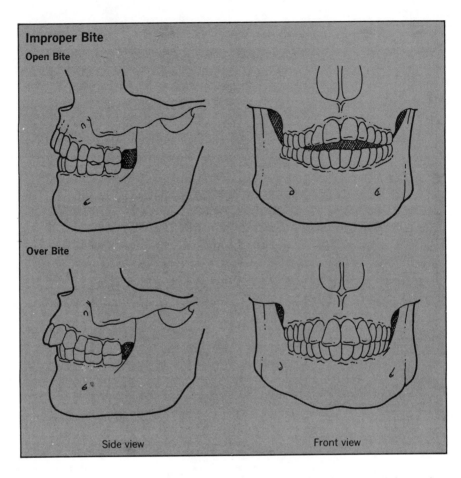

Improper Bite

Open Bite

Over Bite

Side view   Front view

teeth are among other factors that can result in *malocclusion,* or improper bite, and the need for orthodontic treatment.

Diagnosis of Orthodontic Problems

Each child should visit a dentist before the eruption of his permanent teeth for an examination that may determine the need for orthodontic treatment. Because there are many genetic and other influences that help shape the facial contours and occlusion of each individual, there are no standard orthodontic procedures that apply to any or all children. The dentist may recommend what treatment, if any, would be needed to produce normal occlusion and when it should begin; some dentists advise only that necessary procedures for correcting malocclusion be started before the permanent set of teeth (excluding wisdom teeth) has become established, or around the age of 12 or 13. However, there are few age limits for orthodontic care, and an increasing number of adults are receiving treatment today for malocclusion problems that were neglected during childhood.

In the normal or ideal occlusion positions of the teeth, the first and second permanent upper molars fit just slightly behind the same molars of the lower jaw; all of the teeth of the upper jaw are in contact with their counterparts of the lower jaw. In this pattern of occlusion, all of the biting surfaces are aligned for optimum use of their intended functions of cutting, tearing, or grinding.

There are numerous variations of malocclusion, but generally, in simple deformities, the teeth of the upper jaw are in contact with lower jaw teeth once removed from normal positions. Other variations include an *open bite,* in which the upper and lower incisors do not contact each other, or *closed bite,* in which there is an abnormal degree of overlapping (*overbite*) of the front teeth.

Diagnosis is made with the help of X-ray pictures, photographs of the face and mouth, medical histories, and plaster models of the patient's teeth and jaws. The plaster models are particularly important because the dentist can use them to make experimental reconstructions without touching an actual tooth of a patient. For example, the dentist can remove one or more teeth from the plaster model and reorganize neighboring teeth in the jawbones to get an accurate representation of the effects of extracting teeth or forcing teeth into different developmental situations.

Orthodontic Appliances

Once a plan of orthodontic treatment has been determined by the dentist, he may choose from a dozen or more types of bands, braces, or other orthodontic appliances, some removable and some nonremovable, for shaping the teeth and jaws of the patient. A typical orthodontic appliance may include small curved strips or loops of metal cemented to the surfaces of the teeth as anchors for arch wires that pass around the dental arch. Springs and specially designed rubber bands, called elastics, are sometimes used to bring about alignment of the two jaws, or to align teeth within a dental arch.

In addition to the appliances that are attached to and between the upper and lower dental arches, the dentist may prescribe the use of an elastic tape device with a strap that fits around the back of the patient's neck and is attached also to the arch wire inside the mouth, thus providing a force from outside the mouth to bring teeth into alignment.

Orthodontic appliances are custom-designed and built for the individual patient. This requires several

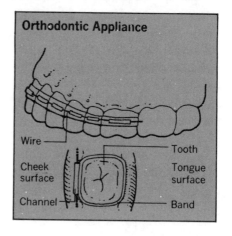

Orthodontic Appliance

Wire

Cheek surface

Channel

Tooth

Tongue surface

Band

rather long sessions or one all-day session in the dental chair while the appliance is being organized and properly anchored. Thereafter, the patient must return at regular intervals spaced a few weeks to a month apart so the dentist can make adjustments in the appliance, determine if any of the bands have pulled away from tooth surfaces, and prevent plaque from building up in places that the braces may make impervious to brushing.

The patient, meanwhile, must follow a diet that prohibits sticky foods or items that may damage the appliance or any of its parts. A conscientious program of oral hygiene, including regular cleaning by the dentist or hygienist, also is necessary because, as indicated above, it is more difficult to do a thorough job of cleaning the teeth when orthodontic appliances are in the mouth.

Orthodontics for Adults

Although orthodontic treatment originally was applied only to children, the technique has been requested with increasing frequency for the correction of a variety of facial and dental disorders. Receding chins, buck teeth, sunken cheeks, sunken mouths, and other abnormalities have been treated successfully in adults beyond the age of 40. Orthodontists have observed that adult patients usually are more patient and cooperative during the long periods of treatment than youngsters.

The upper age limit for orthodontic work has not really been established, but doctors at the National Institute of Dental Research believe it is possible to treat adult patients with protrusion of the upper jaw and related disfigurements until the age of 70.

This is possible because the upper jaw does not completely unite with the frontal bone of the skull, according to the experts, until after the age of 70 in most people.

Orthodontic treatments can be relatively expensive and involve many visits to a dentist's office over a long period of time. Any parent of a prospective patient or a responsible older patient seeking orthodontic work for himself should have a frank discussion with the dentist regarding the time and money to be invested in the corrective procedures before making an agreement to begin the work. In nearly every case some arrangement can be made for covering the costs of dental work that is vital to the health and welfare of a patient.

23

Aches, Pains, Nuisances, Worries

And Other Things You Can Live With But Could Get Along Very Well Without

None of the variety of discomforts discussed in this chapter is a laughing matter. The best thing about most of them is that they will pass, given your commonsense attention, or will disappear if you follow your physician's advice. This includes taking the medications prescribed by your physician exactly as directed. In a few cases, such as allergies or gout, long-term drug therapy may be necessary on a self-supervised basis, once treatment has been established by a physician. Of course, when symptoms of any kind persist or get worse, you should waste no time in seeking a professional diagnosis.

There may be somebody, somewhere, who has never felt rotten a day in his life. But most of us are not so fortunate. Among the most common nuisance ailments are:

- upper respiratory infections

- allergies

- occasional headaches

- backaches

- weight problems

- weather discomforts

- disturbances of normal sleep patterns

- aching feet

- indigestion

The unpleasant feeling associated with any of these common disorders can almost always be banished with a modicum of care and thought. For example, allergic reactions to particular foods can be curtailed by identifying the offending food and avoiding it.

Self-diagnosis and self-discipline can often enable one to cope with weight problems. A backache may be cured by attention to posture, or adjusting your office chair. A sensible approach to clothing and exposure can often do away with weather discomforts.

For many minor disorders and discomforts, particularly those caused by stress, massage may be the answer. Massage is a process that is at least 3,000 years old and has been used to help relieve tension, increase muscle tone, improve blood and oxygen circulation, and aid major body functions. Massage has also helped alleviate aches and pains resulting from exercise, improve posture, and increase joint flexibility. Among the disorders for which massage should not be used are osteoporosis, varicose veins, inflamed joints, herniated discs, tumors, and some cardiovascular problems.

Massage invariably involves kneading, manipulation, and methodical pressure on various body parts. The process should never be painful. The three kinds of massage in most common use are Swedish, a pleasant, muscle-kneading procedure; Shiatsu, or "acupressure," which depends on finger and hand pressure on so-called energy meridians in the body; and reflexology, a system that calls for pressure on various points of the foot.

When symptoms do not respond to self-help—as when sporadic difficulty in sleeping burgeons into a string of near-sleepless nights, or when abdominal pain you interpret as indigestion is intense or frequent in spite of avoiding rich or heavy foods, it's time to see a physician.

The Common Cold and Upper Respiratory Infections

Common cold is the label attached to a group of symptoms that can be caused by one or more of some 20 different viruses. Colds are considered highly contagious, but some physicians think that people don't entirely catch others' colds—in a sense they catch their own. While the viruses that carry the infection are air-borne and practically omnipresent, somebody in good health is usually less susceptible to a cold than someone who is run down. Both environmental factors (such as air pollution) and emotional ones (such as anxiety or depression) seem to increase susceptibility.

Symptoms

Symptoms differ from person to person and from cold to cold with the same person. Generally, a cold starts with sneezes, a running nose, teary eyes, and a stuffed head. Sometimes the nasal membranes become so swollen that a person can breathe only through the mouth; sometimes the senses of smell and taste simply disappear. The throat may be sore; a postnasal drip may cause a constant cough when the person is lying down at night.

When these symptoms are acute and are accompanied by fever and aching joints, the illness is usually referred to as influenza or "the flu." There are many different viruses that cause influenza, and new ones are always turning up. Unfortunately, there is as yet no medicine that can cure either a cold or a flu attack, although many people do get relief from symptoms by taking various cold remedies. Antibiotics are sometimes prescribed by doctors to prevent more serious bacterial diseases, such as pneumonia, from developing, but antibiotics are not effective against the cold viruses.

Treatment

Some people can get away with treating a cold with contempt and an occasional aspirin, and go about their business. Others are laid low for a few days. If you are the type who is really hit hard by a cold, it isn't coddling yourself to stay home for a couple of days. In any event, a simple cold usually runs its course, lasting anywhere from a few days to two weeks.

Discomfort can be minimized and recovery speeded by a few simple steps: extra rest and sleep, drinking more liquids than usual, and taking one or two aspirin tablets every four hours. Antihistamine preparations or nose drops should be avoided unless specifically prescribed by a physician.

A painful sore throat accompanied by fever, earache, a dry, hacking cough, or pains in the chest are symptoms that should be brought to the attention of a physician.

Prevention

Although taking massive doses of vitamin C at the first sign of a cold is said by some authorities to prevent the infection from developing, there is not yet general agreement on the effectiveness of this treatment.

Actually, there are several commonsense ways of reducing the risk of infection, particularly for those people who are especially susceptible to catching a cold. For most people, getting a proper amount of sleep, eating sensibly, avoiding exposure to sudden chill, trying to stay out of crowds, and trying to keep emotional tensions under control can increase resistance to colds and other minor respiratory infections.

Inoculation against particular types of viruses is recommended by many physicians in special cases: for pregnant women, for the elderly, and for those people who have certain chronic heart and lung diseases. Flu shots are effective against a particular virus or viruses for a limited period.

Allergies

Discomforts of various kinds are considered allergies when they are brought on by substances or conditions that ordinarily are harmless. Not too long ago, perturbed allergy sufferers would say things like:

"I can't use that soap because it gives me hives."

"Smelling roses makes me sneeze."

"Eating almonds gives me diarrhea."

Nowadays, such complaints are commonly recognized as indications of allergies.

Symptoms

Allergic symptoms can range from itching eyes, running nose, coughing, difficulty in breathing, welts on the skin, nausea, cramps, and even going into a state of shock, depending upon the severity of the allergic individual's response. Almost any part or system of the body may be affected, and almost anything can pose an allergic threat to somebody.

Allergens

Substances that trigger an allergic reaction are called *allergens.* The system of an allergic individual reacts to such substances as if they were germs, producing *antibodies* whose job it is to neutralize the allergens. But the body's defense mechanism overreacts: in the process of fighting off the effects of the allergens, various chemicals, particularly *histamines,* are dumped indiscriminately into the bloodstream. It is the overabundance of these "good" chemicals that causes the discomforts associated with allergies.

Allergens are usually placed in the following categories:

● Those that affect the respiratory tract, or *inhalants,* such as pollens, dust, smoke, perfumes, and various airborne, malodorous chemicals. These bring on sneezing, coughing, and breathing impairment.

● Food substances that affect the digestive system, typically eggs, seafood, nuts, berries, chocolate, and pork. These may cause not only nausea and diarrhea but also hives and other skin rashes.

● Medicines and drugs, such as penicillin, or a particular serum used in inoculations.

● Agents that act on the skin and mucous membranes, such as insecticides, poison oak, and poison ivy, particular chemical dyes, cosmetics, soaps, metals, leathers, and furs.

● Environmental agents, such as sunlight or excessive cold.

● Microbes, such as particular bacteria, viruses, and parasites.

Treatment

In general, approaches to treatment for allergies fall into three categories:

removing or avoiding as many allergens from the environment as possible; using creams, inhalers, pills, and other medications to control the symptoms; and undergoing immunotherapy (allergy shots) to reduce the allergic response. The type of treatment selected often depends on test findings that indicate what is causing the allergic reaction; the tests may produce such identification quickly or they may have to be continued for weeks or months before the allergen is finally tracked down.

As soon as the source of the allergen is identified, the obvious course is to avoid it, if possible. Avoidance may not, however, be possible. Few persons can avoid breathing pollen in the spring and fall. Giving up a house pet may be almost as difficult, but may be necessary as a health or comfort measure.

New medications that control the symptoms of allergies have been marketed in recent years. Newer antihistamines, for example, relieve allergic reactions but do not cause the drowsiness associated with earlier medications. Other medicines that have been used to treat allergies include adrenaline, ephedrine, and cortisone. Aerosol drugs may be used to attack specific symptoms. Some, for example, may be inhaled to treat the linings of the nose and throat.

In addition to histamines, other body chemicals are released during an allergy "attack." Researchers have found that these chemicals include leukotrienes. Consequently, antileukotrienes have tested as medications.

Direct or specific immunotherapy constitutes the third approach to treatment of allergy. The shots are effective in reducing allergic responses. A person with a substance allergy receives increasing amounts of the substance over a period of years. For example, a person who is allergic to insect stings receives injections of the particular insect's venom.

A life-threatening allergic reaction calls for emergency treatment, usually with adrenalin. Physicians suggest that persons with very intense food allergies or who are allergic to insect stings should carry special kits that include an adrenalin-filled syringe. The allergy victims administer the medication to themselves in case of *anaphylaxis*— an acute, life-threatening response (see "Allergic Shock" in Ch. 35, *Medical Emergencies*).

Persons subject to severe, disabling allergy attacks by a known allergen should also carry a card describing both the allergen and the allergic reactions. Detailed information on the latest developments in allergy treatment is available from the Asthma and Allergy Foundation of America, 1302 18th St., NW, Suite 800, Washington, DC 20036. See also Ch. 24, *Allergies and Hypersensitivities*.

Headaches

The common headache is probably as ancient as primitive man. The headache, a pain or ache across the forehead or within the head, may be severe or mild in character, and can last anywhere from under half an hour to three or four days. It may be accompanied by dizziness, nausea, nasal stuffiness, or difficulty in seeing or hearing. It is not a disease or illness but a symptom.

Causes

Headaches in today's modern world can arise from any of a number of underlying causes. These include excessive drinking or smoking, lack of sleep, hunger, drug abuse, and eyestrain. Eyestrain commonly results from overuse of the eyes, particularly under glaring light, or from failure to correct defective vision.

Treatments for headaches are as varied as the causes of headaches. Diagnosis may take some time, but if you suffer from severe or chronic headaches, it is important to consult your doctor. Headaches may point to an underlying problem, such as high blood pressure.

Headaches that are non-debilitating may be treated with analgesics such as aspirin or ibuprofen. Debilitating headaches such as tension, migraine, or cluster headaches can be treated with prescription drugs if your doctor advises it.

Chronic headaches should be diagnosed so the sufferer does not have to always depend on medication to treat the problem. Long-term solutions may include meditation, relaxation exercises, and exercise to reduce tension and stress. Dietary changes such as eliminating chocolate, caffeine, cheese, alcohol, sugar, or other products may also help.

Migraine

Migraine, also called *sick headache,* is a particularly severe, intense kind of headache. An attack may last several days and necessitate bed rest. Dizziness, sensitivity to light, and chills may accompany a migraine headache.

The exact cause of migraine is unknown, but researchers suspect a hereditary link, since the majority of migraine patients have one or more close relatives with migraine.

Migraine headaches can occur from changes in body hormone balances, sudden body temperature changes, bright light or noise, shifts in barometric pressure, and alcohol and drug use. It may also be caused by a combination of these triggers.

For chronic migraine sufferers, keeping a daily journal of food consumed, activities done, emotional status, and (for women) menstrual cycles, may help provide an indication of why migraines occur.

Migraines can be avoided by eliminating any apparent triggers. The fluctuation in estrogen is believed to be a major cause of migraines. Some foods only bring on headaches during certain times of the menstrual cycle. Hormone replacement therapy, some types of birth control pills, and menopause may increase incidence of migraines, although menopause may also end migraines in women who had them for years.

Tension Headaches

Tension headaches are characterized by a painful pressure in the head. Such headaches can be caused by stress, depression, or poor posture and should be treated with analgesics such as aspirin and ibuprofen, a massage or a cold shower. Tension headaches can occur at any time; you can even wake up with one. The best long-term treatment is learning to reduce or manage the stress in your life.

Cluster Headaches

Cluster headaches cause pain around a specific area of the head, and eye tearing, nasal stuffiness, and a burning sensation on the side of the head affected. The headaches usually last only a few hours but are usually described as excruciating. These headaches usually occur after a person has fallen asleep and typically affect men and heavy smokers. Since the pain is resistant to over-the-counter medicine, cluster headaches can be treated with corticosteroids, such as prednisone, or inhaling 100 percent oxygen.

Backaches

"Oh, my aching back" is probably the most common complaint among people past the age of 40. Most of the time, the discomfort—wherever it occurs, up or down the backbone—can be traced to some simple cause. However, there are continuous backaches that have their origin in some internal disorder that needs the attention of a physician. Among the more serious causes are kidney or pancreas disease, spinal arthritis, and peptic ulcer.

Some Common Causes

Generally a backache is the result of strain on the muscles, nerves, or ligaments of the spine. It can occur because of poor posture, carelessness in lifting or carrying heavy packages, sitting in one position for a long time in the wrong kind of chair, or sleeping on a mattress that is too soft. Backache often accompanies menstruation, and is common in the later stages of pregnancy. Emotional tension can also bring on back pain.

Prevention

In general, maintaining good posture during the waking hours and sleeping on a hard mattress at night—if necessary, inserting a bed board between the mattress and bedsprings—are the first line of defense against backaches. Anyone habitually carrying heavy loads of books or groceries, or even an overloaded attaché case, should make a habit of shifting the weight from arm to arm so that the spine doesn't always get pulled in one direction. Workers who are sedentary for most of the day at a desk or factory table should be sure that the chair they sit in provides firm support for back muscles and is the right height for the working surface.

Treatment

Most cases of simple backache respond to rest, aspirin, and the application of heat, applied by a hot water bottle or heating pad. In cases where the pain persists or becomes more acute, a physician should be consulted. He may find that the trouble is caused by the malfunctioning of an internal organ, or by pressure on the sciatic nerve (*sciatica*). With X rays he may also locate a slipped disk or other abnormality in the alignment of the vertebrae of the spine. See "Back Pain and Its Causes" in Ch. 7, *Diseases of the Skeletal System.*

Weight Problems

A few people can maintain the weight that is right for their body build without ever having to think about it. However, most experts believe that just about half the people in the United States may be risking shorter lives because they are too heavy. By one estimate, approximately one out of five American men and one out of four American women are 10 percent or more overweight, a group that may be called the borderline obese.

There is no longer any reasonable doubt that, if you are overweight, you have statistically a greater chance of high blood pressure, diabetes, and *atherosclerosis* (lumpy deposits in the arteries). And because atherosclerotic heart disease alone accounts for 20 percent of deaths among adults in the United States, it is understandable why physicians consider weight truly a national problem.

Causes

In practically all cases, weighing too much is the result of eating too much and exercising too little. In many cases, the food eaten is of the wrong kind and leisure time is used for riding around in a car rather than walking, or for watching television rather than playing tennis.

Many people like to think that they weigh too much only because they happen to like good food; but the real explanations may be considerably more complicated. In some cases, overeating has been found to have emotional sources: feelings of inadequacy; the need to compensate for a lack of affection or approval, or an unconscious desire to ward off the attention of the opposite sex. Psychological weight problems of this kind can be helped by consulting a psychiatrist or psychologist.

Treatment

There are many overweight people who merely need the support and encouragement that come from participating in a group effort, and for them, joining one of the various weight-control organizations can be extremely beneficial in taking off extra pounds and keeping them off.

Permanent results are rarely achieved by crash diets, faddish food combinations, or reducing pills. Not only are such solutions usually temporary; they may actually be harmful. See "Weight" in Ch. 27, *Nutrition and Weight Control,* for further information about weight problems.

Weather Discomforts

Using good sense about clothing, exercise, and proper diet is probably our best protection against the discomforts caused by extremes of temperature. Sometimes circumstances make this exercise of good sense impossible, with unpleasant but rarely

serious results, if treatment is promptly administered. Following are some of the more common disorders resulting from prolonged exposure to excessive heat or cold, and what you can do to alleviate them.

Heat Cramps

In a very hot environment, a person may drink great quantities of water while "sweating buckets" of salty perspiration. Thus, the body's water is replaced, but its salt is not. This salt–water imbalance results in a feeling of faintness and dizziness accompanied by acute stomach cramps and muscle pains in the legs. When the symptoms

are comparatively mild, they can be relieved by taking coated salt tablets in five-to-ten-grain doses with a full glass of tepid or cool—not iced—water. Salt tablets along with plenty of fluids should be taken regularly as a preventive measure by people who sweat a great deal during hot weather.

Sunburn

If you have not yet been exposed to much sun, as at the beginning of summer, limit your exposure at first to a period of 15 to 20 minutes, and avoid the sun at the hours around midday even if the sky is overcast. Remember, too, that the reflection of the sun's rays from water and beach sand

intensifies their effect. Some suntan lotions give effective protection against burning, and some creams even prevent tanning; but remember to cover all areas of exposed skin and to reapply the lotion when it's been washed away after a swim.

Treatment

A sunburn is treated like any other burn, depending upon its severity. See "Burns" in Ch. 31, *Medical Emergencies*. If there is blistering, take care to avoid infection. Extensive blistering requires a physician's attention.

Heat Exhaustion

This condition is different from heatstroke or sunstroke, discussed below. Heat exhaustion sets in when large quantities of blood accumulate in the skin as the body's way of increasing its cooling mechanism during exposure to high temperatures. This in turn lowers the amount of blood circulating through the heart and decreases the blood supply to the brain. If severe enough, fainting may result. Other symptoms of heat exhaustion include unusual pallor and profuse cold perspiration. The pulse may be weak, and breathing shallow.

Treatment

A person suspected of having heat exhaustion should be placed in a reclining position, his clothing loosened or removed, and his body cooled with moist cloths applied to his forehead and wrists. If he doesn't recover promptly from a fainting spell, smelling salts can be held under his nose to revive him. As soon as he is conscious, he can be given salt tablets and a cool sugary drink—either tea or coffee—to act as a stimulant. Don't give the patient any alcoholic beverages.

Sunstroke or Heatstroke

Sunstroke is much more of an emergency than heat exhaustion and requires immediate attention. The characteristic symptom is extremely high body temperature brought on by cessation of perspiration. If hot, dry, flushed skin turns ashen gray, a physician must be called immediately. Too much physical activity during periods of high temperature and high humidity is a direct contributing cause.

Treatment

See "Heatstroke" in Ch. 31, *Medical Emergencies*, for a description of the emergency treatment recommended for this condition.

Chapped Skin

One of the most widespread discomforts of cold weather is *chapped skin*. In low temperatures, the skin's sebaceous glands produce fewer oils that lubricate and protect the skin, causing it to become dry. Continued exposure results in reddening and cracking. In this condition, the skin is especially sensitive to strong soaps.

Treatment

During cold, dry weather, less soap should be used when washing, a bath oil should be used when bathing, and a mild lotion or creme should be applied to protect the skin from the damaging effects of wind and cold. A night cream or lotion containing lanolin is also helpful, and the use of cleansing cream or oil instead of soap can reduce additional discomfort when cleansing chapped areas. The use of a colorless lip pomade is especially recommended for children when they play out of doors in cold, dry weather for any length of time.

Chilblain

A *chilblain* is a local inflammation of the skin brought on by exposure to cold. The condition commonly affects people overly sensitive to cold because of poor circulation. When the hands, feet, face, and ears are affected, the skin in these areas itches and burns, and may swell and turn reddish blue.

Treatment

The best way to avoid chilblains is to wear appropriate clothing during cold weather, especially warm socks, gloves, and ear coverings. The use of bed socks and a heating pad at night is also advisable. Once indoors, cold, wet feet should be dried promptly, gently, and thoroughly. Rubbing or massaging should be avoided, because these can cause further irritation. People who suffer from repeated attacks of chilblains should consult a physician for diagnosis of circulatory problems.

Frostbite

Frostbite is a considerably more serious condition than chilblains, because it means that a part or parts of the body have actually been frozen. The fingers or toes, the nose, and the ears are most vulnerable. If frostbitten, these areas turn numb and pale and feel cold when touched. The dangerous thing about frostbite is that pain may not be a warning. If the condition is not treated promptly, the temperature inside the tissues keeps going down and eventually cuts off blood circulation to the overexposed parts of the body. In such extreme cases, there is a possible danger of gangrene.

Treatment

In mild cases, prompt treatment can slowly restore blood circulation. The frozen parts should be rewarmed *slowly* by covering them with warm clothing or by soaking them in luke-warm water. Nothing hot should be applied—neither hot water nor a heating pad. Nor should the patient be placed too close to a fireplace or ra-diator. Because the affected tissues can be easily bruised, they should not be massaged or rubbed. If you are in doubt about restoring circulation, a physician should be called promptly or the patient taken to a hospital for emergency treatment.

Sleep and the Lack of It

Until rather recently, it was assumed that sleep was the time when the body rested and recovered from the activities of wakefulness. Although there is still a great deal to learn about why we sleep and what happens when we are sleeping, medical researchers have now identified several different phases of sleep, all of them necessary over the long run, but some more cru-cial than others.

How much sleep a person needs varies a great deal from individual to individual; and the same individual may need more or less at different times. Children need long periods of unbroken sleep; the elderly seem to get along on very little. No matter what a person's age, too little sleep over too long a time leads to irritabil-ity, exhaustion, and giddiness.

Insomnia

Almost everybody has gone through periods when it is difficult or impos-sible to fall asleep. Excitement before bedtime, temporary worries about a pressing problem, spending a night in an unfamiliar place, changing to a dif-ferent bed, illness, physical discom-fort because of extremes of temper-ature—any of these circumstances can interfere with normal sleep pat-terns.

But this is quite different from *chronic insomnia,* when a person con-sistently has trouble falling asleep for no apparent reason. If despite all your commonsense approaches insomnia persists, a physician should be con-sulted about the advisability of taking a tranquilizer or a sleeping pill. Bar-biturates should not be taken unless prescribed by a physician.

The Vulnerable Extremities

Aches and pains in the legs and feet occur for a wide variety of reasons, some trivial and easily corrected, others serious enough to require medical attention. Those that origi-nate in such conditions as arthritis and rheumatism can often be alleviated by aspirin or some of the newer prescrip-tion medications.

Gout

Gout, which is usually a metabolic disorder, is a condition that especially affects the joint of the big toe, and sometimes the ankle joint, causing the area to become swollen, hot, and acutely painful. Although the specific cause of gout is not yet clearly understood, the symptoms can be alleviated by special medication prescribed by a physician. An attack of gout can be triggered by a wide variety of causes: wearing the wrong shoes, eating a diet too rich in fats, getting a bad chill, surgery in some other part of the body, or chronic emotional anxiety, as well as the use of certain medicines, such as diuretics ("waterpills"). See also "Gout" in Ch. 7, *Diseases of the Skeletal System.*

Fallen Arches

Fallen arches can cause considerable discomfort because the body's weight is carried on the ligaments of the inside of the foot rather than on the sole. When the abnormality is corrected by orthopedic shoes with built-in arches for proper support, the pressure on the ligaments is relieved. A physician rather than a shoe salesman should be consulted for a reliable diagnosis. In some cases, the physician may also recommend special exercises to strengthen the arch.

Flat Feet

Flat feet can usually be revealed by a simple test—making a footprint on level earth or hard-packed sand. If the print is solid rather than indented by a curve along the big-toe side of the foot, the foot is flat. Aching ligaments in the area of the instep are often a result, but can be relieved by proper arch supports inside the shoes. Corrective arch supports are particularly important for young children, for anyone who is overweight, and for anyone who has to stand a great deal of the time.

Blisters

Although blisters are sometimes a sign of allergy, fungus infection, or sunburn, they most commonly appear on the feet because of the friction of a shoe or of hosiery that does not fit properly. A *water blister* is a collection of lymph that forms inside the upper level of the skin; a *blood blister* goes down deeper and contains some blood released from broken capillaries. A normal amount of walking in shoes and hosiery that fit comfortably—neither too loose nor too tight—rarely results in blisters. When blisters do appear, it is best to protect them from further friction by the use of a sterile bandage strip.

Treatment

A blister that causes acute pain when one is walking can be treated as follows: after cleaning the area with soap and water, pat it dry and swab it with rubbing alcohol. Sterilize the tip of a needle in a flame, let it cool a little, and then puncture the edge of the blister, absorbing the liquid with a sterile gauze. The loose skin can be removed with manicure scissors that have been sterilized by boiling for ten minutes. The surface of raw skin should then be covered with an adhesive bandage. This procedure is best done before bedtime so that healing can begin before shoes are worn again.

If redness appears around the area of any blister and inflammation appears to be spreading, a physician should be consulted promptly.

Bunions

A *bunion* is a deformation in the part of the foot that is joined by the big toe. The swelling and pain at the joint is caused by inflammation of the *bursa* (a fluid-filled sac) that lubricates the joint. Although bunions often develop because of wearing shoes that don't fit correctly, they most frequently accompany flat feet. Pain that is not too severe can be relieved by the application of heat; the condition may eventually be cured by doing foot exercises recommended by a physician, who will also help in the choice of correct footwear. A bunion that causes acute pain and difficulty in walking can be treated by a simple surgical procedure.

Calluses

A *callus* is an area of the skin that has become hard and thick as a result of constant friction or pressure against it. Pain results when the callus is pressed against a nerve by poorly fitting shoes. A painful callus can be partially removed by rubbing it—very cautiously—with a sandpaper file or a pumice stone sold for that purpose. The offending shoes should then be discarded for correctly fitted ones. Foot care by a podiatrist is recommended for anyone with recurring calluses and corns (see below), and especially for those people who have diabetes or any disorder of the arteries.

Corns

A *corn* is a form of callus that occurs on or between the toes. When the thickening occurs on the outside of the toe, it is called a *hard corn;* when it is located between the toes, it is called a *soft corn.* The pain in the affected area is caused by pressure of the hard inside core of the corn against the tissue beneath it. The most effective treatment for corns is to wear shoes that are the right size and fit. Corns can be removed by a podiatrist, but unless footwear fits properly, they are likely to return.

Treatment

To remove a corn at home, the toes should be soaked in warm water for about ten minutes and dried. The corn can be rubbed away with an emery file, or it can be treated with a few drops of 10 percent salicylic acid in collodion, available from any druggist. Care should be exercised in applying the solution so that it doesn't reach surrounding tissue; it is highly irritating to normal skin. The area can then be covered with a corn pad to relieve pressure. This treatment may have to be repeated several times before the corn becomes soft enough to lift out. Diabetics or those suffering from any circulatory disorder should never treat their own corns.

Bursitis

Bursitis is a pain and swelling in a joint caused when the bursa, a sac-like cushion between the bones and tendons, becomes worn or torn from constant use.

Forms of bursitis include: housemaid's knee, characterized by a swollen kneecap that has become inflamed by injury or constant pressure; bunions, where the joint of the big toe is swollen and inflamed by poorly fitting shoes; and weaver's bottom, where the bursa around the pelvic girdle become damaged from long periods of sitting on hard surfaces.

Bursitis can be treated by resting the inflamed joint, applying heat, taking an anti-inflammatory drug, such as aspirin or ibuprofen, or getting a corticosteroid injection or antibiotic therapy. For chronic bursitis, surgery may be required, and physical therapy to repair the joint may follow treatment.

Tendinitis

Tendinitis is inflammation of a tendon, and tenosynovitis is inflammation of the tendon sheath from injury. These problems tend to occur together. The tendon becomes injured by excessive or unusual use, such as a weekend athlete might experience, or from extreme strain on the tendon by overexertion in lifting, carrying, or moving something heavy. The tendon may also be injured by repetitive movement. The areas most susceptible to tendon injuries are the shoulder, hips, hamstrings, ankles, and heels.

Tendinitis can be treated with aspirin or ibuprofen, corticosteroid injections, elevating the injured limb and applying ice, and using a sling. Tendinitis can be avoided by doing warm-up exercises before engaging in an athletic activity, and by not overexerting.

If the pain is persistent, you should seek professional medical advice. Because rest and then gradually increased exercise of the injured area is required, your doctor will have to help you develop a plan for recovery.

Carpal tunnel syndrome

Carpal tunnel syndrome is caused when a median nerve, which provides feeling in the wrist, thumb and fingers, is compressed and becomes swollen and inflamed. The result is a painful stiffness of the hand, wrist, or fingers. The pain also can reach an arm or shoulder.

The debilitating condition is caused by repetitive motion caused by overusing the wrist. It typically affects people who type, such as secretaries and reporters, and is common among carpenters, meat cutters, gymnasts, and supermarket checkers. Water retention and weight gain in pregnant women often causes them to develop carpal tunnel syndrome which disappears after the baby is born.

Treatments include halting the activity that caused the syndrome, performing the activity differently, and using a splint to keep the wrist from bending while it heals. Antiinflammatory drugs are also used. In severe cases, a carpal tunnel sufferer may be injected with corticosteroid drugs or undergo surgery to cut the bandlike ligament that is pressing on the median nerve.

Unnecessary delays in treating carpal tunnel may cause loss of function, although the condition need not reach such a stage.

The Exposed Integument

Common skin and scalp annoyances such as rashes, itches, dandruff, excessive perspiration, and infections of various kinds (such as athlete's foot and ringworm), as well as acne, wrinkles, and baldness, are discussed in Ch. 21, *Skin and Hair.*

Splinters

If lodged superficially in the hand, a splinter will usually work its own way out, but a splinter of no matter what size in the sole of the foot must be removed promptly to avoid its becoming further embedded by pressure and causing infection. The simplest method of removal is to pass a needle through a flame; let the needle cool; then, after the skin surface has been washed with soap and water or swabbed with alcohol, press the point of the needle against the skin, scraping slightly until the tail of the splinter is visible and loosened. It can then be pulled out with tweezers that have been sterilized in boiling water or alcohol.

Hangnails

Hangnails are pieces of partly living skin torn from the base or side of the fingernail, thus opening a portion of the underskin to infection. A hangnail can cause considerable discomfort. It should not be pulled or bitten off; but the major part of it can be cut away with manicuring scissors. The painful and exposed area should then be washed with soap and water and covered with a sterile adhesive bandage. Hangnails are likely to occur when the skin is dry. They can therefore be prevented by the regular use of a hand cream or lotion containing lanolin.

"Normal" Disorders of the Blood and Circulation

Almost everybody is bothered occasionally by minor disturbances of the circulatory system. Most of the time these disturbances are temporary, and in many cases where they are chronic they may be so mild as not to interfere with good health. Among the more common disturbances of this type are the following.

Anemia

Anemia is a condition in which there is a decrease in the number of red blood cells or in the hemoglobin content of the red blood cells. *Hemoglobin* is the compound that carries oxygen to the body tissues from the lungs. Anemia in itself is not a disease but rather a symptom of some other disorder, such as a deficiency of iron in the diet; excessive loss of blood resulting from an injury or heavy menstrual flow; infection by industrial poisons; or kidney or bone marrow disease. A person may also develop anemia as a result of hypersensitivity (allergy) to various medicines.

In the simple form of anemia, caused by a deficiency of iron in the diet, the symptoms are rarely severe. There may be feelings of fatigue, a loss of energy, and a general lack of vitality. Deficiency anemia is especially common among children and pregnant women, and can be corrected by adding foods high in iron to the diet, such as liver, lean meat, leafy green vegetables, whole wheat bread, and dried peas and beans.

If the symptoms persist, a physician should be consulted for diagnosis and treatment. For more information on anemia, see "Diseases of the Blood" in Ch. 9, *Diseases of the Circulatory System.*

Varicose Veins

Varicose veins are veins that have become ropy and swollen, and are therefore visible in the leg, sometimes bulging on the surface of the skin. They are the result of a sluggish blood flow (poor circulation), often combined with weakened walls of the veins themselves. The condition is common in pregnancy and occurs frequently among people who find it necessary to sit or stand in the same position for extended periods of time. A tendency to develop varicose veins may be inherited.

Even before the veins begin to be visible, there may be such warning symptoms as leg cramps, feelings of fatigue, or a general achiness. Unless the symptoms are treated promptly, the condition may worsen, and if the blood flow becomes increasingly impeded, ulcers may develop on the lower area of the leg.

Treatment

Mild cases of varicose veins can be kept under control, or even corrected, by giving some help to circulation, as follows:

- Several times during the day, lie flat on your back for a few minutes, with the legs slightly raised.

- Soak the legs in warm water.

- Exercise regularly.

- Wear lightly reinforced stockings or elastic stockings to support veins in the legs.

If varicose veins have become severe, a physician should be consulted. He or she may advise injection treatment or surgery. See also "The Inflammatory Disorders" in Ch. 9, *Diseases of the Circulatory System.*

Chronic Hypertension

Hypertension, commonly known as *high blood pressure,* is a condition that may be a warning of some other disease. In many cases, it is not in itself a serious problem and has no one underlying specific cause: this is called *functional, essential,* or *chronic hypertension.* The symptoms of breathing difficulty, headache, weakness, or dizziness that accompany high blood pressure can often be controlled by medicines that bring the pressure down, by sedatives or tranquilizers, and in cases where overweight is a contributing factor, by a change in diet, or by a combination of these.

More serious types of high blood pressure can be the result of kidney disease, glandular disturbances, or diseases of the circulatory system. Acute symptoms include chronic dizziness or blurred vision. Any symptoms of high blood pressure call for professional advice and treatment. See "Hypertensive Heart Disease" in Ch. 10, *Heart Disease.*

Tachycardia

Tachycardia is the medical name for a condition that most of us have felt at one time or another—abnormally rapid heartbeat, or a feeling that the heart is fluttering, or pounding too quickly. The condition can be brought on by strong feelings of fear, excitement, or anxiety, or by overtaxing the heart with sudden exertion or too much exercise. It may also be a sign of heart disease, but in such cases, it is usually accompanied by other symptoms.

The most typical form of occasional rapid heartbeat is called *paroxysmal tachycardia,* during which the beat suddenly becomes twice or three times as fast as it is normally, and then just as suddenly returns to its usual tempo. When the paroxysms are frequent enough to be disturbing and can be traced to no specific source, they can be prevented by medicines prescribed by a physician.

Nosebleed

Nosebleeds are usually the result of a ruptured blood vessel. They are especially common among children, and among adults with high blood pressure. If the nosebleed doesn't taper off by itself, the following measures should be taken: the patient should be seated—but not lying down—clothing loosened, and a cold compress placed on the back of the neck and the nose. The soft portion of the nostril may be pressed gently against the bony cartilage of the nose for at least six minutes, or rolled wads of absorbent cotton may be placed inside each nostril, with part of the cotton sticking out to make its removal easier. The inserted cotton should be left in place for several hours and then gently withdrawn.

Fainting

Fainting is a sudden loss of consciousness, usually caused by an insufficient supply of blood and oxygen to the brain. Among the most common causes of fainting are fear, acute hunger, the sight of blood, and prolonged standing in a room with too little fresh air. Fainting should not be confused with a loss of consciousness resulting from excessive alcohol intake or insulin shock. A person about to faint usually feels dizzy, turns pale, and feels weak in the knees.

Treatment

If possible, the person should be made to lie down, or to sit with his head between his knees for several minutes. Should he lose consciousness, place him so that his legs are slightly higher than his head, loosen his clothing, and see that he gets plenty of fresh air. If smelling salts or aromatic spirits of ammonia are available, they can be held under his nose. With these procedures, he should revive in a few minutes. If he doesn't, a physician should be called.

Troubles Along the Digestive Tract

From childhood on, most people are occasionally bothered by minor and temporary disturbances connected with digestion. Most of the disturbances listed below can be treated successfully with common sense and, if need be, a change in habits.

The Mouth

The digestive processes begin in the mouth, where the saliva begins chemically to break down some foods into simpler components, and the teeth and the tongue start the mechanical breakdown. Disorders of the teeth such as a malocclusion or poorly fitted dentures that interfere with proper chewing, should promptly be brought to the attention of a dentist.

Inflammation of the Gums

Also known as *gingivitis,* inflammation of the gums is caused by the bacteria that breed in food trapped in the spaces between the gums and the teeth. The gums become increasingly swollen, may bleed easily, and be sore enough to interfere with proper chewing. The condition can be prevented by cleaning the teeth thoroughly and frequently, which includes the use of dental floss or the rubber tip on the toothbrush to remove any food particles lodged in the teeth after eating. Because gingivitis can develop into the more serious condition of *pyorrhea,* persistent gum bleeding or soreness should receive prompt professional treatment. See Ch. 22, *The Teeth and Gums.*

Canker Sores

Canker sores are small ulcers inside the lips, mouth, and cheeks. Their specific cause is unknown, but they seem to accompany or follow a virus infection, vitamin deficiency, or emotional stress. They may be additionally irritated by citrus fruit, chocolate, or nuts. A canker sore usually clears up in about a week without special treatment. A bland mouth rinse will relieve pain and, in some cases, speed the healing process.

Coated Tongue

Although a coated tongue is commonly supposed to be a sure sign of illness, this is not the case. The condition may occur because of a temporary lack of saliva.

Glossitis

Glossitis, an inflammation of the tongue causing the tongue's surface to become bright red or, in some cases, glazed in appearance, may be a symptom of an infection elsewhere in the body. It may also be a symptom of anemia or a nutritional deficiency, or it may be an adverse reaction to certain forms of medication. If the inflammation persists and is accompanied by acute soreness, it should be called to a physician's attention.

Halitosis or Bad Breath

Contrary to the millions of commercial messages on television and in print, bad breath cannot be cured by any mouthwash, lozenge, spray, or antiseptic gargle now on the market. These products can do no more than mask the odor until the basic cause is diagnosed and cured. Among the many conditions that may result in bad breath (leaving out such fleeting causes as garlic and onions) are the following: an infection of the throat, nose, or mouth; a stomach or kidney disorder; pyorrhea; respiratory infection; tooth decay; improper mouth hygiene; and excessive drinking and smoking. Anyone who has been made self-conscious about the problem of bad breath should ask his physician or dentist whether his breath is truly offensive and if it is, what to do about it.

Gastritis

Gastritis, one of the most common disorders of the digestive system, is an inflammation of the lining of the stomach that may occur in acute, chronic, or toxic form. Among the causes of *acute gastritis* are various bacterial or viral infections; overeating, especially heavy or rich foods; excessive drinking of alcoholic beverages; or food poisoning. An attack of acute gastritis may be severely painful, but the discomfort usually subsides with proper treatment. The first symptom is typically sharp stomach cramps, followed by a bloated feeling, loss of appetite, headache, and nausea. When vomiting occurs, it rids the stomach of the substance causing the attack but usually leaves the patient temporarily weak. If painful cramps persist and are accompanied by fever, a physician should be consulted about the possibility of medication for bacterial infection. For a few days after an attack of acute gastritis, the patient should stay on a bland diet of easily digested foods, taken in small quantities.

Toxic Gastritis

Toxic gastritis is usually the result of swallowing a poisonous substance, causing vomiting and possible collapse. It is an emergency condition requiring prompt first aid treatment and the attention of a physician. See "Poisoning" in Ch. 31, *Medical Emergencies.*

Chronic Gastritis

Chronic gastritis is a recurrent or persisting inflammation of the stomach lining over a lengthy period. The condition has the symptoms associated with indigestion, especially pain after eating. It can be caused by excessive drinking of alcoholic beverages, constant tension or anxiety, or deficiencies in the diet. The most effective treatment for chronic gastritis is a bland diet from which caffeine and alcohol have been eliminated. Heavy meals should be avoided in favor of eating small amounts at frequent intervals. A tranquilizer or a mild sedative prescribed by a physician may reduce the tensions that contribute to the condition. If the discomfort continues, a physician should be consulted about the possibility of ulcers. See Ch. 11, *Diseases of the Digestive System.*

Gastroenteritis

Gastroenteritis is an inflammation of the lining of both the stomach and the intestines. Like gastritis, it can occur in acute or toxic forms as a result of food poisoning, excessive alcohol intake, viral or bacterial infections, or food allergies. Vomiting, diarrhea, and fever may be more pronounced and of longer duration. As long as nausea and vomiting persist, no food or fluid should be taken; when these symptoms cease, a bland, mainly fluid diet consisting of strained broth, thin cereals, boiled eggs, and tea is best. If fever continues and diarrhea doesn't taper off, a physician should be called.

Diarrhea

Diarrhea is a condition in which bowel movements are abnormally frequent and liquid. It may be accompanied by cramps, vomiting, thirst, and a feeling of tenderness in the abdominal region. Diarrhea is always a symptom of some irritant in the intestinal tract; among possible causes are allergy, infection by virus or bacteria, accidentally swallowed poisonous substances, or excessive alcohol. Brief attacks are sometimes caused by emotions, such as overexcitement or anxiety.

Diarrhea that lasts for more than two days should be diagnosed by a physician to rule out a more serious infection, a glandular disturbance, or a tumor. Mild attacks can be treated at home by giving the patient a light, bland diet, plenty of fluids, and the prescribed dosage of a kaolin-pectin compound available at any drugstore.

Constipation

Many people have the mistaken notion that if they don't have a bowel movement every day, they must be constipated. This is not necessarily so. From a physician's viewpoint, constipation is determined not by an arbitrary schedule of when the bowel should be evacuated but by the individual's discomfort and other unpleasant symptoms. In too many instances, overconcern and anxiety about bowel movements may be the chief cause of constipation.

The watery waste that results from the digestion of food in the stomach and small intestine passes into the large intestine, or colon, where water is absorbed from the waste. If the waste stays in the large intestine for too long a time, so much water is removed that it becomes too solid and compressed to evacuate easily. The efficient removal of waste material from the large intestine depends on wavelike muscular contractions. When these waves are too weak to do their job properly, as often happens in the elderly or the excessively se-

dentary, a physician may recommend a mild laxative or mineral oil.

Treatment

Constipation is rarely the result of an organic disorder. In most cases, it is caused by poor health habits; when these are corrected, the disorder corrects itself. Often, faulty diet is a major factor. Make sure that meals contain plenty of roughage in the form of whole-grain cereals, fruit, and leafy green vegetables. Figs, prunes, and dates should be included from time to time. Plenty of liquid intake is important, whether in the form of juices, soups, or large quantities of water. Scheduling a certain amount of exercise each day strengthens the abdom-

inal muscles and stimulates muscle activity in the large intestine. Confronting the sources of worries and anxieties, if necessary with a trained therapist, may also be helpful.

An enema or a laxative should be considered only once in a while rather than as regular treatment. The colon should be given a chance to function properly without relying on artificial stimulation. If constipation resists these commonsense approaches, the problem should be talked over with a physician.

Hemorrhoids

Hemorrhoids, commonly called *piles,* are swollen veins in the mucous membrane inside or just outside the rectum. When the enlargement is slight, the only discomfort may be an itching sensation in the area. Acute cases are accompanied by pain and bleeding. Hemorrhoids are a very common complaint and occur in people of all ages. They are usually the result of straining to eliminate hard, dry stools. The extra pressure causes a fold of

the membranous rectal lining to slip down, thus pinching the veins and irritating them.

Because hemorrhoids may be a symptom of a disorder other than constipation, they should be treated by a physician. If neglected, they may bleed frequently and profusely enough to cause anemia. Should a blood clot develop in an irritated vein, surgery may be necessary.

Treatment

Advertised cures should be avoided because they are not only ineffective but can cause additional irritation. Laxatives and cathartics, which may temporarily solve the problem of constipation, are likely to aggravate hem-

orrhoids.

If pain or bleeding becomes acute, a physician should be consulted promptly. Treatment can be begun at home. Sitting for several minutes in a hot bath in the morning and again in the evening (more frequently if necessary) will provide temporary relief.

Preventing constipation is of the utmost importance.

Anal Fissure

This is a condition in which a crack or split or ulcerated place develops in the area of the two anal sphincters, or muscle rings, that control the release of feces. Such breaks in the skin are generally caused by something sharp in the stool, or by the passage of an unusually hard and large stool. Although discomfort often accompanies a bowel movement when there is a fissure, the acute pain typically comes afterward. Healing is difficult because the injured tissue is constantly open to irritation. If the condition persists, it usually has to be treated by a minor surgical procedure. Intense itching in this area is called *anal pruritis*.

Minor Ailments in the Air Pipes

In addition to all the respiratory discomforts that go along with the common cold, there are various other ailments that affect breathing and normal voice production.

Bronchitis

Usually referred to as a chest cold, *bronchitis* is an inflammation of the bronchial tubes that connect the windpipe and the lungs. If bronchitis progresses down into the lungs, it can develop into pneumonia. Old people and children are especially susceptible to acute bronchitis. The symptoms include pain in the chest, a feeling of fatigue, and a nagging cough. If the infection is bacterial, it will respond to antibiotics. If it is viral, there are no specific medicines. The attack usually lasts for about ten days, although recovery may be speeded up with bed rest and large fluid intake.

Chronic Bronchitis

Chronic bronchitis is a condition that may recur each winter, or may be present throughout the year in the form of a constant cough. The condition is aggravated by smoking and by irritants such as airborne dust and smog. The swollen tissues and abnormally heavy discharge of mucus interfere with the flow of air from the lungs and cause shortness of breath. Medicines are available that lessen the bronchial phlegm and make breathing easier. People with chronic bronchitis often sleep better if they use more than one pillow and have a vaporizer going at night.

Coughing

Coughing is usually a reflex reaction to an obstruction or irritation in the trachea (windpipe), pharynx (back of mouth and throat), or bronchial tubes. It can also be the symptom of a disease or a nervous habit. For a simple cough brought on by smoking too much or breathing bad air, medicines can be taken that act as sedatives to inhibit the reflex reaction. Inhaling steam can loosen the congestion (a combination of swollen membranes and thickened mucus) that causes some types of coughs, and hot drinks such as tea or lemonade help to soothe and relax the irritated area. Constant coughing, especially when accompanied by chest pains, should be brought to a physician's attention. For a discussion of whooping cough and croup, see the respective articles under the "Alphabetic Guide to Child Care" in Ch. 2, *The First Dozen Years.*

Laryngitis

Laryngitis is an inflammation of the mucous membrane of the larynx (voice box) that interferes with breathing and causes the voice to become hoarse or disappear altogether. This condition may accompany a sore throat, measles, or whooping cough, or it may result from an allergy. Prolonged overuse of the voice, a common occupational hazard of singers and teachers, is also a cause. The best treatment for laryngitis is to go to bed, keep the room cool, and put moisture into the air from a vaporizer, humidifier, or boiling kettle. Don't attempt to talk, even in a whisper. Keep a writing pad within arm's reach and use it to spare your voice. Drinking warm liquids may help to relieve some of the discomfort. If you must go out, keep the throat warmly protected.

Chronic laryngitis may result from too many acute laryngitis attacks, which can cause the mucous membrane to become so thick and tough that the voice remains permanently hoarse. The sudden onset of hoarseness that lasts for more than two weeks calls for a physician's diagnosis.

Hiccups

Hiccups (also spelled *hiccoughs*) are contractions of the diaphragm, the great muscle responsible for forcing air in and out of our lungs. They may be brought on by an irritation of the diaphragm itself, of the respiratory or digestive system, or by eating or drinking too rapidly. Common remedies for hiccups include sipping water slowly, holding the breath, and putting something cold on the back of the neck. Breathing into a paper bag is usually effective because after a few breaths, the high carbon dioxide content in the bag will serve to make the diaphragm contractions more regular, rather than spasmodic. If none of these measures helps, it may be necessary to have a physician prescribe a sedative or tranquilizer.

The Sensitive Eyes and Ears

Air pollution affects not only the lungs but the eyes as well. In addition to all the other hazards to which the eyes are exposed, airborne smoke, chemicals, and dust cause the eyes to burn, itch, and shed tears. Other common eye troubles are discussed below.

Sty

This pimplelike inflammation of the eyelid is caused by infection, which may be linked to the blocking of an eyelash root or an oil gland, or to general poor health. A sty can be treated at home by applying clean compresses of hot water to the area for about 15 minutes at a time every two hours. This procedure should cause the sty to open, drain, and heal. If sties are recurrent, a health checkup may be indicated.

Pinkeye

Pinkeye, an acute form of *conjunctivitis,* is an inflammation of the membrane that lines the eyelid and covers the eyeball, causing the eyes to become red and the lids to swell and stick together while one is sleeping. The condition may result from bacterial or viral infection—in which case it is extremely contagious—or from allergy or chemical irritation. A physician should be consulted.

Conjunctivitis can be treated by washing the eyes with warm water, drying them with a disposable tissue to prevent the spread of infection, and applying a medicated yellow oxide of mercury ophthalmic ointment (as recommended by your physician) on the inner edges of the lids. This should be done upon rising in the morning and upon retiring at night. The eyes should then be closed until the ointment has spread. Apply compresses of hot water three or four times a day for five-minute periods.

Eyestrain

Eyestrain—with symptoms of fatigue, tearing, redness, and a scratchy feeling in the eyelids—can be caused by a need for corrective glasses, by a disorder of the eye, or by overuse of the eyes. One of the most common causes of eyestrain, however, is improper lighting. Anyone engaged in close work, such as sewing or miniature model building, and at all times when reading, should have light come from behind and from the side so that no shadow falls on the book or object being scrutinized. The light should be strong enough for comfort—not dazzling. Efforts should be made to avoid a shiny or highly polished work surface that produces a glare. To avoid eyestrain when watching television, be sure the picture is in sharp focus; the viewer should sit at least six feet from the screen; and see that the room is not in total darkness.

Ear Infections

Ear infections related to colds, sore throats, or tonsillitis can now be kept from spreading and entering the mastoid bone by the use of sulfa drugs and antibiotics. Any acute earache should therefore be called to a physician's attention promptly. Aspirin can be taken for temporary relief from pain; holding a heating pad or a hotwater bottle to the affected side of the face may also be helpful until proper medication can be prescribed.

Earwax

An excessive accumulation of earwax can cause pain and interfere with hearing. A small wad of cotton should be used to gently clean the ear canal, and sharp objects such as hairpins and matchsticks should never be used.

Hardened earwax can be softened by a few drops of hydrogen peroxide. Sometimes a doctor may have to flush out earwax that is deeply imbedded.

Ear Blockage

A stopped-up feeling in the ear can be caused by a cold, and also by the change in air pressure experienced when a plane makes a rapid descent.

The obstruction of the eustachian tube can usually be opened by swallowing hard or yawning.

Ringing in the Ear

The general word for a large variety of noises in the ear is *tinnitus*. Tinnitus can be ringing, buzzing, or other low level continual sounds. Everyone experiences some form of ear ringing on occasion, such as after listening to loud music or noise. However, chronic noise is symptomatic of other problems. Tinnitus can be caused by tension in the jaw muscle from stress, grinding of the teeth, or structural problems with the jaw. It can also be caused by high blood pressure, infec-tions, or as a reaction to chemicals, such as nicotine. If you experience continual or chronic ringing, you should discuss it with your physician.

Tinnitus is treated by avoiding excessive noise, masking irritating ear noises with music or amplified sounds from a hearing aid or cleaning ear wax out of ears. A doctor's opinion should also be sought to determine if the ringing is caused by an inner ear infection. Avoiding caffeine, nicotine and alcohol also helps.

The Path from the Kidneys

Cystitis

Cystitis is the general term for inflam-mation of the bladder caused by var-ious types of infection. It is more common in women than in men. Infecting microbes may come from outside the body by way of the urethra, or from some other infected organ, such as the kidney. When the bladder becomes inflamed, frequent and painful urination results.

Cystitis may also occur as a consequence of other disorders, such as enlargement of the prostate gland, a structural defect of the male urethra, or stones or a tumor in the bladder. Although there is no completely reliable way to prevent cystitis, some types of infection can be prevented by cleansing the genital region regularly so that the entrance of the urethra is protected against bacterial invasion. Cystitis is usually cured by medicines prescribed by a physician. For a detailed discussion of cystitis and related conditions affecting women, see "Disorders of the Urinary System" in Ch. 25, *Women's Health.*

Prostatitis

Prostatitis is an inflammation of the prostate gland (present in males only), caused by an infection of the urinary tract or some other part of the body. It may occur as a result of venereal infection. The symptoms of painful and excessive urination generally respond favorably to antibiotics. *Acute prostatitis* is less common: the patient is likely to have a high fever, as well as a discharge of pus from the penis. These symptoms should be brought to a physician's attention without delay.

Excessive Urination

A need to empty the bladder with excessive frequency can be merely a nuisance caused by overexcitement or tension, or it can be the sign of a disorder of the urinogenital system. A physician should be consulted if the problem persists.

The All-Important Feet

The *podiatrist* is the specialist who treats foot problems. Causes of foot ailments range from lack of cleanliness to ill-fitting shoes and overindulgence in athletic activities (see "Care of the Feet" in Ch. 5, *The Middle Years,* "The Vulnerable Extremities" in Ch. 23, *Aches, Pains, Nuisances, Worries*).

An ache, pain, or other disorder of the foot can be particularly annoying because it usually hampers mobility. A severe problem can keep a person bedridden, sometimes in the hospital, for substantial periods of time. As humans, we move about on our feet. They deserve the best of care from us, as their owners, and from the podiatrist in case a serious problem arises.

Podiatry, the science of foot care, has become more and more important as Americans have taken to athletics and exercises of various kinds. Most of these activities require the use of the feet. Increasing numbers of persons in the adult years are also taking up walking, jogging, or running as diversions or exercises.

Podiatrists believe that some persons "walk old"—they give the appearance, by the way they walk, of greater age than their chronological years. Others "walk young," or walk normally. Those who walk old may be inviting foot problems, and a fact of podiatric science is that every foot problem has its reflection in another part, or other parts, of the body.

By contrast, good foot and body posture often suggests that the owner of the feet enjoys good health in other parts of the body. Foot care may in effect help other body parts to function better. Because many problems with parts of the body remote from the feet make good foot posture and normal walking difficult or impossible, individuals with diverse problems, such as back pains, sometimes go to a podiatrist for treatment. The back pain may disappear when the feet have been brought into good working order.

Diabetes and the Feet

"Care" for the feet of diabetics means prevention. The diabetic tries to keep his feet so healthy that he avoids major problems. He knows that diabetes affects blood circulation, and that the leg and foot are extremely vulnerable to circulatory problems. Where blood cannot reach a limb or member, gangrene becomes a possibility.

Foot Care

What kind of care serves the diabetic best? Effective care means that the diabetic takes steps quickly to treat such problems as abrasions or ulcers that refuse to heal. Other conditions that warn of possible future problems are dry skin, numbness, and dry or brittle nails. Ulcers that appear in the skin of the foot and that appear to have roots in deeper layers of tissue serve as danger signals. Such ulcers may appear on the site of an injury, cut, or scratch. A physician will usually prescribe medication, dietary adjustments, or other measures.

Ulcers may result from neglect of a corn or callus. But such neglect itself indicates the risks that diabetics incur: they may neglect to have a foot problem such as a corn treated because their disease has, over time, reduced the sensitivity of their feet. They may lose much of their ability to feel pain, heat or cold, or stress in the foot. Because of such problems, diabetics generally follow certain rules of foot care, including the following:

- Give the feet a daily examination for cuts, bruises, or other abnormalities

- Use only prescribed medications in caring for the feet—and avoid over-the-counter preparations

- Visit a podiatrist regularly, as often as once a month, and avoid medical "treatment" of one's own feet or even cutting one's own toenails

- Wash the feet daily in warm, not hot, water and dry them carefully, including the area between the toes

- Use a gentle lubricant on the feet after washing and drying—and

never go barefoot

- Avoid the use of items of clothing that may interfere with circulation, including wraparound garters and support hosiery

- Avoid "holey" socks, darned socks, or anything else that may irritate the soles of the feet and

- Avoid constrictive boots or shoes

Jogging and Running

The podiatrist usually tries to learn about a patient's work, his hobbies and sports, and other facts before undertaking treatment. In particular, the podiatrist asks whether the patient runs or jogs or takes part in other strenuous exercises. With such background information, he or she can suggest appropriate treatment.

A podiatrist will advise runners or joggers on the kind of footwear that would be best—especially if problems have been encountered or may be expected. Shoe inserts may be custom-designed if needed. The podiatrist may also advise runners and joggers to run on softer surfaces rather than cement. Jogging or running "in place," without forward movement, is to be avoided if possible; even when jogging inside the home or apartment, the jogger should move from room to room.

Podiatrists point out that even the more serious knee and ankle problems incurred in running and jogging can be treated. "Jogger's ankle," pain resulting from too much jogging and the attendant strain, can be controlled

if the jogger will use moderation. Beginning joggers in particular should start slowly and gradually increase their level of participation. Runners' knee problems may be cured in many cases by treatment that enables the feet to carry the weight of the body properly. In part, the treatment requires practice in throwing the body weight onto the balls of the feet, not on the inner sides of the feet. The remainder of the body, including the knees, can be kept in proper alignment with the feet if the weight falls where it should.

Podiatrists also advise runners, joggers, and others taking part in sports to make certain *all* their clothing and equipment are appropriate. That applies especially in skiing, ice-skating, and other sports requiring extensive foot use.

With proper equipment, including good shoes, and a moderate approach, runners and joggers can avoid physical difficulties that could require podiatric care. These others include fallen arches; corns, calluses, and bunions.

24

Allergies and Hypersensitivities

*A*llergy is a broad term used to describe an unusual reaction of the body's tissues to a substance that has no noticeable effect on other persons. About 17 out of every 100 persons in America are allergic, or hypersensitive, to one or more substances that are known to precipitate an unusual reaction. Such substances, known as *allergens,* include a variety of irritants, among them mold spores, pollens, animal dander, insect venoms, and house dust. Some individuals are allergic to substances in soap, which produce a skin irritation. Others react to the smell of a rose by sneezing. Still others react with an outbreak of hives, diarrhea, or other symptoms to allergens in foods.

How Allergens Affect the Body

Allergic symptoms can range from itching eyes, running nose, coughing, difficulty in breathing, and welts on the skin to nausea, cramps, and even going into a state of shock, depending upon the severity of the particular individual's sensitivity and response. Almost any part or system of the body can be affected, and almost anything can pose an allergic threat to somebody.

The Role of Antibodies

The system of an allergic individual reacts to such substances in the way it would react to an invading disease organism: by producing *antibodies* whose job it is to neutralize the allergen. In the process of fighting off the effects of the allergen, the body's defense mechanism may overreact by dumping a chemical mediator, *histamine,* indiscriminately into the individual's bloodstream. It is the overabundance of this protective chemical that causes the discomforts associated with allergies.

At the same time, the antibodies can sensitize the individual to the allergen. Then, with each new exposure to the allergen, more antibodies are produced. Eventually the symptoms of allergy are produced whenever the allergen is encountered. Most allergic reactions, including hay fever, asthma, gastrointestinal upsets, and skin rashes, are of the type just described; their effect is more or less immediate. A second type, known as the delayed type, seems to function without the production of antibodies; contact dermatitis is an example of the delayed type.

Eosinophils

Some individuals seem to be sensitive to only one known allergen, but others are sensitive to a variety of substances. Persons who suffer acute allergic reactions have abnormally high levels of a type of white blood cell called *eosinophil.* The eosinophil contains an enzyme that may have some control over the allergic reaction, and varying degrees of the enzyme's efficiency appear to account for individual differences in the severity of allergic reactions.

Allergic Symptoms in Children

Many of the common allergies appear during the early years of life. It has been estimated that nearly 80 percent of the major allergic problems begin to appear between the ages of 4 and 9. Allergic youngsters may have nasal speech habits, breathe through the mouth, have coughing and wheezing spells, or rub their eyes, nose, and ears because of itching. A not uncommon sign of allergic reaction in a child may be dark circles under the eyes caused by swelling of the mucous membranes to such an extent that blood does not drain properly from the veins under the lower eyelids. Nose twitching and mouth wrinkling also are signs that a youngster has allergic symptoms.

Common Allergens

The allergens responsible for so many unpleasant and uncomfortable symptoms take a variety of forms too numerous and sometimes too obscure for any book to enumerate. Discussed below are some of the more common types of allergens.

Foods

Foods are among the most common causes of allergic reactions. While nearly any food substance is a potential allergen to certain sensitive individuals, those most frequently implicated are cow's milk, orange juice, and eggs, all considered essential in a child's diet. However, substitute foods are almost always available. Many natural foods contain vitamin C, or ascorbic acid, found in orange juice. Ascorbic acid also is available in vitamin tablets. All of the essential amino acids and other nutrients in cow's milk and eggs also can be obtained from other food sources, although perhaps not as conveniently packaged for immediate use. Other common food offenders are chocolate, pork, seafoods, nuts, and berries. An individual may be allergic to the gluten in wheat, rye, and oats, and products made from those grains.

Inhaled Allergens

Allergens also may affect the respiratory tract, bringing on sneezing, coughing, and breathing impairment. The substances involved can be pollens, dust, smoke, perfumes, and various airborne chemicals.

Mold Spores

A person also can become allergic to a certain mold by inhaling the spores, or reproductive particles, of fungus. In the nose, the mold spores trigger a reaction in cells of the tissues beneath the mucous membranes that line the nasal passages. This in turn leads to the symptoms of allergy. Because they are small, mold spores can evade the natural protective mechanisms of the nose and upper respiratory tract to reach the lungs and bring on an allergic reaction in that site. Usually, this leads to the buildup of mucus, wheezing, and difficulty in breathing associated with asthma.

Less frequently, inhaling mold spores can result in skin lesions similar to those of eczema or chronic hives. In all but the very warmest areas of the United States, molds are seasonal allergens, occurring from spring into late fall. But unlike pollens, molds do not disappear with the killing frosts of autumn. Actually, frost may help increase the activity of molds, which thrive on dying vegetation produced by cold temperatures.

Dust and Animal Hair

House dust and animal hair (especially cat and dog hair) are also responsible for respiratory allergies in many people. Asthma attacks are often triggered by contact with these substances. Symptoms of dust allergy are usually most severe in the spring and fall, and tend to subside in the summer.

Man-Made Allergens

An example of respiratory allergy caused by man-made allergens is the complaint known as "meat wrappers' asthma," which results from fumes of the price-label adhesive on the polyvinyl chloride film used to package foods. The fumes are produced when the price label is cut on a hot wire. When the fumes are inhaled, the result is burning eyes, sore throat, wheezing and shortness of breath, upset stomach, and other complaints. Studies show that exposure to the fumes from the heat-activated label adhesive for as little as five minutes could produce airway obstruction in food packagers.

Another source of respiratory allergy is the photochemical smog produced by motor vehicle exhaust in large city areas. The smog is composed of hydrocarbons, oxides of nitrogen, and other chemicals activated by the energy of sunlight. When inhaled in the amounts present along the nation's expressways, the smog has been found to impair the normal function of membranes in the lungs.

Drugs

Medicines and drugs, such as penicillin, or serums used in inoculations, can cause allergic reactions. Estimates of the incidence of allergy among those receiving penicillin range from one to ten percent. The National Institutes of Health has calculated that just three common drugs—penicillin, sulfonamides, and aspirin—account for as much as 90 percent of all allergic drug reactions. The allergic reactions include asthmatic symptoms, skin rash, shock, and other symptoms similar to tissue reactions to other allergens. Medical scientists theorize that chemicals in certain drugs probably combine with protein molecules in the patient's body to form a new substance that is the true allergen. However, it also has been noted that some persons show allergic reactions to placebo drugs, which may contain sugar or inert substances rather than real drugs.

Insect Venom

Insect stings cause serious allergic reactions in about four of every 1,000 persons stung by bees, fire ants, yellow jackets, wasps, or hornets. A single sting to a sensitive person may lead to a serious drop in blood pressure, shock, and possibly death. There are more than 50 reported fatalities a year, and experts suspect that other deaths occur as a result of insect stings but are listed as heart attacks, stroke, or convulsions.

Sensitivity tests of persons who might be acutely allergic to insect stings have been difficult to develop, because allergic individuals reacted in the same way as nonallergic persons to skin tests performed with extracts from insect bodies. More recently, physicians have found that using pure insect venom produces a reaction that determines whether a person is allergic to the sting. Medical scientists also have isolated the major allergen in an insect venom for use in diagnos-ing and treating patients who are particularly sensitive to stings.

Skin Allergies

Allergies affecting the skin take many forms, the most common being eczema, urticaria (hives), angioedema (swelling of the subcutaneous tissues), and contact dermatitis. Among the most common causes are foods, cosmetics, fabrics, rubber, metals, plants and flowers, plastics, insecticides, furs and leather, jewelry, and many industrial chemicals. Studies of patients who seem to be especially sensitive to skin allergies show that they have higher than average amounts of a body protein called *immunoglobulin E* in their systems.

Contact dermatitis usually is distinguished by skin swelling, hives, or blisters. The area affected is usually the skin that comes in direct contact with the allergen, so a watch band allergy response will appear as a band around the wrist where the watchband touches the skin. Long-term exposure will cause dry, cracked, darkened patches on the skin.

Poisonous Plants

Poison ivy, poison oak, and poison sumac contain an extremely irritating oily resin that sensitizes the body; repeated contact seems to increase the severity of the allergic reactions. About 50 percent of the population who come in contact with the resin will experience a severe form of dermatitis, and up to 10 percent will be temporarily disabled by the effects. Exposure to the resin may come from direct contact with the plant, from contact with other objects or animals that have touched the plant, or from inhaling smoke from the burning plant.

Cosmetics and Jewelry

A wide variety of cosmetics and jewelry can cause allergic reactions through skin contact. Even jewelry that is presumably pure gold can contain a certain amount of nickel that will produce a mild reaction that causes a skin discoloration, sometimes aided by chemical activity resulting from perspiration in the area of jewelry contact. Among cosmetics that may be involved in allergic reactions are certain permanent-wave lotions, eye-lash dyes, face powders, permanent hair dyes, hair-spray lacquers, and skin-tanning agents. Of course, not all persons are equally sensitive to the ingredients known to be allergens, and in most cases a similar product with different ingredients can be substituted for the cosmetic causing allergic reactions. For more information on skin allergies, see "Disorders of the Skin" in Ch. 21, *Skin and Hair*.

Environmental Allergies

Environmental agents such as sunlight, excessive cold, and pressure are known to produce allergic reactions in certain individuals. Cold allergy, for example, can result in hives and may even lead to a drop in blood pressure, fainting, severe shock, and sometimes death. Research into the causes of cold allergy has shown that cold urticaria, or hives, results from a histamine released from body tissues as they begin to warm up after a cold stimulus. Extremely high histamine levels coincide with episodes of very low blood pressure, the cause of fainting.

Although reaction of the body tissues to the invasion of microbes, such as bacteria, viruses, and other microorganisms, generally is not thought of as an allergic situation, the manner in which the body musters its defenses against the foreign materials is essentially the same as the way the antibodies are mobilized to neutralize other allergens. Thus, there is a similarity between infectious diseases and allergies.

Temporary Allergies

Occasionally, a change in the body's hormonal balance may trigger a hypersensitivity to a substance that previously had no effect on the individual. Pregnant women are especially susceptible to these temporary allergies, which almost always disappear after childbirth. Some women during pregnancy, on the other hand, experience complete relief from allergies that have plagued them since childhood.

People who suffer from seasonal allergies, such as hay fever, often have heightened allergic reactions to dust, animal dander, and even certain foods, such as chocolate and pineapple, during the season when ragweed pollen or other airborne allergens are plentiful.

Diagnosis of Allergies

Some allergic reactions are outgrown; some don't develop until adulthood; some become increasingly severe over the years because each repeated exposure makes the body more sensitive to the allergen. In many instances, the irritating substance is easily identified, after which it can be avoided. In other cases, it may take a long series of tests before the offending allergen is tracked down.

Medical History

If a person suspects he may have an allergy, the first thing he should do is consult a physician to see if the help of an allergy specialist should be sought. The physician or allergist will first take a complete medical history and check the patient's general health. Not infrequently the source of an allergy can be found by general questioning about the patient's life style. For example, the reaction may occur only on or immediately after the patient eats seafood. Or a patient may have an apparently chronic allergy but be unaware that it may be related to daily meals that include milk and eggs. A patient who keeps several cats or sleeps every night with a dog in the bedroom may not realize that an asthmatic condition actually is an allergic reaction to dander from the fur of a pet animal.

The history taken by the physician will include questions about other known allergies, allergies suffered by other members of the family, variations in symptoms according to the weather, time of day, and season of the year. The symptoms may be related to a change in working conditions or the fact that the symptoms, if perhaps a result of house dust, diminish during periods of outdoor exercise. A person sensitive to cold may unwittingly exacerbate the symptoms with cold drinks, while another person who is sensitive to heat may not realize that symptoms can be triggered by hot drinks but relieved by cold drinks, and so on.

Skin Testing

If the patient is referred to an allergy specialist, the allergist will continue the detective story by conducting skin tests.

Scratch Test

Based on information in the medical history of the patient and the allergist's knowledge of molds, pollens, and other airborne allergens in the geographical area, "the allergist" will conduct what is called a *scratch test*.

A diluted amount of a suspected allergen is applied to a small scratch on the patient's arm or back. If the results of the scratch test are inconclusive, a more sensitive test may be tried.

Intracutaneous Test

In the *intracutaneous* test, a solution of the suspected allergen is injected into the underlayer of skin called the *dermis*. The intracutaneous test also may be used to verify the results of a positive scratch test. With either test, a positive reaction usually consists of a raised reddish welt, or *wheal*. The welt should develop within 15 or 20 minutes if that particular allergen is the cause of the symptoms.

Culture Plates

If the allergen has been identified, or if the allergist still suspects a substance in the environment of the patient despite negative or inconclusive tests, the patient may be given a set of culture plates to place around his home and office or work area. If the allergen has been identified, the culture plates can help the physician and patient learn where his exposure to the substance takes place. If the allergen is not known, the cultures may pick up samples of less common allergens that the specialist can test.

Mucosal Test

Another kind of approach sometimes is used by allergists when skin tests fail to show positive results despite good evidence that a particular allergen is the cause of symptoms. It is called the *mucosal test.* The allergist using the mucosal test applies a diluted solution of the suspected allergen directly to the mucous membranes of the patient, usually on the inner surface of a nostril or by aerosol spray into the bronchial passages. In some cases, the allergic reaction occurs immediately and medication is administered quickly to counter the effects. Because of the possibility of a severe reaction in a hypersensitive patient, the mucosal test is not employed if other techniques seem to be effective.

Relief from Allergies

Other Tests

Allergists have other ways to test for allergies. They can, for example, use the *prick test,* a kind of skin test in which a physician or nurse pricks the skin as many as 30 or 40 times. On each pricked spot a drop of a watery solution is dropped; the solution contains a small amount of one allergen. A red welt appears on the spot within 15 to 30 minutes if the patient is allergic. Using another approach, an *elimination diet,* an allergist may specify a diet that omits certain foods for stated periods. Improvement in the patient's condition while avoiding certain foods usually indicates that the individual has an allergy to that food.

A variation of the prick test involves injection of small amounts of food in solution under the skin or application of the solution under the tongue. If the injection or drops provoke reactions, an allergy is indicated.

Avoidance

For a patient sensitive to a particular type of allergen, such as molds, complete avoidance of the substance can be difficult, but some steps can be taken to avoid undue exposure. For example, the mold allergy sufferer should avoid areas of his home, business, or recreational areas that are likely spots for mold spores to be produced. These would include areas of deep shade or heavy vegetation, basements, refrigerator drip trays, garbage pails, air conditioners, bathrooms, humidifiers, dead leaves or wood logs, barns or silos, breweries, dairies, any place where food is stored, and old foam, rubber pillows and mattresses.

Medication

To supplement avoidance measures, the allergist may prescribe medications that will significantly reduce or relieve the irritating symptoms of the allergic reaction. Antihistamines, corticosteroids, and a drug called cromolyn sodium are among medications that may be prescribed, depending upon the nature and severity of the patient's reactions to the allergen.

Immunotherapy

If avoidance measures and medications do not control the symptoms effectively, the allergist may suggest *immunotherapy.* Immunotherapy consists of injections of a diluted amount of the allergen, a technique similar to that used in the skin tests. A small amount of a very weak extract is injected once or twice a week at first. The strength of the extract is gradually increased, and the injections are given less frequently as relief from the symptoms is realized. The injections are continued until the patient has experienced complete relief of the symptoms for a period of two or three years. However, some people may have to continue the injections for longer time spans. Even though the treatments may relieve the symptoms, they may not cure the allergy.

Identification Cards

Any person subject to severe disabling allergy attacks by a known allergen should carry a card describing both the allergic reaction and the allergen. Detailed information can be obtained from the Asthma and Allergy Foundation of America, 1302 18th St., NW, Washington, DC 20036. See also "Allergic Respiratory Diseases" in Ch. 12, *Diseases of the Respiratory System,* and "Asthma Attack" in Ch. 31, *Medical Emergencies.*

25

Women's Health

The special health matters that are related to a woman's reproductive system belong to the branch of medicine known as *gynecology*. *Obstetrics* is a closely related specialty associated with pregnancy and childbirth. The distinction is something of a technicality for most patients, since obstetricians usually are quite capable of handling gynecological cases and vice versa. The practice of obstetrics and gynecology is commonly combined in a medical service identified by the contraction *Ob-Gyn*. However, there are medical matters that are specifically concerned with female reproductive organs and related tissues but have little to do with obstetrics. For a discussion of obstetrics, see "Infertility, Pregnancy, and Childbirth" in Ch. 4, *The Beginning of a Family*.

The Gynecological Examination

What should a woman expect on her first visit to a gynecologist? First, the gynecologist will interview her, asking about her family, her medical history, and any fears or apprehensions she may have about her personal health. The woman's answers and comments are written into her medical records for future reference. The information can contain important clues that may help in diagnosing any present or future disorders.

A sample of urine and a sample of blood are usually obtained for laboratory tests. During the ensuing physical examination, the woman lies on a special examination table with her feet in metal stirrups and her knees apart. A nurse will be present to assist the doctor. While she is in the *lithotomy position,* the woman's abdomen will be palpated for lumps or other abnormalities. The breasts also will be palpated for possible lumps. Then an external inspection of the vulva and surrounding areas is made by the physician, followed by internal inspection, in which a speculum is used to spread apart the sides of the vagina so that the cervix is exposed. A digital examination (using the fingers) is made of the walls of the vagina and rectum and the neighboring tissue areas, in a search for possible growths or other abnormal conditions. And a sample of cells and secretions from the cervix is taken for a Pap-smear test.

In addition to the examination of the breasts and reproductive system, the gynecologist usually conducts a general physical examination, recording information about height, weight, blood pressure, heart and lung condition, and so on. The routine physical examination, like the medical history, provides additional clues that, when added to the results of the examination of the breasts and reproductive system, will give a complete picture of the patient's gynecological health.

Following the examination, the gynecologist discusses his appraisal of the woman's condition and answers questions. He will discuss whatever treatment she needs. Medications can be explained at this time, including reasons why certain drugs can or should not be taken. If any surgery or further testing is recommended, those aspects of the health picture also should be discussed in some detail.

Results of some laboratory tests and the Pap smear are not usually available for several days. But the physician or nurse will contact the patient when the results are available and advise if she should return in the near future for follow-up testing. The American Cancer Society and the American College of Physicians and

The Female Reproductive System

Fallopian tube

Fimbria

Ovary

Ovum discharged from ovary moves toward open end of the Fallopian tube

Uterus

Cervix

Vagina

Location of the reproductive organs

Gynecologists agree (1) that all women should have their first Pap smear when they become sexually active or at age 18, whichever occurs first; (2) that every woman should have a yearly Pap smear for the following two years; and (3) that later tests should be administered at the physician's discretion if the first three Pap smears are negative. The woman also should discuss arrangements for future checkups or Pap smear tests rather than wait until signs or symptoms of a serious disorder warrant an immediate visit.

Menstrual Disorders

Among the health concerns of women that specifically belong to gynecology are menstrual disorders. Normally, the first menstrual period (menarche) occurs about age 12 or 13, or sometimes earlier or later. Periods are generally irregular for the first year or two, and then they tend to recur at intervals of 24 to 32 days. Each period begins about two weeks after ovulation, or the release of an egg cell (ovum) from the ovary—unless, of course, the ovum happens to be fertilized in the interval and pregnancy interrupts the whole process.

The menstrual flow, which lasts from three to seven days, is composed mainly of serum, mucus, and dead cells shed from the lining (endometrium) of the uterus. The loss of blood is minimal, usually from two to four ounces. The volume of flow, as well as the time schedule, tends to be fairly regular for most women. When one's menstrual pattern varies noticeably from the expected pattern, and in the absence of pregnancy, it may be a sign of a physical or emotional disorder.

Amenorrhea

Failure to menstruate is called *amenorrhea*. Amenorrhea is a natural effect of pregnancy and of nursing a baby. In an older woman, it may be a sign of menopause. But if a nonpregnant or nonnursing woman after menarche and before menopause (say between the ages of 17 or 18 and 52) fails to menstruate for two or more periods, she should bring it to the attention of a doctor—unless, of course, she has undergone a hysterectomy or other surgical or medical treatment that eliminates menstruation.

Primary Amenorrhea

When menarche has not occurred by the age of 16 or 17, the absence of menstruation is called *primary amenorrhea*. In such a case, a physical examination may show that an imperforate hymen or a closed cervix is obstructing the flow of menses, or a congenital defect may be interfering with menstruation. In almost all cases, menarche can be started with a bit of minor surgery, by treatment of any existing systemic disease, or by the injection of sex hormones; or it will start spontaneously later.

Secondary Amenorrhea

When menstrual periods cease after menarche, the condition is known as *secondary,* or *acquired, amenorrhea.* Secondary amenorrhea may involve missing a single menstrual period or many periods in consecutive months. Among possible causes of interrupted menstruation are certain medications, drugs of abuse, emotional stress, normal fluctuations in ovarian activity in the first few years after menarche, and a number of organic diseases. Medicines that can disrupt normal menstrual activity include tranquilizers and other psychotropic (mind-affecting) drugs that apparently influence hormonal activity in the brain centers, amphetamines, and oral contraceptives. When a particular medication is found to be the cause of amenorrhea, the medical treatment may be judged to be more important than maintaining normal menstrual cycles. When the use of oral contraceptives is followed by amenorrhea for six or more months, normal menstrual activity may resume eventually, but it can often be started sooner by a prescribed medication. Among drugs of abuse known to cause amenorrhea are alcohol and opium-based drugs.

Just as the mind-altering effects of psychotropic drugs involve the hypothalamus and pituitary glands in the brain, which control the hormones that regulate menstrual functions, emotional stress seems to have a parallel influence on the incidence of amenorrhea. *Anorexia nervosa,* a disorder associated with emaciation resulting from an emotional disturbance, also can result in an interruption of menstruation.

Other factors contributing to secondary amenorrhea are measles, mumps, and other infections; cysts and tumors of the ovaries; changes in the tissues lining the vagina or uterus; premature aging of the ovaries; diabetes; obesity; anemia; leukemia; and Hodgkin's disease. In many cases, normal or near-normal menstrual function can be restored by medical treatment, such as administration of hormones, or by surgery, or both. In one type of amenorrhea, marked by adhesion of the walls of the uterus, curettage (scraping of the uterus) is followed by insertion of an intrauterine contraceptive device (IUD) to help hold the uterine walls apart.

Menorrhagia

Almost the opposite of amenorrhea is *menorrhagia,* an excessive menstrual flow. The causes of menorrhagia are as varied as those associated with amenorrhea. They include influenza and other infectious diseases, emotional stress, polyps of the cervical or uterine tissues, hypertension, congestive heart failure, leukemia, and blood coagulation disorders. Menorrhagia may occur during the early stages of a young woman's re-productive life soon after reaching puberty, and medical treatment may be necessary to control the excessive loss of blood. In some cases, dilation and curettage is recommended in addition to the administration of hormones and other medications, such as iron tablets to correct anemia resulting from the loss of red blood cells.

Dilation and Curettage

Dilation and curettage, generally referred to as *D and C,* is a procedure in which the cervix is dilated and the cavity of the uterus is cleaned out by a scooplike instrument, a curette. The same procedure is sometimes used to abort an embryo or to remove a tumor or a polyp.

Although it takes only a few minutes to perform a D and C, the procedure is done in a hospital while the patient is anesthetized. There is no afterpain, only a dull discomfort in the lower pelvic region similar to menstrual awareness.

A physical examination is usually made to determine if there are tumors anywhere in the reproductive organs. Except where tumors are found to be a causative factor, most women will resume normal menstrual cycles after treatment of menorrhagia with medications and D and C. For women beyond the age of 40, the physician may recommend a hysterectomy to prevent recurrence of excessive menstrual blood loss.

Polymenorrhea and Metrorrhagia

These medical terms refer to two other ways in which menstrual periods may depart from typical patterns. *Polymenorrhea* is abnormally frequent menstruation, so that menstrual periods occur at intervals of less than 21 days. This short interval may be the natural established pattern for some women. If it is not, the cause may be physical or emotional stress. *Metrorrhagia* is marked by menstrual bleeding that occurs erratically at unpredictable times. It may be the result of a cyst in the lining of the uterus, a tumor in the reproductive tract, polyps, or some hormonal imbalance, including a disorder of the thyroid gland.

Dysmenorrhea

Abdominal or pelvic pain occurring just before or along with the onset of menstruation is known as *dysmenorrhea.* The symptoms include severe colicky abdominal cramps, backache, headache, and, in some cases, nausea and vomiting. As with amenorrhea, there are two general types of dysmenorrhea, primary and secondary.

Primary Dysmenorrhea

This type includes all cases in which no organic disorder is associated with the symptoms, which are presumed to be a result of uterine contractions and emotional factors. More than 75 percent of all cases are of this type. Primary dysmenorrhea generally begins before age 25, but it may appear at any time from menarche to menopause. It frequently ends with the birth of the first child.

Since primary dysmenorrhea by definition occurs in the absence of organic disease, the diagnosis can be made only after a careful medical history is compiled and a special study of the reproductive organs is made to ensure that no disorder has been overlooked. In some cases, oral contraceptives may be prescribed because of the effect such drugs have in suppressing ovulation; the contraceptives prevent the natural production of the hormone progesterone, which is responsible for certain tissue changes associated with the discomfort of dysmenorrhea. Analgesic drugs to relieve pain and medications that help to relax muscles may be prescribed. Medication is often less beneficial, however, than emotional support—including the easing of any stress at home, school, or work, and reassurance about the worries sometimes associated with menstruation.

Secondary Dysmenorrhea

This condition comprises all menstrual pain that is a result of or associated with an organic disease of the reproductive organs, such as endometriosis, to cite just one example. Secondary dysmenorrhea can occur at any age.

Premenstrual Syndrome

Premenstrual syndrome (PMS) has emerged in recent years as a major challenge to the medical profession. PMS clinics have begun to offer specialized counseling, physical examinations, and treatment for women unable to cope with the disorder. Treatment regimens or therapies range from aspirin to large doses of sex hormones, diet programs, and exercise.

A group of related symptoms, PMS involves both psychological and physical changes. Among the psychological are lethargy, tension, irritability, depression, and feelings of aggression. The physical signs may include headache, bloating, asthma, and more exotic problems, such as recurrent herpes or hives. In all, more

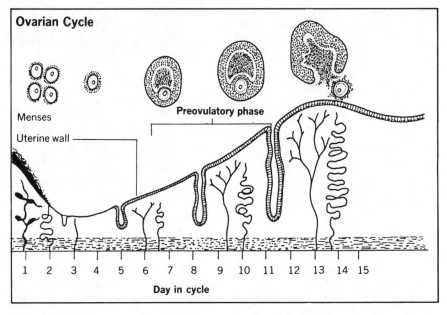

Ovarian Cycle

Menses

Uterine wall

Preovulatory phase

1 2 3 4 5 6 7 8 9 10 11 12 13 14 15

Day in cycle

than 300 different symptoms have been attributed to PMS.

The symptoms, gynecologists warn, should become "disturbing" before they are labeled PMS. Restlessness, minor cramps, and other premenstrual problems may indicate that menstruation is about to start but do not necessarily point to PMS. Such minor problems are called *menstrual molimina.* Cramping and other painful conditions occurring during menstruation are referred to as *dysmenorrhea* (see above).

Of the many treatments for PMS, none has proved uniformly effective. This is because the cause or causes of PMS are not totally understood. Most commonly, physicians believe the disorder represents some basic imbalance in the major female hormones, estrogen and progesterone. Thus one treatment calls for administration of "natural" progesterone to correct the supposed imbalance.

Another common treatment suggested for PMS is vitamin B_6, although the treatment remains partly experimental. Some researchers and physicians, however, have reported disturbing neurological side-effects.

Other theories and treatments exist. Some physicians who have studied PMS and its symptoms believe *prolactin,* a pituitary hormone that stimulates milk secretion, and PMS are associated. A diet and nutrition theory has evolved out of findings that some women report improvement after going on a hypoglycemic diet.

Treated over a substantial period, PMS victims often find that diagnostic tests combined with diet and exercise regimens and vitamin therapy bring good results. If such initial attempts fail, the physician may prescribe medications. In all cases of PMS, according to researchers, psychological support for the sufferer may be important to treatment effectiveness.

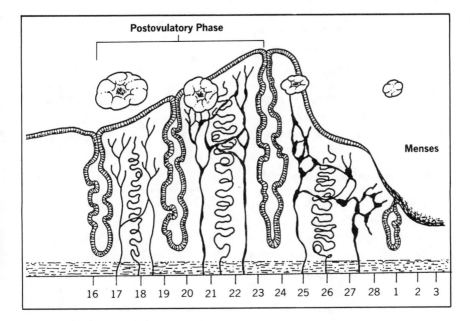

Minor Menstrual Problems

Blood Clots

There is not usually any cause for alarm if blood clots are expelled during menstruation. Ordinarily, the menstrual flow is completely liquefied, but a few clots tend to appear when the flow is profuse. However, if many clots appear and the flow seems excessive, medical advice is recommended, since these conditions may be a sign of fibroid tumors in the uterus.

Oral Contraceptives

Women on combination birth-control pills can expect to see a changed menstrual pattern. The flow becomes slighter than before and very regular. For a discussion of oral contraceptives, see "Birth Control" in Ch. 4, *The Beginning of a Family.*

Odor

The menstrual flow of a healthy woman generally has a mild odor that develops when it is exposed to the air or to the vulva. Some women are concerned about this odor, although it usually is not offensive. When it is, it tends to be associated with inadequate bathing. Detergents are added to some commercial tampons and pad products, and special deodorants have been developed to mask the odor. However, such materials produce allergic reactions in some women, and they can have the unfortunate effect of masking an odor that may be the sign of an abnormal con-

dition.

Onset of Menopause

Menstrual irregularities almost always precede the natural cessation of menstrual function. For a full discussion of menopause, see Ch. 5, *The Middle Years.*

Postmenopausal Bleeding

Bleeding that occurs after the final cessation of menstrual activity should be seen as an urgent signal to seek medical advice. The bleeding may be painless or painful and may range from occasional spotting that is brownish or bright red to rather profuse bleeding that continues for several days or more. The various signs and symptoms should be noted carefully because they can help suggest to a physician the possible cause of bleeding. Bleeding after the menopause is often a sign of cancer of the cervix or the lining of the uterus, but there is a wide variety of other possible causes, including polyps, ulcers, hypertensive heart disease, an ovarian tumor, or infection. In many cases, the problem can be treated by dilation and curettage or withdrawal of any hormone medications, such as estrogens prescribed for menopausal symptoms, or both. In these cases, if D and C and treatment and discontinuance of hormone therapy fail, the physician may advise a hysterectomy.

Infections of the Reproductive Tract

Vaginal and other reproductive tract infections are among the most common gynecological problems, and among the most stubborn to treat successfully.

Leukorrhea

A whitish, somewhat viscid discharge from the vagina, which is known medically as *leukorrhea,* may be quite normal, especially if it is not continual but occurs only intermittently—prior to menstruation, for example, or associated with sexual excitation. It may also be increased when oral contraceptives are used.

Constant leukorrhea, on the other hand, often is a symptom of an abnormality. Leukorrhea resulting from disease can occur at any age. It is generally associated with an infection of the lower reproductive tract. The discharge may occur without any discomfort, but in some cases there is itching, irritation, and *dyspareunia*—or painful intercourse.

Laboratory tests of vaginal secretions may be needed to help identify the precise cause of the discharge. Leukorrhea can result from vaginal ul-

cers; a tumor of the vagina, uterus, or fallopian tubes; gonorrhea; or infection by any of various disease organisms of the vulva, vagina, cervix, uterus, or tubes. It may also result from an abnormality of menstrual function, or even emotional stress.

Treatment, of course, depends on the cause. If the discharge is because of an infection, care must be taken to avoid being reinfected or transmitting the disease organism through sexual contact or possibly contaminated underclothing, etc.

Moniliasis

Moniliasis, also known as *candidiasis,* is an infection by a yeastlike fungus that invades mucous membrane and sometimes skin in various parts of the body. Inside the mouth, the organism causes thrush, most commonly in babies. When the organism invades the vaginal area, it causes a scant white discharge of a thick consistency resembling that of cottage cheese. There is itching, burning, and swelling of the labial and vulvar areas. The symptoms tend to worsen just before the menstrual period. The occurrence

of the disease is thought by some researchers to be fostered by oral contraceptives. Antibiotic therapy may increase the moniliasis organism because it destroys many of the benign organisms that regularly share the same environment.

Moniliasis is treated with suppositories, creams, and other medications. The woman's partner should be treated at the same time to prevent a cycle of reinfection because the fungus will otherwise spread to the genital tissues of the man.

Trichomoniasis

A type of leukorrhea that consists of a copious yellow to green frothy and fetid discharge is caused by infection by the *Trichomonas* organism. The organism causes an irritating itching condition that tends to set in or

worsen just after a menstrual period. The condition is diagnosed by a test similar to a Pap smear, made with a specimen taken from the vagina. Trichomonas organisms, if present, are easy to identify under a microscope;

they are pear-shaped protozoa with three to five whiplike tails.

The organism favors warm, moist areas, such as genital tissues, but it can also survive in damp towels and washcloths, around toilet seats, and on beaches and the perimeters of swimming pools. Thus it can spread from one member of a family to other members and from one woman to other women. *Trichomoniasis* is not technically a venereal disease, but it can be transmitted by sexual contact. When one partner is infected with trichomoniasis, both must be treated at the same time and a condom must be worn during intercourse.

Several drugs are available for treating trichomoniasis, including tablets taken orally and suppositories inserted in the vagina. The tablets are taken for ten days, then an examination is made to determine if any *Trichomonas* organisms are still present. Medication may be continued for several months if the infection resists the drug—studies show that the organism appears to survive in about 10 percent of treated cases.

Herpes Simplex Virus Type 2

Herpes is acquired by contact with the mucous membranes of an infected person. The mucous membrane of the mouth and lips, the genitals, or the rectum may be affected. The causative agent is known as *herpes simplex virus Type II,* or *HSV-II*. It is similar to but not the same as the virus that causes fever blisters, or cold sores, which is Type *I* (HSV-I). The virus is associated with some sponta-neous abortions. If the mother has blisters at the time of delivery, the virus can be transmitted to the baby as he or she passes through the vagina. The central nervous system, including the brain, may be damaged by the virus if the baby becomes infected. To avoid exposure to the virus, a caesarian delivery is recommended.

Symptoms

Patients with their first HSV-II infection usually complain of intense itching, painful blisterlike eruptions, and ulcerated patches with a discharge. Other symptoms may include genital pain and vaginal bleeding. Fever, swelling, difficult urination, and a gen-eral feeling of ill health and lack of appetite may accompany the infection.

Symptoms may subside after a few weeks, but recurrences are common, though they are less painful and of shorter duration. There is no known cure for the viral infection.

Treatment

No drug has been found to attack the viruses while they are "hibernating" in cells at the base of the spine. But one antiviral drug, *acyclovir,* has been found to reduce recurrent outbreaks and to block flareups for up to several months. Taken orally in pill form, acyclovir is ingested daily. Some patients can stop taking acyclovir and still have no further flare-ups. Researchers have discovered that the capsules kill or neutralize the herpes viruses only when they are active. Because of evidence that the virus may be related to the subsequent development of cervical cancer, women sufferers should have Pap-smear tests at intervals of six months instead of the usual twelve.

Pelvic Inflammatory Disease

Pelvic inflammatory disease, or PID, is on the increase in the female population. Commonly caused by bacteria from other diseases such as chlamydia or gonorrhea, PID may go for years without detection. Frequently symptomless, PID infects and destroys the interior of the reproductive system. It attacks the fallopian tubes and uterine lining, leaving permanent scarring. The increase in the number of ectopic pregnancies (fallopian tube pregnancies) is believed to stem from the increase in women who have scarring from PID. The increase in sterility in the population is also linked directly to PID scarring.

One is seven women in the United States has been infected with PID. Treatment for both partners involves antibiotics to kill the bacteria, and treatment of any original disease that may have caused it. Douching should be avoided if PID is suspected. Symptoms include abdominal tenderness or pain, vaginal discharge, or dull ache or twitching in the uterine cavity.

Blood tests and cultures for chlamydia or other diseases should be done. Two-thirds of PID cases are from sexual transmission. If left untreated, PID can cause sterility, miscarriage, ectopic pregnancy, blood infection, and eventually death.

Disorders of the Urinary System

B oth men and women are subject to disorders of the urinary system. There are, however, a few disorders that affect women chiefly or women only, for reasons related to anatomical structure. See also Ch. 17, *Diseases of the Urinogenital System.*

Inflammation of the Bladder

Any inflammation of the bladder is known medically as *cystitis*. Factors such as urinary tract stones, injury, and obstructions to the normal flow of urine can aggravate or cause cystitis in either sex. Cystitis resulting from infectious organisms, however, is much more common in women than in men. This is understandable in view of the relative shortness of the female urethra—the tube through which urine is discharged from the bladder and through which infectious organisms can reach the bladder from the outside. In addition, the anus and the vagina, both of which may frequently be sources of infection, are situated relatively close to the external opening of the female urethra.

In women generally, the symptoms of cystitis may include a burning sensation around the edges of the vulva. There is usually a frequent urge to urinate and difficulty or pain (*dysuria*) associated with urination. Urinary retention and dehydration, which are generally under the control of the individual, can contribute to the spread of infection once it begins. The lining of the urinary bladder is relatively resistant to infection by most microorganisms as long as the normal flow of liquids through the urinary tract is maintained. In cases that do not yield quickly to copious fluid intake, there are medications that may be prescribed to cure the infection. Where urinary frequency or difficulty is accompanied by the appearance of blood in the urine, a physician should be consulted immediately.

Honeymoon Cystitis

One type of cystitis tends to occur mostly in young women during the first few weeks of frequent sexual activity, to which it is attributed. Sexual activity may result in swelling of the urethra and the neck of the bladder, making urination difficult. The inflammation of these tissues can in turn make them more susceptible to infection. A treatment recommended specifically for honeymoon cystitis is to drink large quantities of water or other fluids and to empty the bladder before and after engaging in sexual intercourse. Adequate lubrication, such as K-Y Jelly™ or a water-soluble product, is also important. Medical care should be sought if the condition persists.

Urethral Disorders

The urethra is perforce involved in the inflammation of cystitis because it is the route by which infectious organisms reach the bladder. In addition, there are disorders that are essentially confined to the urethra.

Urethral Caruncle

Urethral caruncle is a rather uncommon urinary tract disorder that tends to be confined to women after the menopause. A *caruncle* (not to be confused with *carbuncle*) is a small, red, fleshy outgrowth. It may be visible near the opening of the urethra. A caruncle growing from the cells of the urethra may be a sign of a bacterial infection, a tumor, or any of several other possible conditions. Symptoms may include vaginal bleeding, pain, tenderness, painful sexual intercourse (dyspareunia), a whitish, viscid discharge, and difficulty in urinating. A physician should be consulted when such symptoms are present. A tissue biopsy and Pap smear may be taken to diagnose the condition. Caruncles are easily treated and of no long-term consequence.

Urethral Diverticulum

Another disorder of the urethra is a *urethral diverticulum,* or outpocketing of the urethra. The problem can be caused by a developmental malformation, an injury, inflammation, a cyst, a urinary stone, or a venereal disease. Stones are a common cause, and in some patients there may be more than one diverticulum. The symptoms may include discomfort and urinary difficulty, as well as dyspareunia. The disorder can be diagnosed with the help of X-ray photographs of the region of the urethra and bladder after they have been filled with a radiopaque substance that flows into any diverticula that may be present.

Treatment of a urethral diverticulum includes antibiotics to stop infection, medications to relieve pain and discomfort, and douches. In some cases, surgery is needed to eliminate the diverticula.

Structural Anomalies

Various kinds of injury may be sustained by the female reproductive system and other abdominal organs, chiefly as a result of childbearing. The structural damage can generally be repaired by surgical measures.

Fistula

An abnormal opening between two organs or from an organ to the outside of the body is known as a *fistula*. Fistulas may involve the urinary and reproductive systems of a woman. Damage to the organs during pregnancy or surgery, for example, can result in a fistula between the urethra and the vagina, causing urinary incontinence. A similar kind of fistula can develop between the rectum and the vagina as a result of injury, complications of pregnancy, or surgery. Disorders of this sort must be repaired surgically.

Prolapsed Uterus

The uterus normally rests on the floor of the pelvis, held in position by numerous ligaments. Damage to the ligaments and other supporting tissues causes the uterus to descend, or *prolapse*, into the vagina. There are various degrees of prolapse, ranging from a slight intrusion of the uterus into the vagina to a severe condition in which the cervix of the uterus protrudes out of the vaginal orifice. Prolapse of the uterus resembles a hernia but is not a true hernia, because the opening through which the uterus protrudes is a normal one.

Backache and a feeling of heaviness in the pelvic region may accompany the condition. Many women complain of a "dragging" sensation. An assortment of complications may involve neighboring organ systems; bleeding and ulceration of the uterus are not uncommon. Coughing and straining can aggravate the symptoms.

Like the various types of hernia, a prolapsed uterus does not improve without treatment but tends instead to worsen gradually. The only permanent treatment is surgical repair. In mild cases, a woman may get relief from symptoms through exercises intended to strengthen the muscles of the pelvic region. Supporting devices,

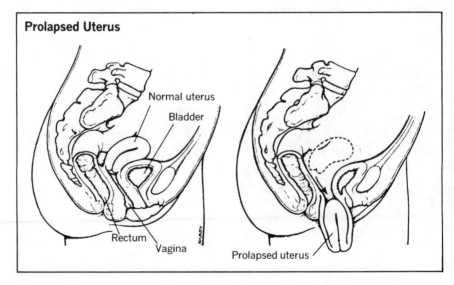

Prolapsed Uterus

Normal uterus
Bladder
Rectum
Vagina
Prolapsed uterus

such as an inflatable, doughnut-shaped pessary, are available as temporary methods of correcting a prolapse. Preventive exercises may be recommended for childbearing women who want to avoid weakened muscles and ligaments leading to prolapse.

Tipped Uterus

The uterus may be out of its normal position without being prolapsed. A malpositioned uterus may be "tipped" forward, backward, or otherwise be out of alignment with neighboring organs. A malpositioned uterus may cause no symptoms, or it may be associated with dysmenorrhea or infertility. If a malpositioned uterus causes pain, bleeding, or other problems, the condition can be corrected surgically, or a pessary support may relieve the symptoms. Displacement of the uterus occasionally is the result of a separate pelvic disease that requires treatment.

Hernias of the Vaginal Wall

The wall of the vagina may be ruptured in childbirth, especially in a mul-

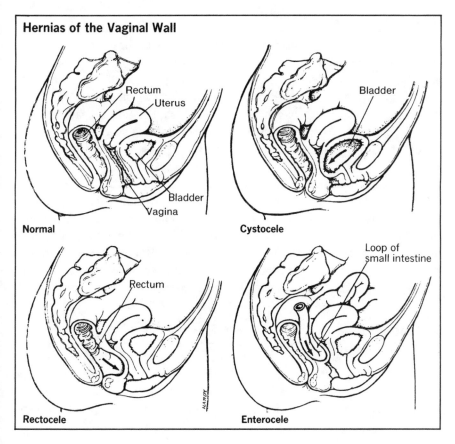

Hernias of the Vaginal Wall

Normal — Rectum, Uterus, Bladder, Vagina

Cystocele — Bladder

Rectocele — Rectum

Enterocele — Loop of small intestine

tiple delivery or birth of a larger-than-average baby. The kind of hernia depends on the exact site of the rupture and what organ happens to lie against the vaginal wall at that point. The condition may be further complicated by a prolapsed uterus. Careful examination of the patient and X-ray pictures may be necessary to determine whether just one or several of the urinary, reproductive, and gastrointestinal organs in the pelvic cavity are involved.

Cystocele

Cystocele is a hernia involving the bladder and the vagina. Structurally, part of the bladder protrudes through the wall of the vagina. The symptoms, in addition to a feeling of pressure deep in the vagina, may be urinary difficulties, such as incontinence, a frequent urge to urinate, and inability to completely empty the bladder. Residual urine in the bladder may contribute to infection and inflammation of the bladder. Treatment includes surgery to correct the condition, pessaries if needed to support the structures, and medications to control infection.

Rectocele

A hernia involving the tissues separating the vagina and the rectum, behind the vagina, is called a *rectocele*. The symptoms are a feeling of fullness in the vagina and difficulty in defecating. Enemas or laxatives may be needed to relieve constipation because straining, or even coughing, can aggravate the condition. Surgery is the only permanently effective treatment. Special diets, laxatives, and rectal suppositories may be prescribed pending surgery.

Enterocele

A herniation of the small intestine into the vagina is called an *enterocele*. Some of the symptoms are similar to those of other hernias involving the vaginal wall, and in addition, a patient with an enterocele may experience abdominal cramps shortly after eating. An enterocele can be dangerous, as well as uncomfortable, because a segment of the small bowel can become trapped and obstructed, requiring emergency surgery.

Varicose Veins

Varicose veins of the vulva, vagina, and neighboring areas are another possible effect of pregnancy, although the legs are more often affected. Obesity, reduced physical activity during pregnancy, and circulatory changes associated with pregnancy can contribute to the development of varicose veins. The symptoms generally are limited to discomfort, although there can be bleeding, particularly at the time of childbirth. Varicose veins that occur in the vulva and vagina during pregnancy and cause discomfort can be treated surgically during the early months of pregnancy. Some drugs and supportive therapy can be used to help relieve symptoms. But many physicians recommend that surgical stripping of veins be delayed until after the pregnancy has been terminated. A complication of untreated varicose veins can be development of blood clots in the abnormal blood vessels. For a discussion of varicose veins of the legs during pregnancy, see "Leg Cramps and Varicose Veins" in Ch. 4, *The Beginning of a Family.*

Benign Neoplasms

T he word *neoplasm* refers to any abnormal proliferation of tissue that serves no useful function. There are numerous kinds of neoplasms but just two main groups—cancerous, or *malignant;* or noncancerous, or *benign.* In ordinary speech the word *benign* suggests some positive benefit, but a benign neoplasm, though noncancer-

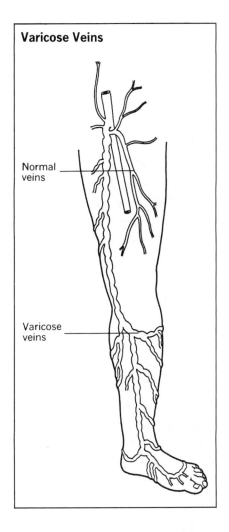

Varicose Veins

Normal veins

Varicose veins

ous, may in fact be harmful to health or at least worrisome. Benign neoplasms that are of particular concern to women are discussed below.

Cysts

A *cyst* is a sac containing a gaseous, fluid, or semisolid material. (Certain normal anatomical structures, like the urinary bladder, are technically known as cysts—hence the term *cystitis* for

inflammation of the bladder.) Abnormal, or neoplastic, cysts can develop at several sites within the urinary and reproductive systems.

Vaginal Cysts

A cyst may develop in a gland at the opening of the vagina as a result of infection with a venereal or other disease. Such a cyst can block the flow of secretions from the gland and produce swelling and pain. Dyspareu- nia, or painful intercourse, is some- times a symptom. A vaginal-gland cyst usually is treated with antibiotics and hot packs. In some cases, it may be necessary for a physician to make an incision to drain the cyst.

Ovarian Cysts

Cysts in the ovaries may be caused by a malfunction of physiological pro- cess or by a pathological condition. Some pathological cysts are malig- nant. The cysts in the ovaries gen- erally are filled with fluid that may range in color from pale and clear to reddish brown, depending upon the source of the fluid. Some cysts are too small to be seen with the naked eye, whereas others may be four or five inches in diameter when symp- toms begin to cause discomfort. There are several different kinds of ovarian cysts.

Follicular Cyst

A *follicular,* or *retention,* cyst is a physiological cyst and is one of the most common types. It develops in an old follicle in which an ovum for some reason has failed to break out of its capsule during the ovulation process. Ordinarily, the contents of such a fol- licle are resorbed, but sometimes a cyst develops. It rarely grows larger than about two inches in diameter. It may rupture but usually disappears after a few months. The symptoms may include pain with some uterine bleeding and dyspareunia. Treatment consists of warm douches, analgesics, and hormone therapy designed to re- store normal ovarian activity. If the symptoms persist or the cyst contin- ues to increase in size, or if serious complications occur, the physician may recommend exploratory surgery.

Occasionally such cysts, whether or not they rupture, produce symp- toms that mimic those of appendicitis, with severe abdominal pain. The ab- domen may become so tender that a physician cannot palpate the organs in order to distinguish between an ovar- ian cyst and appendicitis, particularly if the right ovary is involved. The symptoms occur at the time that ovu- lation would be expected. If the phy- sician cannot be certain that the cause of the abdominal pain is indeed a cyst, for which surgery is not needed, he may recommend surgery anyway— just to be on the safe side.

Multiple follicular cysts, involving the ovaries on both sides (*bilateral polycystic ovaries*) can result in a syn- drome (or group of symptoms) that includes infertility, obesity, and ab- normal growth of body hair. All of these effects are related to a disrup- tion of normal sex-hormone activity; they generally occur in young women, from teenagers to those in their 20s. The therapy includes both medical and surgical efforts to restore normal menstrual function, a diet to control obesity, and the use of various depilatory techniques to remove unwanted body hair.

Corpus Luteum Cyst

This kind of cyst may develop in the ovary following ovulation or during the early part of a pregnancy. The corpus luteum is a small, temporary gland that forms in the empty follicle after the ovum has been released from the ovary. Its function is to produce the hormone progesterone, which is important in preparing the endometrium, the lining of the uterus, to receive a fertilized ovum. The corpus luteum, however, also can be overproductive of a brownish fluid that fills the former follicular space, causing it to swell to a diameter of two or three inches. The cyst causes symptoms of pain and tenderness and may also result in a disruption of normal menstrual cycles in a woman who is not pregnant.

Most corpus luteum cysts gradually decrease in size without special treatment, except to relieve the symptoms. There may, however, be complications, such as torsion, or painful twisting of the ovary, or a rupture of the cyst. A ruptured corpus luteum cyst can result in hemorrhage and peritonitis, requiring immediate surgery.

Chocolate Cyst

So called because of their brownish-red color, chocolate cysts consist of misplaced endometrial tissue growing on the ovary instead of in its normal position lining the uterus. Chocolate cysts are among the largest of the ovarian cysts, ranging up to five or six inches in diameter. They cause symptoms associated with a variety of disorders of the reproductive system, including infertility, dyspareunia, and dysmenorrhea. Surgery usually is a favored method of therapy, the precise procedure depending upon the amount of ovarian tissue involved. A small chocolate cyst can be cauterized, but a large cyst may require removal of a portion of the ovary. See also "Cancer of the Ovary" later in this chapter.

Cysts of the Breast

Cysts may form in the milk glands or the ducts leading from the glands. They are caused by imbalances in ovarian hormones and they tend to develop in mature women approaching the menopause. The cysts tend to fluctuate in size, often enlarging just before or during menstruation, and there may be a discharge from the nipple. Pain and tenderness are usually present, although painless cysts are sometimes discovered only when a woman examines her breasts for possible lumps. Cysts may be almost microscopic in size or as large as an inch or more in diameter. It is not uncommon for more than one cyst to occur at the same time in one breast or both.

A medical examination is recommended when any kind of lump can be felt in the breast tissue. This is particularly important for women who have passed menopause. The physician frequently can determine whether a lump is a result of a cyst or cancer by the patient's history and

by physical examination, especially when repeated at intervals of several weeks. Mammography and biopsy study of a small bit of tissue are used to confirm the diagnosis.

Women who are troubled by breast cysts may be helped by wearing a good brassiere at all times, even during sleep, to protect tender areas. The only medications available are those that relieve pain and discomfort—symptoms that usually subside when the menopause is reached.

Other Noncancerous Masses

A benign lump in the breast can be caused by either a fat deposit or an abscess. A fatty mass frequently forms if an injury to the breast damages adipose tissue. Because of a similarity of the symptoms to those of breast cancer, a biopsy is usually required to distinguish the lesion from a cancer. The involved tissue may in any case be removed surgically.

An abscess of the breast as a result of an infection, although a rare prob-

lem, may produce a lump that requires treatment with antibiotic medications or by an incision to drain the pus. Breast infections leading to abscesses are most likely to occur in nursing mothers but can also develop in women who are not lactating. When an infection develops in a breast being used to nurse a baby, nursing has to be discontinued temporarily while the infection is treated. See also "Cancer of the Breast" later in this chapter.

Polyps

A *polyp* is a strange-looking growth, even for an abnormal growth of tissue. It has been described as having the appearance of a tennis racket or a small mushroom. Polyps are found in many parts of the body, from the nose to the rectum. Usually they are harmless. But a polyp can result in discomfort or bleeding and require surgical excision. A polyp on the breast, for example, can become irritated by rubbing against the fabric of a brassiere. Although polyps gen-

erally are not cancerous, it is standard procedure to have the polyp tissue, like any excised tissue, tested in the laboratory. If malignant cells accompany a polyp, they are usually found at the base of the growth, which means that some of the tissue around the polyp must be excised along with the growth itself. Once a polyp is removed it does not grow again, although other polyps can occur in the same region.

Cervical Polyp

Polyps in the cervix are not uncommon, occurring most frequently in the years between menarche and menopause. A cervical polyp may be associated with vaginal bleeding or leukorrhea; the bleeding may occur after douching or sexual intercourse. In some cases, the bleeding is severe. Cervical polyps can usually be located visually by an examining physician and removed by minor surgery.

Endometrial Polyp

Endometrial polyps, which develop in the lining of the uterus, usually occur in women who are over 40, although they can develop at any age after menarche. They are frequently the cause of nonmenstrual bleeding. They tend to be much larger than polyps that grow in other organs of the body: an endometrial polyp may be rooted high in the uterus with a stem reaching all the way to the cervix. Such a polyp is usually located and removed during a D- and C- procedure. As in the case of a cervical polyp, the growth and a bit of surrounding tissue are studied for traces of cancer cells.

Benign Tumors

Tumors are rather firm growths that may be either benign or malignant. In practice, any tumor is regarded with suspicion unless malignancy is ruled out by actual laboratory tests. Even a benign tumor represents a tissue abnormality, and if untreated can produce symptoms that interfere with normal health and activity.

Fibromas

Among the more common of the benign tumors is the *fibroma,* commonly known as a *fibroid tumor,* composed of fibrous connective tissue. About one of every 20 ovarian tumors is a fibroma, and a similar growth in the uterus is the most common type of tumor found in that organ. Fibromas also occur in the vulva.

Ovarian Fibroma

Ovarian fibromas are usually small, but there are instances in which they have grown to weigh as much as five pounds. A large fibroma can be very painful and produce symptoms such as a feeling of heaviness in the pelvic area, nausea, and vomiting. The growth may crowd other organs of the body, causing enlargement of the abdomen and cardiac and respiratory symptoms. The only treatment is surgical removal of the tumor, after which there is usually a quick and full recovery.

Uterine Fibroma

Fibroid tumors of the uterus can also grow to a very large size, some weighing many pounds. Like ovarian fibromas, they can press against neighboring organs such as the intestine or the urinary bladder, producing constipation or urinary difficulty. More commonly, there is pain and vaginal bleeding, along with pelvic pressure and enlargement of the abdomen. It is possible in some cases for a fibroid tumor to grow slowly in the uterus for several years without causing serious discomfort to the patient. If the tumor obstructs or distorts the reproductive tract, it may be a cause of infertility.

Treatment of fibroid tumors varies according to their size, the age of the patient and her expectations about having children, and other factors. If the tumor is small and does not appear to be growing at a rapid rate, the physician may recommend that surgery be postponed as long as the tumor poses no threat to health. For an older woman, or for a woman who does not want to bear children, a hysterectomy may be advised, especially if symptoms are troublesome. If the patient is a young woman who wants to have children, the physician is likely to advise a *myomectomy,* a surgical excision of the tumor, since a fibroid tumor of the uterus can cause serious complications during pregnancy and labor. It can result in abortion or premature labor, malpresentation of the fetus, difficult labor, and severe loss of blood during childbirth. While fibroid tumors of the uterus are not malignant, special tests are made of the endometrial tissue as part of any myomectomy or hysterectomy to rule out the possibility that cancer cells may be involved in the disorder.

Endometriosis

Endometriosis is the medical term for a condition in which endometrial tissue, the special kind of tissue that lines the uterus, grows in various areas of the pelvic cavity outside the uterus. Endometrial cells may invade such unlikely places as the ovaries (the most common site), the bladder, appendix, Fallopian tubes, intestinal tract, or the supporting structure of the uterus. The external endometrial tissue may appear as small blisters of endometrial cells, as solid nodules, or as cysts, usually of the ovary, which may be four inches or more in diameter, like the chocolate cysts of the ovaries. Such a mass of sometimes tumorlike endometrial cells is called an *endometrioma.*

The misplaced endometrial tissue causes problems because it goes through menstrual cycles just as the endometrium does within the cavity of the uterus. The endometrial tissue proliferates after ovulation and may cause almost constant pain, wherever it is located, for a few days before the start of menstruation. The symptoms subside after the menstrual flow begins. The effects may include dyspa-

ANTERIOR CHEST
CAVITY
1. Clavicle
2. Manubrium
3. Body of sternum
4. Xiphoid process
5. Rib
6. Floating rib
7. Cartilage
8. Anterior super-
   ior iliac spine

© C. S. HAMMOND & Co., N. Y.

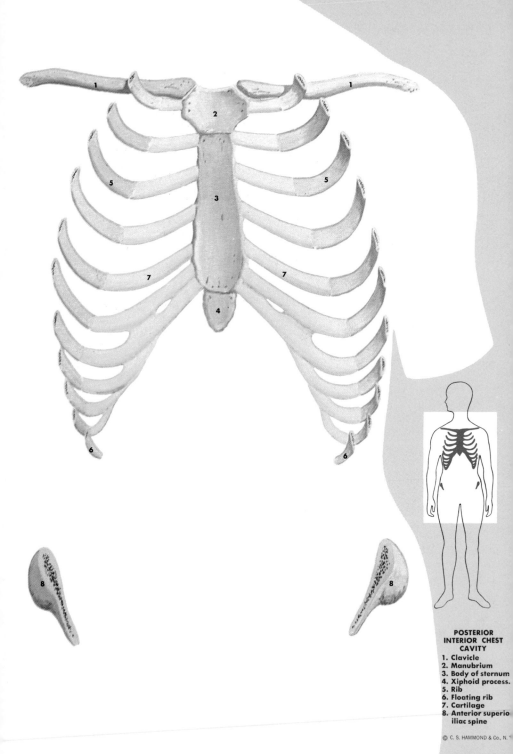

POSTERIOR INTERIOR CHEST CAVITY

1. Clavicle
2. Manubrium
3. Body of sternum
4. Xiphoid process.
5. Rib
6. Floating rib
7. Cartilage
8. Anterior superio
   iliac spine

© C. S. HAMMOND & Co., N. Y

ANTERIOR STOMACH, COLON, AND ORGANS OF REPRODUCTION

23. Esophagus
24. Stomach (cardia)
25. Stomach (fundus)
26. Stomach (body)
27. Stomach (pylorus)
28. Duodenum
31. Ileum
32. Ileocolic junction
33. Caecum
34. Ascending colon
36. Descending colon
37. Sigmoid colon
39. Vermiform appendix
40. Taenia coli
45. Spleen
49. Superior mesenteric artery
50. Superior mesenteric vein
51. Pancreas (head)
52. Pancreas (tail)
80. Bladder
81. Urachus
82. Pubic symphysis
83. Inguinal ligament
100. Uterus
102. Vagina (cross section)
103. Fallopian tube
104. Ostium of fallopian tube
105. Ovary

LACTATING BREAST

97. Pectoralis major muscle
117. Areola
118. Nipple
119. Fat
120. Lactiferous (milk producing) glands and ducts
120a. Cross section of gland and duct
121. Tissue separating and supporting glandular tissue

STRUCTURE OF THE MAMMARY GLANDS

The mammary glands are composed of three major elements:
1. Their skin covering and special structures (nipple, areola).
2. The lactiferous glands or functional units of the breast.
3. The supporting structures, the connective tissue "ligaments" and the fat tissue that makes up the mass of the breast.

The breast is supported by the "suspensory ligaments." These are anchored to the sheet of connective tissue surrounding the pectoralis major muscle, and extend in a complex network separated by the fat tissue outward to the skin. The lactiferous glands are buried in the supporting tissues and empty outward onto the surface of the nipple. These glands at first are very small and clustered just beneath the nipple and areola. In pregnancy they enlarge and push downward into the mass of the breast causing it to enlarge in turn. The enlargement continues through the period of breast feeding, following which the glands gradually grow smaller and the entire breast returns to normal size.

MMOND & Co., N. Y.

101. Cervix
108. Myometrium
109. Endometrium
111. Placenta
113. Amniotic sac
114. Umbilical cord
116. Fetus

THE FETUS AT 3 1/2 AND 6 MONTHS

Most of the definitive development of the fetus occurs during the first 3½ months, and the remaining 5½ months is primarily concerned with gradual increase in size and maturation of organs already begun. The fetus receives all of its nourishment through the placenta and umbilical cord. There is no direct contact between fetal and maternal blood in the placenta. During its entire development, the fetus floats in a fluid (amniotic fluid) contained within a sac (the amniotic sac) attached to the placenta. This sac is in turn surrounded by the uterine cavity, the endometrium and the muscle or myometrium of the uterus.

101. Cervix	111. Placenta
108. Myometrium	113. Amniotic sac
109. Endometrium	114. Umbilical cord
116. Fetus	

THE FETUS AT 8 AND 9 MONTHS

Until birth, the fetus is surrounded by the amniotic sac and fluid, and attached to the placenta by the umbilical cord. The fetus continues to increase in size and the uterus stretches to accommodate it. Usually before the eighth month the fetus assumes a head-downward position. At birth, the amniotic sac ruptures, the fluid escapes, and the child is slowly pushed out of the uterine cavity by the contractions of the myometrium. Shortly after birth of the child, the placenta is similarly expelled having been detached from the endometrium.

X-RAY OF THE HUMAN BODY
SHOWING THE
BONE STRUCTURE

reunia, rectal bleeding, backache, and generalized pain in the pelvic region as sensitive tissues throughout the pelvic cavity are irritated by monthly cycles of swelling and bleeding.

Because infertility is associated with endometriosis, which can become progressively worse, young women who want to bear children are sometimes encouraged to begin efforts to become pregnant as early as possible if they show signs or symptoms of the disorder. Treatment includes hormone medication and surgery to remove the lesions of endometriosis or the organ involved. For patients with extensive spread of endometrial tissue outside the uterus, the physician may recommend removal of one or both ovaries. Destruction of the ovaries surgically or by radiation therapy may be employed to eliminate the menstrual cycle activity that aggravates the symptoms of endometriosis. These procedures cause sterility and premature menopause, but some women prefer this to the discomfort of endometriosis. The hormone therapy inhibits the ovulation phase of the menstrual cycle. Without ovulation, the endometrial tissue does not proliferate. For this reason, pregnancy often eliminates or eases the symptoms of endometriosis during parturition and for a period of time thereafter.

Dyspareunia

Dyspareunia, or painful intercourse, is often associated with endometriosis and is attributed to irritation of nerve fibers in the area of the cervix from the pressure of sexual activity. There are many other possible causes of painful intercourse, some functional and some organic in nature. In addition to endometriosis, the problem may be owing to a vaginal contracture, a disorder involving the muscles of the pelvic region, inflammation of the vagina or urethra, prolapsed or malpositioned uterus, *cervicitis* (inflammation of the cervix), or a disorder of the bladder or rectum. A cause of dyspareunia in older women may be a degeneration of the tissues lining the vagina, which become thin and dry. Temporary therapy for dyspareunia may include water-soluble lubricants, anesthetic ointments, steroid hormones, analgesics, and sedatives. In appropriate cases, surgery is effective in correcting an organic cause of painful sexual intercourse. Functional or psychogenic (of psychological origin) causes of dyspareunia usually require psychological counseling for the patient and her sexual partner.

Backache

Still another effect of endometriosis that can suggest other disorders is backache. When endometrial tissue invades the pelvic region, there may be a fairly constant pain in the back near the tailbone or the rectum. Usually the backache subsides only after the cause has been eliminated. Temporary measures include those advised for other kinds of backache: sleeping on a firm mattress, preferably reinforced with a sheet of plywood between springs and mattress; application of dry heat or warm baths; sedatives to relieve tension, and analgesics to relieve the pain.

A backache that radiates down the back and into a leg, following the path of a sciatic nerve, can be the result of a disorder of the ovaries or uterus. An ovarian cyst or infection of the Fallopian tubes can produce a backache that seems to be centered in the lumbosacral area of the spinal column. Such backaches, sometimes called gynecologic backaches, tend to occur most frequently during a woman's childbearing years and more often af-fect women who have had several children than women who have not been pregnant. Tumors also can produce backache symptoms. X-ray pictures, myelograms, and laboratory studies may be required in order to rule out the possibilities that the back pain may be caused by a tumor, a herniated or "slipped" disk, or a deformity of the spinal column that might have been aggravated by one or more pregnancies. Most backaches, however, relate to poor posture or muscle tension. Anxiety or other kinds of emotional stress can aggravate the symptoms. See also "Backaches" in Ch. 23, *Aches, Pains, Nuisances, Worries,* and "Back Pain and Its Causes" in Ch. 25, *Women's Health.*

Cancers of the Reproductive System

Cancer of the Cervix

The cervix of the uterus is the ninth most common site of cancers affecting women. As compared with all cancers of the reproductive organs of women, it rates third, after uterine cancer and ovarian cancer. It has been estimated that about 13,000 cases of cervical cancer are found among American women each year, and approximately 4,500 deaths ev-ery year are a result of this disease.

The number of cases of pre-invasive cervical cancer is down because of the increased number of women who undergo regular gynecological examination. When cancer is diagnosed early, the survival rate increases tremendously for the patient.

The actual causes of cervical cancer are still unknown. Current medical thinking suggests that there is no causal relationship between cervical cancer and the use of oral contraceptives.

Preinvasive Stage

The earliest signs of cervical cancer tend to appear between the ages of 25 and 45. At this early, *preinvasive* stage, the cancer is described as *in situ*—confined to its original site. If the cancer is not treated at this stage, the disease spreads and becomes a typical invasive cancer within five to ten years. Signs of bleeding and ulceration usually do not appear until this has occurred. However, because of the relatively slow growth of cervical cancer in the early stage, the disease usually can be detected by a Pap smear test before it becomes invasive.

Invasive Cancer

Cancer that has spread beyond the cervix is far more difficult to treat. Surgery, radiation or chemotherapy, and regular examinations to catch any recurrence of cancer will probably be necessary. It is unusual for anyone to develop invasive cancer without knowing it, if she has undergone regular, routine pelvic exams.

Diagnostic Methods

Pap Smear Test

The *Pap smear* test (named for Dr. George Papanicolaou, who developed the technique in 1928) is a quick and simple method of detecting cancerous cells in secretions and scrapings from mucous membrane. It requires the collection of small samples of cells from the surface of the cervix and from the cervical canal. Such samples are obtained by inserting a plastic spatula or a brush-tipped tube into the vagina, into which a speculum has been placed previously. The device is scraped gently over the area of the cervix. The physician may collect also a sample of vaginal secretions, which may contain possibly cancerous cells not only from the cervix but from the ovaries and uterus as well. (This is the only way a Pap smear test can be done if a woman has had a complete hysterectomy and has no cervix.) All cell samples are placed (smeared) on microscope slides and treated with a chemical preservative. The slides are sent to a laboratory for study and a report is made to the examining physician, usually within a few days, on the findings.

Results from the Pap smear are reported as: normal, inadequate sampling, showing infection, or showing cell abnormalities. Except for the normal results, Paps will be done again to ensure accuracy. No one should wait more than six months for a follow-up reading on an infectious diagnosis and treatment. For all others, follow-up should be immediate. Cell abnormalities are divided into at least three categories: low-grade lesions (non-cancerous), high-grade lesions (non-cancerous), and cancer.

Other Diagnostic Tests

When a report of positive findings is returned by the laboratory, the physician immediately arranges for further studies. These involve examination of the cervix visually by a special microscopic technique known as *colposcopy,* and the removal of small tissue samples. These studies are usually done in a physician's office. In some cases a biopsy is necessary. The biopsy sample is taken when possible from the same location on the cervix as the Pap smear that resulted in positive findings. The Loop Electrosurgical Excision Procedure (LEEP) is a method of combining the biopsy and the excision of the diseased tissue. An electrified loop removes the abnormal tissue from the cervix. The small circle that is removed can then be examined for signs of cancer. The electrical charge of the loop cauterizes the cut to prevent infection and bleeding. Treatment ordinarily is not started until all of the studies have verified that there is cancer in the tissues of the cervix; other disorders, such as cervicitis, venereal infection, and polyps, can mimic symptoms of cervical cancer.

Therapy

The kind of treatment recommended for a case of cervical cancer generally depends upon several factors, such as the stage of cancer development and the age and general health of the patient. For a young woman who wishes to have children despite cancer *in situ,* which is limited to the cervix, surgeons may excise a portion of the cervix and continue watching for further developments with frequent Pap smears and other tests. The treatment of choice for cervical cancer in the early stage, however, is surgical removal of the body of the uterus, as well as of the cervix—a procedure called a *total hysterectomy.* This is the usual treatment for women over the age of 40 or for those who do not wish to have children. Sometimes more extensive surgery is necessary.

Radiation treatment may be advised for women who are not considered to be good surgical risks because of other health problems. Radiation may be recommended along with surgery for women with advanced cervical cancer in order to help destroy cancer cells that may have spread by metastasis to other tissues.

The five-year cure rate for cervical cancer is about 99 percent when treatment is started in the early, pre-invasive stage. The chances of a cure drop sharply in later stages, but the five-year cure rate is still as high as 65 percent if treatment is started when the cancer has just begun to spread to the vagina or other nearby tissues.

Cancer of the Body of the Uterus

Cancer of the body of the uterus, or *endometrial cancer,* is more common than cancer of the cervix. Uterine cancer is the most common type of cancer of the reproductive organs. Cervical cancer primarily affects women before middle age; uterine cancer occurs more frequently among women beyond the menopause, with its highest rate occurring among women between the ages of 50 and 70. Survival rate for cancer of the uterus is high, with 82 percent living 5 years after diagnosis. Risk factors for uterine cancer include obesity, diabetes, and ovarian cysts. Other potential risks are for women who have taken estrogen-only pills for menopausal symptoms and women who have taken tamoxifen for breast cancer.

Diagnostic Methods

Early symptoms usually include bleeding between menstrual periods or after menopause, and occasionally a watery or blood-stained vaginal discharge. Most patients experience no pain in the early stages, although pain is a symptom in advanced uterine cancer or when the disease is complicated by an infection. Unfortunately, there is no simple test, like the Pap smear for cervical cancer, that provides a good diagnostic clue to the presence of endometrial cancer. The Pap smear does occasionally pick up cells sloughed off by the endometrium, and laboratory tests can tell if they might be malignant. The best chance for early diagnosis is for a woman to report to her gynecologist or physician any signs of abnormal bleeding between periods, or post-menopausal bleeding. Unusual bleeding should be followed up by the doctor with examination of the uterine lining.

A physician who is suspicious of symptoms of endometrial cancer must depend upon direct methods to confirm or rule out the disease. The usual method is a dilatation and curettage (D and C), during which a small sample of uterine lining will be removed for biopsy, or a sample may be withdrawn by suction (aspirated) from the uterine cavity. The cervix is dilated (opened) and the uterine lining scraped with a curette. Aspiration can be done in the physician's office with local anesthesia of the cervix or with no anesthesia. There is little or no discomfort following aspiration.

Therapy

If the diagnostic D and C is done when the abnormal bleeding associated with uterine cancer first begins, the chances of a cure are very good. The first step, if the general health of the patient permits surgery, is complete removal of the uterus, ovaries, and fallopian tubes—a procedure called a *radical hysterectomy.* Radiation may also be administered to control the spread of cancer cells.

A hysterectomy should not affect a woman's normal sexual activity. Sexual relations usually can be resumed about six to eight weeks after the operation, or when the incision has healed. If the incision is made through the pubic region or vagina, there should be little or no visible scar. See "Family Planning," in Chapter 4.

Estrogen and Cancer

There is a higher incidence of cancer of the uterus among women who have tumors of the ovary that produce estrogen, as well as among women whose menopause begins later than the usual age (and hence who have produced estrogen naturally for a longer-than-usual period). Because of the statistical associations between uterine cancer and estrogen-producing tumors, as well as other factors, the American Cancer Society has cautioned that physicians should exert "close supervision of women on estrogen, with an awareness that sustained use [of estrogens] may stimulate dormant factors in the body and lead to development of endometrial cancer." For women who are prescribed estrogen for menopause, it is recommended that the estrogen be given in combination with a synthetic progestin. Unopposed estrogen increases the growth of cancerous tumors already present, and is suspected of increasing the risk of new cancer growths.

Among the conditions for which estrogen has been prescribed for women of middle age and beyond are uncomfortable effects of menopause, such as itching and irritation caused by dryness of the vagina, and what is commonly referred to as "hot flashes." See *The Middle Years,* Ch. 5, "Menopause" for more information.

Diethylstilbestrol

An estrogenlike synthetic compound has definitely been implicated in the development of a type of cancer, *adenocarcinoma,* which primarily affects epithelial tissue. The synthetic hormone known chemically as *diethylstilbestrol* (DES) or stilbestrol was taken for the most part in the late 1940s and through the 1960s by pregnant women for the treatment of such complications as bleeding and threatened miscarriage. Around 1971, physicians became aware that some of the daughters whose mothers had taken DES during their pregnancy had developed an unusual cell formation in vaginal tissue, vaginal and cervical cancers, and some anatomical abnormalities. Cancers have been discovered in daughters as young as seven years of age. An unknown but substantial number of women in the United States alone received DES while pregnant, but approximately 1 in 1000 have been found to be afflicted with cervical or vaginal cancers. The National Cancer Institute has urged that all mothers and daughters who may have been exposed to DES during the mother's pregnancy arrange to be examined by a physician for possible effects of the drug.

The use of DES for pregnant women has been discontinued, although the compound is still available for treating certain cases of breast cancer and menopausal symptoms in nonpregnant women.

Cancer of the Ovary

Ovarian cancer is the fifth most common type of cancer in women, with an average of 21,000 new cases each year. It is second to uterine cancer in the number of cases of cancer of the reproductive system. It has, however, a much lower survival rate. Because of the difficulty in diagnosing ovarian cancer, the cancer is more likely than other forms to go unchecked until it has spread to other areas of the body. Less than 2 in 5 women will survive five years after diagnosis. There are several different kinds of malignant tumors of the ovary; some originate in the ovaries and others are caused by cells that have metastasized from a cancer at some other site, such as the uterus.

There are no age limits for cancer of the ovary, although most cases are detected in women between 50 and 70. A physician at a routine pelvic examination may notice a lump or other abnormal growth in the abdominal region. The symptoms reported by patients usually include abdominal discomfort or digestive problems, possibly because ovarian cancers often grow large enough to press on neighboring organs and cause urinary difficulties, constipation, or other digestive disorders. A clue is given in some cases by endometrial bleeding as a result of abnormal hormone production by the affected ovary. However, the more common kinds of ovarian cancers do not produce hormones. Occasionally, cancer cells from an ovarian tumor will be found in a Pap smear sample. But there are no direct, simple tests for cancer of the ovary.

Treatment for ovarian cancer varies with the individual case. As with cancer at other sites, surgery is generally necessary. The extent of the surgery depends upon the type of lesion and other factors. In an advanced case of an older woman, total hysterectomy along with removal of the ovaries and fallopian tubes would be the treatment of choice. But if the patient is a young woman and the cancer is not extensive, the surgeon may excise the affected ovary and leave the remainder of the reproductive system intact. Radiation and chemotherapy are commonly applied in addition to surgery. The most important risk factor is having relatives who have had ovarian cancer. If a mother, grandmother, or sibling have been diagnosed with ovarian cancer, then the woman is recommended to undergo regular blood tests to check for malignancy. Let your doctor know if you have a family history of ovarian cancer.

Cancer of the Breast

Cancer of the breast is one of the oldest and best-known types of cancer. It is described in an ancient Egyptian papyrus of 5,000 years ago. The hormonal factors involved in the physiology of breast cancer have been studied by physicians for more than 100 years. But it remains the most common of cancers affecting woman. It kills more women than any other kind of cancer, except lung cancer. About 150,000 women in the United States develop breast cancer each year, and 35 percent die of the disease. Nearly everyone knows a friend or relative who has been stricken by breast cancer. Yet the cause of breast cancer is still unknown.

Women whose female relatives have had breast cancer are more likely to be victims than women from families in which breast cancer is not present. The disease appears to be linked statistically also to women who do not have children before their 30s or who do not have any children; to mothers who do not nurse their babies; to women who reach the menopause later than normal; and to women who began menstruation earlier in life than normal. There is increasing evidence also that ovarian activity may play an important role in the development of breast cancer. Women with ovarian tumors and women who use supplementary estrogen have been shown by some studies to be at increased risk, while the process of having many children and nursing them, which suppresses estrogen hormone activity, is associated with a decreased risk of developing breast cancer. However, 55 percent of the diagnosed cases are for women who have no known risk factors.

Cancer of the breast may occur as early as the teens, but this is rare. It is generally not found before the age of 30, and the incidence peaks around the time of menopause. Then there is a second period after the age of about 65 when the incidence of breast cancer rises again.

Breast cancer usually begins in the ducts of the milk glands; the first noticeable sign is a lump in the breast. The lump may appear anywhere in the breast, but the most common site is the upper, outer quadrant. Most lumps are not usually cancerous, but a biopsy (described below) must be performed to check the tissue involved.

In a typical case of breast cancer, a small tumor half an inch in diameter, large enough to be detected during careful self-examination, can grow to a cancer two inches in diameter in six months to a year. The lump generally causes no pain; pain is rarely associated with early breast cancer. If the tumor is allowed to grow unchecked, it may cause pulling of the skin from within. This effect may appear as a flattening of the breast or a dimpling of the skin, or a sinking, tilting, or flattening of the nipple. Less frequently, the tumor begins in a duct near the nipple, causing irritation of the skin of the nipple and a moist discharge. In such cases a scab eventually forms at that site. In time, cancer cells spread to the nearby lymph nodes and the danger becomes very serious of metastasis to any part of the body.

Detection of Breast Cancer

Fortunately, breast cancer can be treated effectively if it is detected early enough. Some 95 percent of breast cancers are discovered by the patient herself when she notices a lump. In all too many cases the discovery is made by chance and the lump may be quite large. The cure rate for breast cancer could be greatly improved if all women made a routine of monthly self-examination and then consulted a physician immediately if they found the least indication of a thickening or lump. Most such lumps are benign, but it is most important that the ones that are malignant be identified without delay.

The American Cancer Society and the National Cancer Institute recommend that every woman follow a prescribed method of self-examination just after the menstrual period, continuing every month after the menopause. The procedure consists of carefully looking at and feeling the breasts, and takes only a few minutes. A detailed description of the proper procedure is available in pamphlet form from the Superintendent of Documents, U.S. Government Printing Office, Washington, D.C. 20402. Ask for Public Health Service Publication No. 1730. A film entitled *Breast Self-Examination,* produced by the American Cancer Society and the National Cancer Institute, is also available.

If a tumor can be detected as even a small lump, it must have been developing for some time. There is a truism about breast cancer to the effect that a cancer that is undetectable is curable—leaving unspoken the implication that a cancer that is detectable may not be curable. In recent years, methods of early detection have been refined to the point that tumors once undetectable can now be detected before any lump becomes palpable.

Thermography

One early warning detection technique involves the use of *thermography,* which is based on the fact that tumor cells produce slightly more heat than normal tissue. Hence a device that is sufficiently heat sensitive can detect and pinpoint the location of an incipient tumor. A harmless tumor, too, would have a higher-than-normal temperature. Further tests would be needed to determine the true cause of the "hot" tissue-reading.

Self-examination of the Breasts

Step 1   Step 2

Step 3

Self-examination of the breasts as recommended by the American Cancer Society. *(Step 1)* Examine breasts during a shower or bath; hands glide easier over wet skin. With fingers flat, move the left hand gently over every part of the right breast, then the right hand over the left breast. Check for any lump, hard knot, or thickening. *(Step 2)* Before a mirror, inspect the breasts with arms at the sides, then with arms raised. Look for any changes in the contour of each breast, a swelling, dimple of skin, or changes in the nipple. Then rest palms on hips and press down firmly to flex the chest muscles. Left and right breasts will not match exactly — few women's breasts do. But regular inspection will show what is normal for you. *(Step 3)* While lying down with a pillow or folded towel under the right shoulder and with the right hand behind the head, examine the right breast with the left hand. With fingers flat, press gently in small circular motions around an imaginary clock face. Begin at 12 o'clock, then move to 1 o'clock, and so on around back to 12. A ridge of firm tissue in the lower curve of each breast is normal. Next, move in an inch toward the nipple and keep circling to examine every part of the breast, including the nipple. This requires at least three more circles. Then repeat the procedure slowly on the left breast with the pillow under the left shoulder and left hand behind the head. Notice how the breast structure feels. Finally, squeeze the nipple of each breast gently between thumb and index finger. Any discharge, clear or bloody, should be reported to a physician immediately.

Mammography

Mammography is an X-ray technique developed specifically for examination of breast tissue. A tumor shows up on a mammogram as an opaque spot because of mineral concentrations associated with the growth. However, like thermography, mammography cannot determine whether a tumor is benign or malignant or if the opaque spot on the film is because of some other mineral-rich tissue rather than a tumor. The examining physician uses mammography only as one among other diagnostic tools.

Guidelines from medical groups such as the American Medical Association and the American Cancer Society are as follows:

- Physical breast exams by doctors once a year, and monthly self-exams for all age groups from puberty to 40 onward.

- No known risk factors, ages 40-49, physical breast exam by doctor every year, mammogram every one to two years

- Risk factors ranked medium to high, ages 40-49, physical breast exams and mammograms once a year or more frequently with the advice of a physician

- Age 50, with or without risk factors, mammogram and physical breast exam every year

Some gynecologists recommend a mammogram at the age of 35 so that there is an opportunity for comparison when mammograms are done after the age of 40. Consult with your physician about his or her personal recommendations. Some insurance companies will pay for yearly mammograms; others pay for biannual mammogram exams. Some states require insurance companies by law to pay for at least one exam. Check with your insurance company about their policy. Medicare covers mammograms for women over the age of 65.

Xeroradiography

Xeroradiography is a method that, like mammography, uses X rays, but it entails only about half the exposure to radiation. The pictures are developed by xerography, the process made familiar by Xerox copying machines. The picture consists of dots in varying shades of blue. The process produces a sharp picture, making interpretation simpler and more accurate than is possible with X-ray photographs. When performed by experienced medical technicians, xeroradiography can detect from 85 to 95 percent of all breast cancer, including those too small to be located by palpation. The xeroradiography examination and the physician's examination of the breast usually take only about 20 minutes.

Other Methods

Other diagnostic tools have come into use. *Ultrasound* and *diaphanography,* for example, have reportedly proved their value, especially when combined with other techniques, including mammography. Ultrasound depends on sound waves that vibrate at frequencies beyond the range of human hearing; transmitted into the breast, ultrasound can distinguish between lumps that are cystic and fluid-filled — and therefore benign — and those that are solid. Other tests, however, may be needed to differentiate between benign solid and malignant solid lumps. In diaphanography, or transillumination, a technician or physician shines an ordinary white light through the breast in the dark. An overhead camera takes pictures with infrared film. Diaphanography can determine whether breast lumps are fibrous, benign, or malignant.

Fine needle aspiration has also proved useful in diagnosing breast cancer. The surgeon uses a needle to draw out a sample approximately 0.5 cm in size. Microscopic examination of the sample follows.

Biopsy

When a physician believes there is good evidence of a cancer in a breast as a result of thermography, xeroradiography, mammography, palpation of lumps, and other factors, the next step is a biopsy study. An entire nodule of breast tissue is removed for microscopic examination of the tissue cells. It is sent to the pathology department, which usually reports within 90 minutes whether the tissue is noncancerous or malignant.

If the lesion is not cancerous—and between 60 and 80 percent of biopsies of breast lumps are not—the patient is taken back to the recovery room and, as soon as possible, reassured that the tumor was benign. The incision made for the biopsy leaves an almost indiscernible scar. In some cases, a hollow needle may be used to withdraw tissue, leaving no scar. This is called a *needle biopsy*.

The Two-Step Procedure

Because of the psychological and physical problems associated with breast cancer, the test and operation can take place in two separate stages. In many cases, it may be necessary to perform both operations on the same day.

Presurgical Staging involves administration of various tests that are carried out before a mastectomy. The tests show whether the cancer has already spread, or metastasized, to parts of the body other than the breast and local lymph node regions. Staging is widely regarded as a necessary procedure in all cases of breast cancer. A mastectomy has the single purpose of preventing the spread of cancer; the patient has to know, for her own peace of mind, whether it has already spread.

A two-step procedure involves other choices. Where the biopsy is to be carried out separately, the patient may ask to have it done under local anesthesia, as an outpatient. That possibility can be explored with the surgeon. If a general anesthetic appears preferable, the patient may have to spend a night in the hospital. But the *diagnostic biopsy*—involving surgical removal of the entire tumor—and mastectomy can still be performed separately. After a biopsy specimen is removed, the specimen may be subjected to an estrogen-receptor assay. The assay tells the surgeon whether or not the cancer depends on the female hormone estrogen for its growth. That information provides a clue to possible future treatment.

For many women, the one- to two-day wait for the results of a biopsy is worth the time involved, especially because it may be possible to perform the biopsy under local anesthesia on an outpatient basis.

Following the biopsy, the patient receives the pathologist's report on whether the finding is positive or negative. If positive, precise information will usually be given on the type of cancer and where it is located in the breast. Then the patient may want to obtain a second opinion on the permanent-section pathology report and slides. The second opinion is also given by a pathologist. It helps in making decisions on surgery.

The striped areas show the tissue removed in a radical *(above)* and a simple *(below)* mastectomy, including the axillary lymph nodes in the former case.

Mastectomy

If the lesion is malignant, the surgeon proceeds with the mastectomy. Depending upon the seriousness of the case and the procedure recommended by the surgeon and the pathologist, the operation may remove just the breast tissue, leaving the skin and nipple for reconstructive surgery; remove the skin tissue as well; or remove breast tissue and tissue from around the breast area. The type of surgery is determined by the type and size of the cancerous growth, the risk of further growth, and other factors. The physician and the patient should discuss the reasons for each type of surgery before deciding which to perform. In the United States until recently, radical mastectomy was the usual procedure for breast cancer treatment.

Today, at least five different types of mastectomy may be performed. The five:

- *Simple mastectomy*: The breast tissue is removed, but the surrounding muscles and lymph nodes remain.

- *Radical mastectomy*: The breast, lymph nodes, and surrounding muscle are removed.

- *Modified radical mastectomy*: The underlying muscle stays intact while the breast, lymph nodes, and surrounding tissue are removed.

- *Subcutaneous mastectomy*: The breast is removed but not the nipple and skin. This procedure usually is done to allow the most natural looking reconstructive surgery.

- *Lumpectomy or segmental mastectomy*: Only the cancer and surrounding tissue are removed. No reconstructive surgery is usually necessary.

Survival rates depend as much on timely use of pre- and postoperative radiotherapy and postoperative chemotherapy as on the type of operation. But the kind of operation may determine whether the patient will be able to function normally in a relatively short period of time.

Some surgeries allow reconstruction of the breast either during or after a mastectomy, using artificial material to create a breast to match the natural one.

Breast implants

Breast implants for reconstruction are the same types used for cosmetic breast enlargement. There are two basic types: silicone-gel and saline filled. The saline sacs duplicate the natural breast's shape. The sac is inserted under the skin and then filled slightly larger than the final size. After the skin has adjusted to the enlarged sac, some of the liquid is drained to give the breast a natural sag, in most cases closely matching the remaining breast.

Although silicone-gel implants have been widely discouraged for cosmetic use since 1992, they are still considered an important rehabilitation option for women with breast cancer or women with premalignant conditions requiring mastectomies, according to the American Cancer Society. The silicone implant is carefully inserted under the skin tissue and the body forms a scar tissue seal around the sac.

Reactions to silicone-gel implants may include side effects such as hardening of scar tissue around the implant, ruptured silicone sacs, and obscured diagnostic X rays. The link between silicone and diseases of the immune system is still under study. In addition, implants also may block the results of mammographic X rays. However, studies show that implants do not increase the risk of breast cancer or cancer in other parts of the body.

According to the United States Food and Drug Administration, women should only consider removing implants if they are experiencing difficulties. Women should have periodic exams to check for ruptures. Those who want implants for cosmetic purposes should know the importance of detecting early cancer through mammography and the chance of having results obscured by implants.

Postoperative Therapies

The type of surgery recommended in any given case of breast cancer has significance for postoperative therapy. Breast surgery may be extensive where the cancer has spread to the lymph nodes or to other parts of the body; the use of chemotherapy and radiation therapy may be aggressive.

Options include:

- surgery only;

- surgery with radiation; chemotherapy; or hormone therapy

- surgery with a combination of these treatments; or

- radiation or chemotherapy without surgery.

The choices of alternative therapies should be made with an eye to still other factors.

Radiation

A lumpectomy, or segmental mastectomy, is usually followed by radiation therapy. Radiation treatments are typically given five days a week for five weeks. A "booster" treatment may follow completion of the initial series of treatments. Side effects from radiation therapy include fatigue; reddened, moist, or dry skin at the site of the radiation; decreased or heightened sensitivity; enlarged pores; and sometimes changes in breast size.

Chemotherapy

Adjuvant (auxilliary) chemotherapy, which follows surgery, is the usual treatment where breast cancer has spread to the lymph nodes and the patient has not entered menopause. Postmenopausal women may be given tamoxifen, an antiestrogen drug, or may undergo chemotherapy. Except for some high-risk patients, adjuvant chemotherapy is not recommended for women with noncancerous nodes.

Hormone Therapy

Less toxic than chemotherapy, hormone treatments are normally given to those women whose cancer has not spread to the underarm nodes and whose tumors were hormone-dependent. This is especially the case if a patient is postmenopausal. For these women tamoxifen would also be a standard treatment if the cancers had spread to the lymph nodes.

The Rape Victim

The woman who has been raped faces special problems. Authorities agree that long-term health threats can be minimized if the victim takes certain precautions. Complications arising from sexual assault include contracting sexually transmitted disease (STD) or other diseases; becoming pregnant; and experiencing the aftereffects of contusions and abrasions. In general, the experts suggest that women take steps to protect themselves against rape and follow certain procedures in the event that a rape occurs.

Precautions

Because rapists generally attack without warning, the woman who feels that she is at risk can sometimes do little more than exercise vigilance in protecting herself. There are precautions, however, that women may take. Self-defense or martial-arts courses may be the answer for some. Although weapons may impart a sense of security, authorities are divided on the issue of their value. Additionally, the weapons themselves may be illegal in some cities or states. Noisemakers, including whistles and siren devices, may or may not be either available or effective, depending upon the circumstances.

Among the possible nonviolent methods of self-protection are the following:

- If you are being followed by a man who is more than 20 or so feet away, you can scream or use a noisemaker.

- Where possible, if followed, you should go into a store and tell the proprietor or clerk that you want to use a telephone.

- Again where possible, bring third parties into the situation—a chance pedestrian, perhaps another woman, or a passing group.

- Remain out of doors if your choice lies between entering a hallway or lobby or staying outside.

- Never go home if you know there is no one home. Instead ring all the door bells on apartment doors or go to a neighbor you know will be home.

- If you find it necessary to walk alone at night, walk in the street—again if possible and safe.

- Take a taxicab home if you have to travel late at night, and ask the driver to wait until you get indoors.

- Even when entering your own building, check the entrance and both sides before going inside.

- If you live alone, pretend you don't.

If a Rape Occurs

The rape victim may face a long period in which recovery and normal living seem impossible. The ability to enjoy life, sex, love, and work may appear to be elusive, even nonexistent. Six months or a year may pass without bringing relief from bad dreams, feelings of guilt, insomnia, and many other physical and psychological aftereffects. But authorities say that what a victim does after experiencing rape may make the transition to normal living easier while also protecting her against recurring health problems.

The Sympathetic Ear

Preferably before, but certainly after reporting to the police, the victim should confide in another person—whether husband, lover, close woman friend, counselor, pastor, hotline volunteer, or someone else trustworthy. The person confided in should go to the police station with the victim—if not the first time, then on any later occasions. The person confided in should be able to provide support, to make sure the victim's rights are protected, and to listen sympathetically to the victim's story.

Going to the Hospital

The rape victim should go as soon as possible to a hospital and undergo the pelvic and other examinations that physicians administer in such cases. If the woman goes to the hospital immediately, she should not wash herself or change clothes. A shower can remove valuable medical evidence. The pelvic examination is designed to find evidence of abrasions or internal damage, and for collection of any semen left by the rapist. Physicians will also examine for any of the rapist's hair, blood, skin, or semen. Any such evidence may be important in court later.

The hospital visit has other purposes. A physician can also administer preventive injections for sexually transmitted diseases and, if desired, an antipregnancy medication. The latter medication must be taken within three days if it is to be effective.

Importantly, the hospital visit may or may not bring the rape case automatically to the attention of the police. That would be true in some areas but not in all. Ultimately, the victim has to report the crime.

Reporting to the Police

Failure to report a rape immediately or after a few days probably means the rapist will not be apprehended. Even so, as many as nine out of ten rapes go unreported simply because most victims cannot face the added trauma of being questioned in detail and, possibly, rude treatment. The woman who does report to the police should, however, do so as soon as possible; each passing day increases the possibility that the police will want to know the reasons for the delay. But reporting late, experts stress, is better than not reporting at all. Reporting a rape does not mean that the victim has to press charges later.

Rape Crisis Centers

Rape crisis centers operate in most communities of any size. The staffs of these centers include many rape victims who have decided to devote time to helping other victims. To find help or advice, or an experienced person to accompany you to the police station, you can:

● Check the front of your telephone directory for the number of a rape hotline.

● Call Women Against Rape (WAR) if the group has an office in your area. WAR should be listed in the telephone book under "Women."

● Failing the other alternatives, the local YWCA or women's center should have a rape crisis center number.

26

Physicians and Diagnostic Procedures

Many people dislike going to the doctor; many fear going to the hospital. And many are overwhelmed by the enormity of the health care industry; much of its costs and procedures seem incomprehensible to us and out of control. Too often, these people put off seeing a doctor until they develop a debilitating problem. Yet many people overlook the one very important way they can alleviate some of their anxiety over their own medical care: choosing a doctor. Having a doctor you trust and with whom you can communicate well not only makes it more likely that you will make appointments for regular checkups, tests, and immunizations, but you will feel comfortable reporting any symptoms that may be the first signs of serious illness, many of which, when diagnosed early, can be treated successfully.

Your Primary Care Physician

Your primary care physician is your regular doctor, the person you see for checkups, and the first person you call when signs of illness appear. More than likely, he or she will be a *general practitioner,* a *family practitioner,* or an *internist* (see below). In selecting a primary care physician you should try to get a few recommendations from other patients, doctors, nurses, or hospital workers. Don't hesitate to make an appointment for an informational interview to meet the doctor in person and ask any questions about his or her methods, background, and philosophy that may be important to you.

Another important thing to check is the doctor's training—how much and from where. Check the American Medical Association's *The Directory of Medical Specialists* and other such directories in the library to find out whether the doctor has graduated from a fully accredited medical school and where he or she received further training.

In addition, remember that good communication is often the key to good health care. Make sure your doctor understands your questions and concerns and make sure you understand your doctor's answers and instructions. Don't hesitate to ask why you're being given a particular medication, or what is the purpose of any tests that are recommended. There are alternatives to some medications, and many tests are very expensive and not always necessary. If you are ever uncomfortable with what your doctor has ordered, seek a second opinion; your doctor should be happy to recommend someone. If not, find out why.

General Practitioner

All doctors must complete four years of schooling at an approved medical school, receive one year of postgraduate training in a supervised clinical setting, and pass a state board examination to become licensed to practice medicine. At this point in his or her training a doctor qualifies as a *general practitioner*. Like the stereotypical old-time country doctor, they treat just about everything from warts to measles, set broken bones, deliver babies, and dispense antibiotics and painkillers.

Family Practitioner

The general practitioner has largely been replaced by the *family practitioner*. Family practitioners must complete a three-year residency that covers certain aspects of internal medicine, pediatrics, obstetrics, and orthopedics, and then pass an exam. They treat the same things that general practitioners treat.

Internist

Like the family practitioner, the *internist* must complete a three-year residency and then pass an exam. Generally, they choose to specialize further in such problems as heart disease, cancer, or diabetes.

Osteopath

A doctor of osteopathy (D.O.) or *osteopath* has similar qualifications as a doctor of medicine. Osteopathy was founded by Andrew Taylor Still (1828-1917) on the principle that the body possesses a natural ability both to defend itself against disease and to heal itself as long as it is intact physically and physiologically and has adequate nutrition and favorable environmental conditions. Osteopaths place great emphasis on the importance of normal body mechanics and use of the hands for detecting and correcting problems.

Medical Specialties

There are 23 major specialties that are recognized by the American Medical Association.

Allergy and Immunology: *Allergists* and *immunologists* diagnose and treat allergies and specialize in the reactions of tissues of the immune system to stimulation by antibodies.

Anesthesiology: An *anesthesiologist* decides which types of pain killers will be used, administers it during surgery, and monitors its effects after surgery.

Colon and Rectal Surgery: A *proctologist* is concerned with disorders of the rectum and anus. A *gastroenterologist* studies problems of the digestive tract, including the lower part of the large intestine.

Dermatology: A *dermatologist* diagnoses and treats diseases of the skin, hair, and nails.

Emergency Medicine: An *emergency medicine specialist* practices emergency medicine in a trauma center.

Family Practice: The role of the *family practitioner* is discussed above.

Internal Medicine: The role of the *internist* is discussed above. An internist may specialize in any of the following: *cardiology*, the study of diseases of the heart; *endocrinology*, the study of diseases of the glands; *gastroenterology*, the study of disorders of the digestive tract; *hematology*, the study of blood and blood-forming tissues; *infectious diseases; medical oncology*, the study of tumors; *nephrology*, the study of the anatomy, physiology, and pathology of the kidneys; *pulmonary diseases*, the study of disorders of the lungs and respiratory system; and *rheumatology*, the study of connecting and supporting tissues.

Neurological Surgery: The *neurological surgeon* deals with the diagnosis, treatment, and surgical management of disorders and diseases of the brain, spinal cord, and nervous systems.

Nuclear Medicine: The *nuclear medicine specialist* is concerned with the use of radioactive material in the diagnosis and treatment of disease.

Obstetrics and Gynecology: An *obstetrician* specializes in the treatment of pregnant women and delivers babies. A *gynecologist* specializes in the treatment of women and their particular diseases, especially the reproductive system. Often, physicians specialize in both areas.

Ophthalmology: An *ophthalmologist* specializes in the medical and surgical treatment of the eye. They also treat eye diseases.

Orthopedic Surgery: An *orthopedist* diagnoses, treats, and surgically corrects disorders and injuries associated with the bones, joints, muscles, cartilage, and ligaments.

Otorhinolaryngology: An *otorhinolaryngologist* treats and performs surgery on the ears, nose, and throat.

Pathology: A *pathologist* investigates the course and causes of diseases.

Pediatrics: A *pediatrician* specializes in all medical aspects of child care. Subspecialties of pediatrics include: *pediatric cardiology, pediatric endocrinology, pediatric hematology/oncology, neonatal/perinatal medicine,* and *nephrology.*

Physical Medicine and Rehabilitation: A *physiatrist* deals with the full or partial restoration of use and function to body parts that have been injured or diseased, or have been defective at birth.

Plastic Surgery: A *plastic surgeon* performs operations designed to restore features to their former appearance following a disfiguring accident or correct features that the owner feels are unsightly.

Psychiatry and Neurology: A *psychiatrist* treats behavior disorders, often with psychotherapy, but also with drugs. A *neurologist* diagnoses and treats disorders of the brain and nervous system as well as of the muscles.

Radiology: A *radiologist* uses X rays in the diagnoses and treatment of diseases.

Surgery: A *general surgeon* specializes in the diagnosis and surgical treatment of a wide range of diseases, although most surgeons choose to specialize further.

Urology: A *urologist* diagnoses and treats disorders of the urinary-tract organs, and in men, problems of the reproductive system.

The Physical Examination

One of the first questions many people have about the physical exam is "How often should I have one?" Visits for infants from birth to 18 months are typically scheduled at 2, 4, 6, 15, and 18 months. Visits for children from 2 to 18 are typically scheduled once a year. Visits for individuals aged 19 to 65 are recommended every 1 to 3 years, for most people beginning on the low side (every 3 years) and progressing to every year as one approaches age 65. After age 65 annual visits are recommended.

A typical physical examination will include a careful health appraisal by an examining physician, including a detailed health history of the patient and study of the patient's body appearance and functions. Because no two persons are alike and the differences among patients are likely to increase with advancing years, the examining

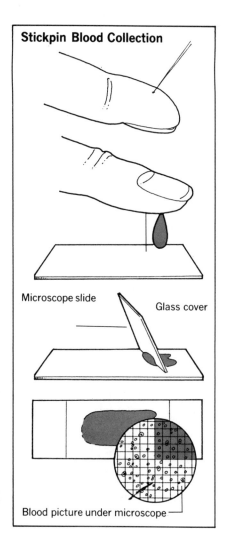

Stickpin Blood Collection

Microscope slide

Glass cover

Blood picture under microscope

any medications the patient is allergic to or currently taking, and any incidence of family illnesses that may make the patient more susceptible to such things as heart disease, cancer, and so on.

The physician may begin the exam with a simple, obvious question like, "Why are you here?" or "What seems to be the matter?" Even if you feel fine and are just in for a routine physical, don't underestimate the importance of even the slightest *symptoms* you may be experiencing; things like aches, pains, headaches, a bloated feeling, gas, bad breath, and so on may not sound very important in and of themselves, and in fact are often only temporary annoyances, but any symptom experienced regularly over a period of time should be reported.

The physician will also want to know something about your lifestyle—whether or not you smoke, drink, exercise regularly, and so on.

After the medical history has been recorded or updated, the physician may begin a general inspection of the patient's body, beginning with the head and neck and working down to the feet. The physician looks for possible deformities, scars or wounds, including insect bites, or pulsations or throbbing areas. Bruises, areas of skin peeling or flaking, areas of heavy skin pigmentation or loss of pigmentation, hair distribution, perspiration or goose bumps, firmness or slackness of the skin, warts, calluses, and other features are noted.

The physician usually checks the exterior of the body by a method

physician's interest in a set of signs and symptoms may vary with different patients as he or she pieces evidence together to come up with a complete evaluation of a particular patient.

The patient's *medical history* is important because the physician needs to know any medical problems the patient may have had in the past, including any operations or pregnancies, known as *palpation,* which means feeling with the fingers and hands. Rough vibrations from a disorder in the respiratory system, the trembling sensation of blood encountering an obstruction, or the grating feeling of a bone deformity can be detected during palpation. In addition to palpation, the physician may apply *percussion,* or tapping, of certain body areas. Tapping the chest, for example, gives the physician some information about the condition of the lungs. A related technique, *auscultation,* involves listening to sounds within the body through a stethoscope. During percussion, the physician listens for changes in sounds that range from resonance over hollow spaces to dullness over solid or muscular areas. Lack of resonance over a normally resonant area of the lung might indicate fluid, pneumonia, or perhaps an abnormal mass. Percussion may also give the first sign of enlargement of organs, such as the liver, heart, or spleen. During auscultation, the physician listens for normal or abnormal breathing sounds. He or she can usually detect specific aberrations in lung function by noises made as the air rushes in and out of the lungs through the bronchi. In auscultation of the heart, the physician listens for extra heartbeats, rubbing sounds, the rumbling noises of a heart murmur, or the sounds of normally

functioning heart valves opening and closing.

The physician may also use the stethoscope to listen to sounds beyond the chest area. He or she may listen to the sounds of blood flowing through vessels of the neck, bowel sounds through the wall of the abdomen, and the subtle noises made by joints, muscles, and tendons as various limbs are moved.

Weight and height are checked as part of any routine examination. These factors are especially important in a health examination for children to determine the rate of growth, even though youngsters of the same age can vary considerably in height and weight and still be within the so-called normal range. Sudden changes in the rate of growth or abnormal growth may be signs that special attention should be given to possible problems. Adults also can vary greatly in weight and height, but special concern may be indicated by the physician if the individual is exceptionally tall, short, fat, or skinny. Posture also provides clues to the condition of a patient; one who has a slouch or holds one shoulder higher than the other may have an abnormal spinal curvature. The physician may watch the patient's manner of walking because a person's gait can suggest muscle, bone, or nervous-system disorders.

Common Screening Tests

A variety of tests may be given in a routine physical exam, depending on

the patient's age, family history, current state of health, the length of time between the last visit, and so on. Some of the following tests will be done each time the patient visits the doctor and some are necessary only when specific complaints or concerns are raised or when an individual reaches a certain age or risk category. Some tests have remained the same for years, and some change or are replaced with newer tests. Your doctor should explain any new test to you.

Blood Pressure and Pulse Rate

The patient's blood pressure and pulse rate are checked on every office visit, no matter what the reason is for the visit. Blood pressure is measured with a *sphygmomanometer* and a stethoscope. The sphygmomanometer has attached to it an inflatable cuff, which is wrapped around the upper arm; a rubber bulb is used to inflate the cuff and increase pressure in it so that it can control the blood flow in the arm. The physician locates the pulse with the stethoscope and increases the cuff pressure until the pulse (heartbeat) can no longer be heard. Then the physician slowly deflates the cuff and lets the reading on the gauge fall gradually until he hears the first beat of the heart. The reading on the gauge at that point is recorded as the systolic pressure (the first number). The physician continues to relax the pressure in the cuff and watches for the reading at the point where the thumping of the heart disappears again. That number is recorded as the *diastolic pressure* (the second number).

The pulse is checked for rate and quality, which means the force of the pulse beat and the tension between beats. The pulse rate for small children may be well over 100 beats per minute and still be considered normal. But in an adult who is relaxed and resting, any pulse rate over 100 suggests that something is wrong. An adult pulse rate of less than 60 in a nonathlete might also indicate an abnormal condition.

Eyes, Mouth, Nose, and Ears

Inspection of the eyes is usually done with the aid of an *ophthalmoscope,* by means of which the physician can visualize the retina on the back inner surface of each eye, and its associated arteries, veins, and nerve fibers. Distended retinal veins may be a sign of a variety of disorders, including diabetes or heart disease; signs of hardening of the arteries also may be observed in the eyes before other indications are found elsewhere. The condition of retinal blood vessels may also signal the development of hypertension.

A device called an *otoscope* is inserted in the outer ear to examine the external auditory canal and the eardrum. In addition, the condition of the tongue, teeth, and gums can reveal much about health habits of the individual.

Cholesterol Measurement

The blood cholesterol level is an important risk factor for coronary artery disease. For most people a blood cholesterol level above 200 mg/dl should be cause for concern, indicating a need for further tests and perhaps a change in life-style. It's a good idea to have your blood cholesterol checked at age 25 and then once every 3 to 5 years thereafter.

Blood Tests

Complete Blood Count

A CBC requires a sample of less than two teaspoons of blood. Four common measurements are taken from it: *Hemoglobin concentration* indicates the level of this substance that transports oxygen to all the cells in the body. A low *red blood cell count* may indicate anemia, as well as be a potential early warning sign for leukemia, kidney malfunction, internal bleeding, or sickle cell anemia. A too high red blood cell count could be an early clue to congenital heart disease, respiratory disease, or polycythemia vera. The *hematocrit* measures the ratio of red blood cells to the plasma in the blood. Like the hemoglobin concentration, the hematocrit can indicate anemia, and all three tests are generally given in order to help diagnose the specific type and cause of anemia. A high *white blood cell count* can indicate the presence of an infection, stress, a major injury, or even leukemia. A low count can be a sign of poor diet, certain infections, or another type of leukemia. If taken in the presence of a fever, the white blood cell count can help distinguish between a bacterial and a viral infection.

Blood Glucose

The glucose test determines the amount of sugar in the blood. Individuals who experience symptoms of diabetes mellitus (such as excessive thirst or urination), hypoglycemia (lightheadedness or fainting), or who are pregnant will most likely be given a blood glucose test. A very high level of blood sugar can indicate diabetes, while a very low level can indicate hypoglycemia. In either case or in border-line cases an *oral glucose tolerance test* is given. This test requires that the individual fast for 12 to 14 hours before the test. The patient is then given a concentrated sugar solution to drink, and blood is drawn at regular intervals over the next several hours. This test now replaces the urine test for sugar.

Blood Urea Nitrogen (BUN) and Blood Creatinine

Blood urea and creatinine are products of protein metabolism. A high level of either in the blood means that the kidneys are not filtering them properly from the blood, and thus may indicate kidney damage.

Blood Electrolytes

The four blood electrolytes are sodium, potassium, chloride, and bicarbonate, and they play important roles in the blood pH, the cells' water balance, kidney function, and so on. Most often this test is given to patients who are taking diuretics, those with liver, kidney, or heart disease, or those who may be experiencing dehydration or excessive vomiting or diarrhea.

Urinalysis

The urinalysis is a simple and important test that can indicate much about a person's overall health and identify potential problems, such as kidney disease, diabetes, and urinary tract infections. For a routine urinalysis a sample can be taken at any time of day, although the physician may specify the first morning's urine, or may give special instructions about food and water intake before taking the urine sample.

In the lab the technician will test the urine for its *specific gravity,* which can indicate whether the kidneys can effectively conserve body fluid; its *pH,* which is an indication of how well the kidneys are able to excrete acids from the body; its *protein content,* which in pregnant women can indicate toxemia of pregnancy and in others is a clue to the condition of the kidneys and the prostate; its *glucose content,* which could suggest diabetes; and its *bilirubin content,* which indicates a potential problem in the liver or bile ducts. The technician will also examine the urine under a microscope, looking for such things as pus cells, bacteria, or too many red blood cells, all of which could indicate potential problems.

Routine blood work and a urinalysis are both simple, common tests that can catch many potential problems early. When these tests do indicate abnormalities, other, more specific—and often more expensive—tests are required for confirmation before treatment can begin. Given the fact that any test can give a false result, whether through human error or through individual variations, the question of whether or not healthy feeling individuals should even have these tests is a much-debated point in the medical community and one best discussed with one's primary care physician.

Electrocardiogram

An *electrocardiogram* is a kind of picture of the heart created by attaching electrodes to the chest, arms, and legs. The wires from the electrodes pick up electrical impulses produced by the heart. The wires are connected to the machine, which translates the impulses into a picture. The

Electrocardiogram

Electrocardiographic lead

test is simple, safe, and takes five to ten minutes to perform.

Since a normally beating heart produces a similar pattern of waves in everybody, abnormal waves can indicate a number of potential problems, such as irregular heart rhythms, damage to the heart muscle, enlargement of the heart's chambers, mineral imbalances in the blood, and whether the patient has had, or is having, a heart attack. The EKG is not foolproof, however, and can produce false results. It is perhaps overused as a screen for coronary artery disease. A "baseline" EKG is recommended at age 35 (when the patient is presumably in a good state of health) to give a pattern with which to compare all future EKGs.

Mammogram

A *mammogram* is an X ray of the breast done to detect breast cancer. It is estimated that yearly mammograms for women over 50 could lead to a one-third reduction in the number of deaths from breast cancer.

To be the most effective, the mammogram must be done on a machine designed especially for this purpose. The patient must remove all clothing from the waist up and either stands or sits with the breast placed on a small shelf that extends out from the machine. The patient is then pushed forward so that the edge of the shelf presses into the chest just below the breast. The compression device is brought down onto the breast, and pressure is applied for about a minute. This is the most uncomfortable part of the test, as much pressure is necessary in order to get the most detailed picture possible. Many women find that eliminating caffeine and foods that tend to cause water retention two weeks prior to the exam makes the breasts less sensitive.

The American Cancer Society recommends a baseline mammogram for women aged 35 to 40. Between the ages of 40 and 49 a mammogram is recommended every 1 to 2 years, and after age 50 an annual mammogram is essential. Regular breast exams before the age of 40 have not been proven to be of value.

Pap Smear

The *pap smear* tests for cervical cancer by the microscopic examination of cells from the vaginal walls and cervix. About 2 percent of all women over 40 develop cervical cancer, but 95 percent of these can be cured if the cancer is caught early.

The procedure can be done any time except during the menstrual period. The patient undresses from the waist down and lies down on her back with her legs spread apart and her feet in special stirrups. The gynecologist inserts a lubricated *speculum* into the vagina and opens it to expose the cervix and its os (mouth). The doctor then inserts a small applicator through the speculum and rubs it gently against the cervix and sometimes the os. The applicator is removed and rubbed onto a glass slide (the smear). The speculum is then removed.

The first pap smear should be done when a woman turns 18 or becomes sexually active (whichever occurs first), and should be followed by pap smears for 2 consecutive years. Providing these tests are negative and there are no risk factors present, tests can be done less frequently at the discretion of one's doctor, although an annual pap smear for women between 25 and 60 is common.

Occult Blood Test

Colon cancer is the second most common form of cancer in the United States. An early warning sign of colon cancer is blood in the stool. It is called *occult,* or hidden, blood because it cannot be detected by sight. It is recommended that everyone over age 50 be tested for occult blood annually.

Home tests are available for occult blood, but because of the seriousness of the results it is often wise to at least discuss the results with a physician or have the physician do the test. Before collecting stool samples the patient must avoid eating red meat, turnips, horseradish, and high doses of vitamin C and consume more fruits, vegetables, and fibrous foods beginning three days before the first test and until the last sample is taken. A sample from three consecutive stools is necessary. Two tests are available and it is best to discuss with your physician which one to use. The *Guaiac test* uses a chemical that turns bluish in the presence of blood. Usually reliable, the test nevertheless fails for a number of reasons to detect colon cancer in about one third of patients who have it. The *HemoQuant* is another test that is better able to detect occult blood even after bacteria have altered it.

Sigmoidoscopy

Another, more expensive procedure for detecting colon cancer is *sigmoidoscopy,* the use of a sigmoidoscope to examine the lower segment of the large intestine. To ensure a clean lower bowel, the patient must eat a soft diet the day before the test, have a liquid dinner, and than take an enema. A light breakfast is permitted, and another enema will be given an hour before the test. The patient removes clothing from the waist down and lies on the left side with the knees drawn up to the chest. A thin, lubricated tube (there are two kinds, flexible and rigid; the flexible one is easier to tolerate and is a better optical tool) is inserted into the rectum and slowly advanced along the large intestine. The tube contains optical filaments and small instruments that allow the doctor to view the interior of the intestine and take samples if necessary. Air may be forced through the tube to expand the intestine, which can cause a feeling of discomfort. The procedure takes from 15 to 30 minutes. The American Cancer Society recommends a baseline sigmoidoscopy for everyone at age 50 (or 40 if there is a family history of colon cancer) and once every three years after that.

Sexually Transmitted Diseases

The prevalence of sexually transmitted diseases (STDs), such as syphilis, gonorrhea, chlamydia, genital herpes, and AIDS, makes regular tests for these diseases in sexually active people who are not involved in monogamous relationships vitally important. Tests are typically blood tests or swab tests and should be done every year or two.

Tuberculosis

Tuberculosis is normally tested for with a simple *skin test.* Either the forearm is pricked with a small device with four prongs or a subcutaneous injection is used. In either case, the patient is asked to observe the area after 48 to 72 hours for signs of redness, raised bumps, or swelling. Individuals who regularly come into close contact with many people, such as those in education or health care, are advised to be tested often.

Stress Test

Stress tests are often given to older people who are about to begin an exercise program. The test is similar to the resting EKG, only instead of just lying still while hooked up to the machine, the patient exercises on a treadmill or stationary bicycle. Because the size of the opening in the vessels of the heart can decrease more than 60 percent before anything abnormal is apparent, the stress test allows the doctor to get a picture of the heart with an increased workload in order to see if it's getting a good supply of oxygen. If it's not, this could indicate a build-up of plaque on the arteries, or coronary artery disease. A routine stress test is often recommended at age 45, and as early as 35 if you have at least one risk factor for coronary artery disease.

Chest X ray

The *chest X ray* was once a routine part of the physical exam. Its expense, potential danger, and limited results in the absence of symptoms has made it less popular. (An individual X ray in and of itself is not harmful, but because exposure to radiation is cumulative throughout your life, a series of X rays over a lifetime can result in increased risk of cancer.)

If you are advised to have a chest X ray, you will be asked to remove all clothing from the waist up and to wear a gown. Depending on the particular area to be X rayed, you will either sit, stand, or lie down. The X-ray beam is centered on the target area, activated, and the film between you and the beam is exposed. Generally two or three exposures are taken for each target area.

Immunizations

Nearly everyone knows the importance of having their children immunized, but many people may not realize that it is important for adults to have regular immunizations as well. When a patient is immunized, he or she receives a shot of modified microbes (bacteria or viruses) or toxins. Although not strong enough to actually give the patient the disease, the dose of microbes does stimulate the patient's own immune system to build up antibodies against the disease, thus making him or her immune to future exposures. Vaccines do wear off, however, and it is best to keep a record of all immunizations and receive scheduled booster shots.

Diphtheria

Diphtheria is a disease that is spread by airborne bacteria that release toxins that can attack the heart and other internal organs. Adults should receive a booster shot every ten years.

Tetanus

Tetanus is spread by bacteria that enter the body through a contaminated wound. Adults should receive a booster shot (often combined with the diphtheria shot) every ten years. If you sustain a contaminated wound, your doctor may recommend a tetanus booster is you have not had one in 5 years.

Influenza

The risk of death from the *flu* increases with age, and people over 65 are strongly advised to receive annual flu shots in the fall. In 1976 about 500 cases of a rare paralytic condition called Guillain-Barre syndrome were associated with a swine flu vaccine. No influenza vaccines since have been associated with the development of Guillain-Barre.

Pneumococcal Pneumonia

Again, those at risk of death from influenza should also be immunized against *pneumonia*. Like the flu shot, the pneumonia shot is about 70 percent effective, so although being immunized against them is no guarantee against coming down with either one, any common form of flu or pneumonia the patient might get will at least be non-life threatening.

Measles and Mumps

Many people born after 1957 have both not had and not been immunized against *measles* and *mumps* and thus are particularly susceptible. In addition, those vaccinated between 1963 and 1967 may have gotten a short-lasting killed-virus vaccine and should be revaccinated. Anyone born between 1957 and 1967 should be revaccinated unless 1) they had a case of measles confirmed by a physician's diagnosis, 2) they are immune, as demonstrated by a blood test, 3) they have a record of receiving live vaccine no earlier than their first birthday.

Hepatitis B

Hepatitis B infects only about 1 in 20 Americans in the course of a lifetime, and most of these will fight the virus off successfully. However, about 10 percent of those infected are unable to rid themselves of the virus and will develop chronic hepatitis, which can lead to cirrhosis or liver cancer. Hepatitis B immunization is recommended for health care workers who frequently handle blood, homosexually active men, users of illicit injectable drugs, hemodialysis patients, recipients of blood products to control bleeding disorders, prison occupants, workers at institutions for the mentally retarded, and household and sexual contacts of hepatitis B carriers.

Children

The standard immunizations for children are 1) combined vaccines for diphtheria, pertussis, and tetanus (DTP); 2) a triple oral polio virus vaccine or TOPV; 3) vaccines for measles, mumps, and rubella (MMR); 4) HIB, hemophilus b for influenza. The Centers for Disease Control recommends the following schedule:

- 2 months: DPT, TOPV, HIB

- 4 months: DPT, TOPV, HIB

- 6 months: DPT and HIB

- 15 months: MMR (also at 12 mos)

- 18 months: DPT and TOPV

- 4 to 6 years: DPT, MMR, and TOPV

- 14 to 16 years: tetanus and diphtheria booster (Td)

Other Tests You May Encounter

If a definite diagnosis cannot be made on the basis of the medical history, preliminary physical exam, and routine diagnostic tests, more specialized tests may be required. What follows is a description, grouped by body system, of some of the other diagnostic tests.

The Skeletal System

The skeletal system includes the bones and cartilage, and the specialist is the orthopedic surgeon. Problems with the nervous system and joints often overlap skeletal problems and may necessitate tests by a neurologist or rheumatologist.

X rays are the most important diagnostic tool for special investigations of the bones. They can reveal a hairline fracture of a major bone, a bony deposit, or abnormal alignment.

Synovial aspiration, or a *synovial fluid exam,* involves the withdrawal of a tiny amount of synovial fluid with a needle inserted into a joint. The laboratory analysis of the fluid can help diagnose such problems as gout and some forms of arthritis.

Magnetic resonance imaging, or *MRI,* is a way of creating an image of a body part by taking advantage of the way protons behave in a magnetic field when exposed to a radiofrequency pulse: the way they line up and the form of the radiowave that they emit produces the image. The patient lies down on a table, and a surface coil (it comes in a variety of forms, depending on the body part to be examined) is applied. The surface coil is the device that emits the radiofrequency pulse. The patient's heartbeat and respiration are monitored, usually by a small band placed around a finger. Next the table moves the patient so that the area to be examined is inside the magnet. The magnet is in the form of a tunnel and may make some people feel claustrophobic. At this point the noise level increases and may be uncomfortable.

The Human Skeleton

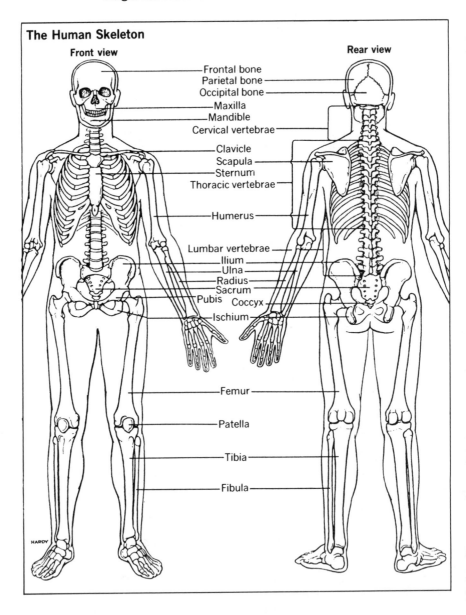

Front view

Rear view

Frontal bone
Parietal bone
Occipital bone
Maxilla
Mandible
Cervical vertebrae
Clavicle
Scapula
Sternum
Thoracic vertebrae
Humerus
Lumbar vertebrae
Ilium
Ulna
Radius
Sacrum
Pubis Coccyx
Ischium
Femur
Patella
Tibia
Fibula

HARDY

Several images are taken, with the table moving slightly between each. MRI is safer than X rays because there is no exposure to radiation; however, pregnant women and people with implanted stimulatory devices, such as pacemakers, should not have MRI.

Nuclear imaging involves the injection, swallowing, instillation, or inhalation of a *radioactive isotope* (a marker, or tracer) into the body that goes where the problem is. The iso-tope is then located by a special cam-era, and an image is produced. Two uses of this technique for skeletal ex-ams are the bone scan and the bone density test. These tests are more sensitive than X rays and can often identify a problem months before it shows up on the X ray. They are used when the X ray comes back normal, but symptoms persist.

In the *bone scan* the patient re-ceives an injection of a bone-seeking nuclide in a vein. Scanning begins two to four hours later. Either the entire body or just the part concerned is im-aged. Injuries, infections, and tumors can all be located with this technique.

The *bone density test* is used to di-agnose osteoporosis, the decrease in bone density that is the major cause of fractures in the elderly. The patient lies on a table while two L-shaped de-vices (an emitter above the table and a detector below the table) pass over him. The emitter emits energy and the detector detects it. Because the energy has to go through your body before it is detected by the detector, the amount that your body absorbs is an indication of your bone density. This procedure is called *absorptiome-try.*

Ultrasonography is most often em-ployed in skeletal exams to determine whether a "lump" or "bump" is solid or fluid-filled. Ultrasonography fol-lows the same principle behind radar and sonar: Sound waves emitted by a transducer are directed at a particular part of the body, bounce back, and are translated into an image. Tissues, bones, water, air, and so on all vary consistently in the way they reflect the sound wave, thus making possible the interpretation of the reflected im-age.

Arthroscopy is a way of seeing in-side the body by using an optical in-strument equipped with lenses and lights (an arthroscope) which is in-serted in a small opening. Anesthesia is generally required, and the area most often studied by this method is the knee. If a problem is found during the exam the doctor may opt to go ahead and take care of it then, a pro-cedure for which the patient's prior permission is required.

The Muscles and Joints

The human body has more than 600 muscles of all sizes and shapes that, attached to the skeletal system, en-able us to move as they contract. The joints are the spaces between two coupled bones that allow the bones to move in more than one direction. Muscles and joints are the domain of the rheumatologist.

The synovial fluid exam, X rays, MRI, nuclear imaging, and ultra-sonography described under the skel-etal system are used to examine the muscles and joints as well. When there is a problem with muscle con-trol, inability to relax a muscle, or weakness in commonly used muscles, another test that may be ordered is the *electromyogram*. This test measures a muscle's electrical potential, which should be zero if the muscle is relaxed. An electrode is attached to the skin over the target muscle and another electrode, in the form of a small needle, is inserted in the muscle. Lead wires from the two electrodes are attached to a monitor, and measurements of the muscle's electrical activity are made while the patient contracts and relaxes it. This test helps determine whether the problem is with the muscle itself or with the nerves controlling it. If the problem points to the nerves, then an electroneurogram is in order.

Joints are prone to stiffness and damage from swelling of the surrounding bursa and tendons. X rays and MRIs will detect damage to the bursa and tendous.

Skin

The dermatologist specializes in treating skin disorders. Many problems specific to the skin can be diagnosed by physical exam and questioning of the patient.

Skin tests are commonly done on allergy sufferers to determine what they are allergic to. In a *prick test* the forearm is cleansed and a drop of up to 35 different solutions is placed in rows on the arm. The doctor then takes a small needlelike object and pricks the center of each drop. After 15 minutes any of the solutions to which the patient is allergic will produce a slight swelling much like a mosquito bite. A *scratch test* is similar except a small scratch is made on the arm and then the drop is applied. In the *intradermal test* the solution is injected. A *patch test* is done when the patient has a rash, probably caused by something that touches the skin. Patches of possible allergens are placed on the back, and the patient returns in two days for a reading.

Sores that refuse to heal, change in the shape, color, and texture of warts or moles, and pimples that itch and recur are all considered symptoms of skin cancer and should be checked by your doctor. Because of the small size of most of these skin eruptions, they are commonly removed entirely and then a biopsy is performed on the tissue. They can be cut out (excised), removed with an electric needle, or frozen (cryosurgery).

The Nervous System

The brain, spinal cord, and network of nerves make up the nervous system. The neurosurgeon and the neurologist are the specialists.

In a *spinal tap*, or *spinal fluid exam*, the doctor inserts a needle into the lower back and removes a small amount of spinal fluid, which is then examined in the lab. The test usually causes severe headaches; it is used to diagnose infections, brain hemorrhages, tumors, polio, meningitis, and other conditions. *Myelography* is a similar study, much more painful, in which a small amount of spinal fluid is removed, dye injected in its place,

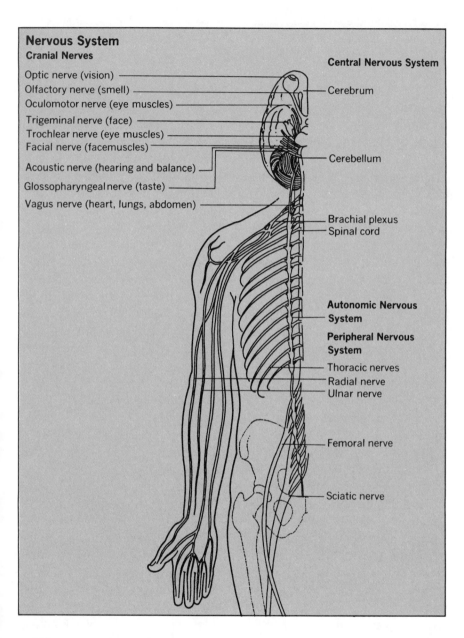

Nervous System

Cranial Nerves

Central Nervous System

Optic nerve (vision)
Olfactory nerve (smell)
Oculomotor nerve (eye muscles)
Trigeminal nerve (face)
Trochlear nerve (eye muscles)
Facial nerve (facemuscles)
Acoustic nerve (hearing and balance)
Glossopharyngeal nerve (taste)
Vagus nerve (heart, lungs, abdomen)

Cerebrum

Cerebellum

Brachial plexus
Spinal cord

**Autonomic Nervous
System**

**Peripheral Nervous
System**

Thoracic nerves
Radial nerve
Ulnar nerve

Femoral nerve

Sciatic nerve

and X rays are taken while the patient lies on a table. Slipped disks, some types of arthritis, and different types of tumors are commonly diagnosed this way, although the use of MRI (see skeletal system) and computer- ized axial tomography (CT) are also used and are often done first.

The CT exam is a noninvasive procedure that takes a series of X-ray pictures of "slices" of the targeted body part. The patient removes all removables from the area being studied and lies on a table (called a gantry) which is then moved into the machine. Several exposures are taken, with the table moving slightly between each. For some studies it is necessary to inject a special "dye," which could cause mild discomfort. Some people experience a claustrophobic reaction while inside the machine. CT is about 100 times more sensitive than conventional X rays and is good for detecting calcium deposits, tumors, cysts, and abscesses. Because of its sensitivity to tissue density, it can sometimes distinguish benign from malignant tumors.

The *brain scan* continues to be an important diagnostic tool. Areas of the brain can be "mapped," patterns are being discovered that allow diagnosis of such things as Alzheimer's disease, and the diagnosis of stroke can be validated days sooner than with CT.

The brain scan involves the injection in the arm of a radioactive isotope and the scanning of the brain by either a single photon emission computed tomography camera (SPECT) or a positron emission tomography camera (PET). The SPECT scanner uses gamma rays to create images, and the camera rotates around the stationary patient (thus there is no sensation of claustrophobia as with CT). The PET scanner uses positrons, which are a type of subatomic particle found in the nucleus of an atom, to create images. The PET scanner looks like a wall with a hole in the middle of it. The patient lies on a table, and the table is positioned so that the patient's head is in the opening of the wall. The scan is able to read through different depths, so problems deeply buried in tissue can be detected without surgery.

When the blood supply to the brain is limited by the blocking of the carotid arteries (in the neck) a condition known as transient ischemic attack (TIA), momentary loss of brain function, can occur and can eventually lead to a stroke. Thus, examining the carotid arteries is important if the patient possesses symptoms or significant risk factors. This can be done by X ray and also by ultrasound. In the ultrasound test two techniques are generally used. The first creates images (called duplex) and the second measures the rate and quality of blood flow (called Doppler). Both involve the gentle movement of the transducer slowly over each side of the neck. The Doppler phase, however, is very noisy. The procedure takes about 30 minutes.

Patients who have experienced TIA, stroke, or vertigo often routinely undergo *ocular plethysmography* (OPG) to detect narrowing of the ophthalmic artery. The patient is seated in a chair with a headrest, blood pressure is taken in each arm, and EKG leads are placed on the chest. The chair is semireclined and anesthetic drops are placed in each eye. The technologist then places tiny plastic cups into the corner of each eye. The cups are attached to wire leads connected to the machine. The patient is instructed to keep the eyes wide open. The machine then produces a slight suction on each eye and measures its pressure.

When epilepsy is suspected, following certain head injuries, or when the patient is experiencing confusional states, sleep problems, and even impotence, an *electroencephalograph* (EEG) may be ordered. The patient sits in a chair while a technologist attaches 16 to 22 electrodes to his head. EKG leads are also placed on the chest. The patient then lies down and may even fall asleep. The technologist may instruct the patient to open and close his eyes while a strobe light flashes. The test takes about two hours.

The electromyogram was discussed under the section on muscles. If the muscle is not the problem, the nerves connected to it may be and a *nerve conduction study,* or *electroneurogram,* is ordered. This test measures the speed of the electrical impulse across a nerve and the speed of the muscle's response. Electrodes are affixed to the skin over the target muscle. The target nerve is then given a mild electric shock. The electrode over the muscle both measures the time between the shock and the response (the muscle will twitch) and the intensity of the response. The corresponding nonaffected muscles are also tested for comparison. There is no hazard, and the shock feels like a mild sting or burn.

The Circulatory System

The cardiologist specializes in diseases of the heart and circulatory system. Coronary artery disease is the most common form of heart disease and involves the blocking of the arteries to the heart. There can also be problems with the heart muscle itself, problems with the heart valves, or congenital problems resulting from birth defects.

The electrocardiogram and the stress test have already been discussed. Nuclear imaging, ultrasound, and X rays are also used to detect coronary artery disease. In order to detect exactly how bad the arteries are and determine the necessary correctional procedure, an *angiograph,* or *arteriograph,* is done.

The angiograph begins with the insertion of a special needle in a major artery (usually in the groin area, but other sites are the armpit, the hollow of the elbow, and the neck). A sudden spurt of blood indicates correct positioning. A wire is then inserted through the needle, which stops the bleeding. The wire is advanced to the target area, and the needle is removed. A catheter is then slid over the wire and advanced to the target area. The wire is then withdrawn. The next step is the injection of a special dye to the target area. To prevent its being diluted it must be injected at high velocity and in large quantity. For most people the injection is extremely uncomfortable, with some reporting severe pain, a feeling of heat, headache, chest pain, or dizziness. The next step involves the rapid imaging of the target area, either by a

The Circulatory System

Arteries

(Carrying blood from the heart
to the rest of the body)

Veins

(Carrying blood from all parts
of the body toward the heart)

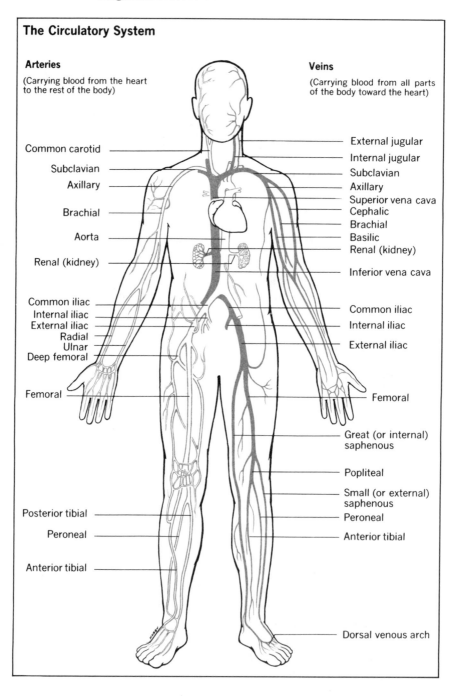

Arteries (left side):
Common carotid
Subclavian
Axillary
Brachial
Aorta
Renal (kidney)
Common iliac
Internal iliac
External iliac
Radial
Ulnar
Deep femoral
Femoral
Posterior tibial
Peroneal
Anterior tibial

Veins (right side):
External jugular
Internal jugular
Subclavian
Axillary
Superior vena cava
Cephalic
Brachial
Basilic
Renal (kidney)
Inferior vena cava
Common iliac
Internal iliac
External iliac
Femoral
Great (or internal) saphenous
Popliteal
Small (or external) saphenous
Peroneal
Anterior tibial
Dorsal venous arch

series of X-ray pictures or by X-ray
movies (both noisy). Often different
views are needed of the targeted
area, which means that the catheter

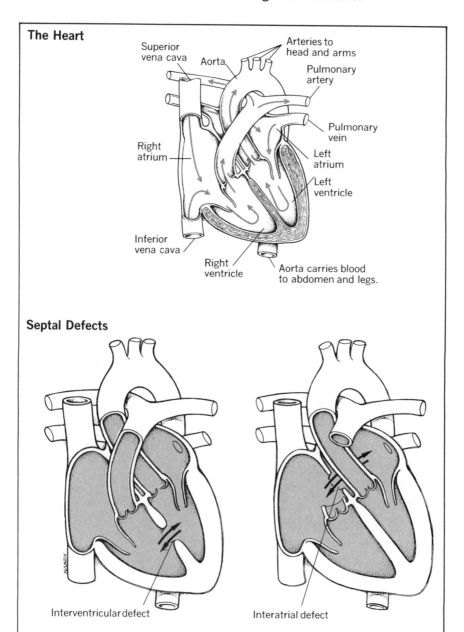

The Heart

Superior vena cava

Aorta

Arteries to head and arms

Pulmonary artery

Pulmonary vein

Right atrium

Left atrium

Left ventricle

Inferior vena cava

Right ventricle

Aorta carries blood to abdomen and legs.

Septal Defects

Interventricular defect

Interatrial defect

A normal heart in cross section (top), shows the circulation of the blood. An interventricular defect (bottom left) allows blood to pass directly between the left and right ventricles. An interatrial defect (bottom right), with the aorta seen in cross section over the left atrium, allows blood to pass freely between the two atria. Any septal defect interferes with the effectiveness of the pumping action of the heart.

must be repositioned and the dye re-injected. Once the pictures are fin-

ished the catheter is slowly removed and pressure is applied, either by the doctor himself or by a mechanical device, to the hole to seal the artery. The pressure involved is intense and lasts for 10 to 15 minutes. Because it is necessary for the patient to be conscious during the procedure, the entire process may cause extreme anxiety, which in turn increases the risk of heart attack. The patient is normally given a sedative to relax him. An overnight stay in the hospital following the procedure is routine. *Venography* is a similar study of the veins.

Not all people who experience sudden and severe chest pain are having a heart attack. A technique called *infarct detection* can confirm the diagnosis. Normally performed within the first 12 to 24 hours after the onset of the pain, the test involves the injection of an isotope (thallium-201) into a vein. The patient is then positioned under a gamma camera and an image is created of the heart that will make evident any occluded (blocked) vessels. A similar nuclear imaging process (under less duress) is used to obtain information about the heart's *wall motion* (how well the muscle relaxes and contracts) and *ejection fraction* (how much blood leaves a chamber of the heart when it contracts). Both tests give valuable information about the heart's health.

While X rays provide more detail, nuclear imaging can also be used to check *circulatory integrity,* or how open the veins and arteries are. Again, an isotope is injected into a vein near the target area and images are produced via a gamma camera.

Examination of the ejection fraction, valve function, and excessive pericardial fluid (the pericardial membrane surrounds the heart) can also be done with ultrasound. In a process similar to that described earlier for the carotid arteries, *echocardiography* produces an image of the working heart.

The Digestive System, the Liver, and the Pancreas

The gastroenterologist specializes in disorders of the digestive tract—the esophagus, stomach, duodenum, and intestine. The proctologist treats disorders of the large intestine, rectum, and anus.

As in many other systems, X rays are the traditional diagnostic tool for gastrointestinal problems. Nuclear imaging, however, may be used for some specific complaints. For example, if you're having trouble with heartburn an *esophageal reflux* test may be done to determine whether or not you have a hiatus hernia. The patient eats nothing the night before the exam. A small balloon is placed over the stomach, held in place by a special inflatable belt. The patient then stands in front of a gamma camera and drinks a glass of orange juice to which an isotope has been added. Pictures are taken as the fluid moves to the stomach. The patient then lies down on a table, and the cuff is inflated, causing the balloon to apply pressure to the stomach. Pictures are taken to see if this pressure causes the liquid

The Digestive System

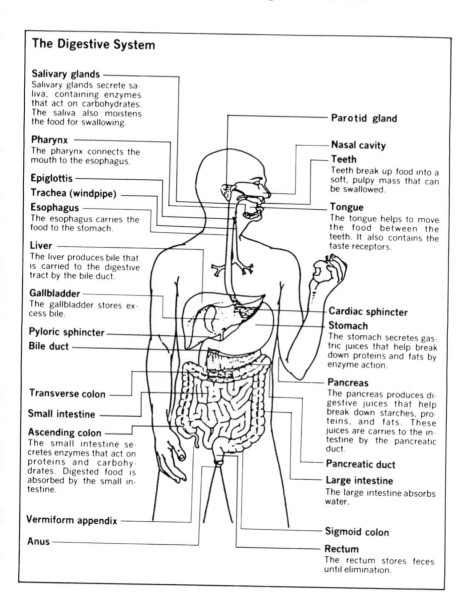

Salivary glands
Salivary glands secrete saliva, containing enzymes that act on carbohydrates. The saliva also moistens the food for swallowing.

Pharynx
The pharynx connects the mouth to the esophagus.

Epiglottis

Trachea (windpipe)

Esophagus
The esophagus carries the food to the stomach.

Liver
The liver produces bile that is carried to the digestive tract by the bile duct.

Gallbladder
The gallbladder stores excess bile.

Pyloric sphincter

Bile duct

Transverse colon

Small intestine

Ascending colon
The small intestine secretes enzymes that act on proteins and carbohydrates. Digested food is absorbed by the small intestine.

Vermiform appendix

Anus

Parotid gland

Nasal cavity

Teeth
Teeth break up food into a soft, pulpy mass that can be swallowed.

Tongue
The tongue helps to move the food between the teeth. It also contains the taste receptors.

Cardiac sphincter

Stomach
The stomach secretes gastric juices that help break down proteins and fats by enzyme action.

Pancreas
The pancreas produces digestive juices that help break down starches, proteins, and fats. These juices are carries to the intestine by the pancreatic duct.

Pancreatic duct

Large intestine
The large intestine absorbs water.

Sigmoid colon

Rectum
The rectum stores feces until elimination.

in the stomach to back up into the esophagus. If it does, a hiatus hernia is the diagnosis.

An *endoscopy,* like the sigmoidoscopy and the arthroscopy, is a way of seeing inside the body, this time inside the gastrointestinal tract to the duodenum. X rays are usually done first, and the endoscopy is done if they are not definitive or if a tissue sample is needed for biopsy. The patient eats nothing the night before the exam. After undressing and putting on a gown, the patient lies down and drinks a bad-tasting liquid, the local anesthetic. The patient may opt for no other medication, thus remaining completely conscious, or having an injection that makes him drowsy, but conscious, or having a general anesthetic, which puts him to sleep altogether. The second of the three is recommended. The first is the most painful; the third has a higher risk factor and requires hospitalization afterward.

The patient lies on his left side with the mouth open. The gastroscope is then put in the mouth and advanced down toward the stomach. The physician pauses at the places he needs to look at. Photographs are commonly taken, and samples of tissue or gastric juice may also be taken. The exam takes about 2 to 3 hours.

An *upper GI* may be in order if your doctor suspects an ulcer or tumor. No food is allowed for 8 hours before the test. An injection of glucagon (which may cause nausea or dizziness) is normally given to slow down the movements of the stomach. Next, the patient swallows a small cupful of granular material, which produces gas and causes the stomach to distend. Finally, the patient is given a glass of barium and stands with his back to the X-ray table. A fluoroscopic screen is positioned in front of the patient, and the radiologist instructs him to take small swallows of the barium. A series of pictures are taken, with the patient changing position several times. If the entire small intestine is being studied, the patient is next taken to a waiting area and returns every 15 to 30 minutes for more pictures. A stomach—duodenum study

takes about a half hour. The longer study takes from 1 to 3 hours.

A *lower GI,* often called simply a *barium enema,* is much more involved. It is used when there is a suspicion of diverticulitis, bowel obstruction, colon polyps, colitis, and so on. A strict diet is prescribed, along with laxatives, for several days before the test. Two enemas are given on the morning of the study. For this exam the patient lies down on the X-ray table. The doctor inserts a lubricated, gloved finger into the patient's rectum to make sure there are no obstructions and then inserts the enema tip. The tip has a built-in balloon that can be inflated if the patient feels he cannot retain the enema. Like the upper GI, an injection of glucagon is often given to counteract the feeling of "fullness" felt by most people. The fluoroscope is then positioned, and the technologist begins the enema: a solution of barium is pumped into the rectum until it fills the large intestine. Air may then pumped into the rectum for greater contrast. Both the enema and the air can cause a feeling of fullness and discomfort. The patient retains the enema and the air until all the pictures are taken.

The gall bladder, an organ in the upper right abdomen responsible for storing the bile necessary for fat digestion, is a frequent site of infection and may also develop calculi or stones. Examination of the gall bladder can be done with X rays, ultrasound, or nuclear imaging. Most routine gall bladder studies are done with ultrasound. An 8-hour fast is required before the test. The patient is given a gown to wear, may be asked to drink a white liquid, and then lies down on the couch. The doctor applies a special lubricant to the abdominal area and moves the transducer over it. The patient can watch the results on a monitor.

If stones develop in the gall bladder and block the flow of bile, infection results, and the condition is called acute cholecystitis. Nuclear imaging is considered the most specific diagnostic tool for this condition. The patient fasts for 4 hours before the exam. An isotope is injected and the patient lies down under a gamma camera. Pictures are taken every 5 to 10 minutes for a half hour and then every 15 minutes for one and a half hours.

The liver makes the bile necessary for fat digestion, and the pancreas makes the enzymes necessary for fat digestion. Neither the entire liver nor the entire pancreas can be seen with X rays. X rays of the blood supply and ductal structures, however, enable the skilled specialist to make accurate assumptions about the condition of either. CT imaging can give a full picture of both organs and is much easier on the patient than X rays. Ultrasound is also useful.

If the results of lab tests suggest liver disease or if the organ is enlarged, a special *needle biopsy* may be done. The patient is normally asked to avoid eating the night before the test. Medication by mouth or injection may be given. The gastroenterologist feels the lower edge of the liver, selects a spot, and injects a small amount of local anesthetic under the skin. Next a larger needle with a syringe is inserted. There will be pressure and even a dull pain. The plunger of the syringe is pulled back, and liver cells are sucked inside. The needle is then removed and pressure is applied to the puncture site.

The Respiratory System

The respiratory system includes the pharynx, trachea, bronchi, and the lungs.

The routine chest X ray (described earlier) is commonly the first test done when symptoms indicate a possible problem in the respiratory system. When the bronchi must be seen in more detail, a *bronchogram* may be done. This requires the disabling of the "coughing reflex" by spraying a local or topical anesthetic in the patient's mouth and back of the throat. Then a thin metal tube shaped like a candy cane (a cannula) will be placed in the mouth with the curved end over the back of the tongue. Anesthetic is injected into the cannula, which then runs down the back of the throat, down into the bronchi. A rubber tube (catheter) is passed through the patient's nose, down the back of the throat, through the voice box, the trachea, and then into the bronchi of one or both lungs. A special dye is then instilled into the catheter, which runs down and fills the tubes. The dye highlights the bronchi, making them easier to see on the X ray displaying blockage and tight areas.

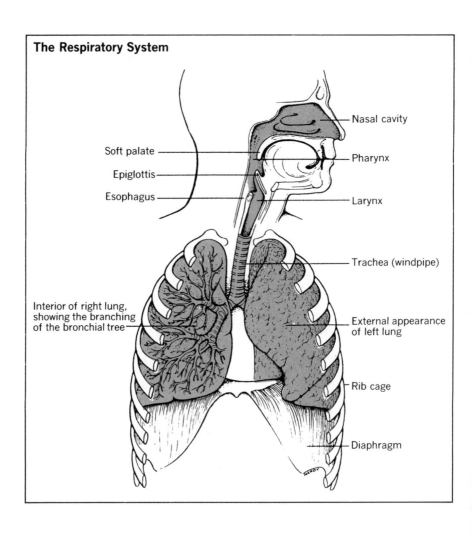

The Respiratory System

- Nasal cavity
- Soft palate
- Pharynx
- Epiglottis
- Esophagus
- Larynx
- Trachea (windpipe)
- Interior of right lung, showing the branching of the bronchial tree
- External appearance of left lung
- Rib cage
- Diaphragm

A *bronchoscopy* may be in order if X rays or CT reveal potential problems and the physician needs a closer look or a tissue sample. The process is similar to the bronchogram except a bronchoscope is inserted for viewing and the taking of tissue samples.

A group of tests called *pulmonary function tests* help the physician determine if certain symptoms may be due to either restrictive or obstructive lung disease. The test measures how much air can be forcibly exhaled after inhaling as deeply as possible, how much air remains in the lungs after a forcible exhalation, how much air is expired with each normal breath, and how well the lungs stretch with each breath in and how well they collapse with each breath out. The patient is put in a pressurized plexiglass cabin called a body box, which looks like a large phone booth. The patient's nose is closed off with a nose clip and a special mouthpiece is inserted in the mouth. The patient is positioned in front of a special apparatus that will measure and record the results. Once comfortable, the patient performs a series of breathing maneuvers on the instructions of the technologist. The tests take 15 to 45 minutes and may involve some straining as the maneuvers can get quite demanding.

The Endocrine System

There are 7 endocrine glands that make up the endocrine system: pituitary, thyroid, parathyroids, adrenals, pancreas, ovaries (women), and testicles (men). The glands secrete hormones that produce a specific effect or regulate a certain action of other body organs. Laboratory tests of blood and urine are important diagnostic tools for the glands, and all can be visualized with X rays, CT, nuclear imaging, and ultrasound if lab tests indicate a potential problem. Some tests may necessitate the injection of a special dye to highlight the target area.

The Kidneys and the Urinary System

Laboratory tests of the urine are the most obvious way of beginning a diagnosis of kidney or urinary system problems. A resting EKG may also be done as well as nuclear imaging, ultrasound, and X rays. If a kidney biopsy is needed, the patient is normally given an anesthetic to make him drowsy and then lies face down on a table. The procedure is similar to that of the liver biopsy. First the anesthetic is injected, then the aspirating needle is inserted. This generally hurts a great deal but takes only a minute or so. An overnight stay is required for observation. A mild backache will last about a week.

An intravenous urography is a common test for urinary tract problems. Colon cleansing (strict diet, laxative, enemas) is often done before the test. A large amount of dye is injected into the patient's arm (or may drip in gradually from a diluted bottle of fluid). X ray exposures are taken at timed intervals. A compression cuff (like a large blood pressure cuff) may be put around the abdomen to apply pressure just below each kidney, and more pictures are taken until the radiologist is satisfied that enough information has been obtained. The patient voids his bladder, another picture is taken, and the test is over.

Ears, Nose, and Throat

The otorhinolaryngologist specializes in treating problems of the ears, nose, and throat. Difficulty hearing, faulty balance or vertigo, pain, and ringing in the ears (tinnitus) are common ear complaints. Congestion, discharge from the nose, postnasal drip, itching and sneezing, headaches over the eyes and top of the head, pain over the upper teeth and unexplained fever are complaints associated with the nose and sinuses. Problems with

A Guide to Some Home Medical Tests

Kind	Function	How It Works	Time Required
Blood glucose monitoring	Measures the level of glucose (a kind of sugar) in blood	Wash your hands thoroughly. Prick a finger or earlobe to obtain a drop of blood, then follow instructions.	1 to 2 minutes
Ovulation monitoring	Measures the quantity of luteinizing hormone (LH) in urine	A chemically treated strip is dipped in urine specimen and compared with a color guide.	20 minutes to 1 hour
Pregnancy	Detects human chorionic gonadotropin, produced by a developing placenta, in urine	Chemicals are mixed with a urine specimen in a small test tube. A ring formation or color change indicates pregnancy.	20 minutes to 2 hours
Urinary tract infections	Detects nitrite in urine	Chemically treated test strip is dipped in urine specimen on three consecutive mornings.	30 to 40 seconds
Occult fecal blood	Detects hidden blood in stools	A color change, appearing when stool specimen is brought into contact with peroxide and guaiac, indicates hidden blood.	30 seconds to 16 minutes
Gonorrhea	Detects the bacteria causing gonorrhea in the specimen of pus from the penis	Specimen, collected on a slide, is allowed to air-dry. Then follow directions.	Several days
Blood pressure	Measures the pressure of blood on the walls of the arteries	The center of a cuff is placed on the pulse point of the upper arm. With or without a microphone, the user listens for artery sounds.	2 to 5 minutes
Impotence	Detects, measures the rigidity of erections during sleep	Soft fabric band or stamps are placed around the penis before the subject goes to bed at night. The strips break at different degrees of pressure.	Overnight
Vision	Screens for visual acuity problems	Using three different tests, you read special eye charts.	2 to 3 minutes

the voice, sore throat, or difficulty swallowing are common throat complaints.

An *audiogram* evaluates and measures the ears' ability to hear. The patient is seated in a booth, instructions about communicating with the technician are given, and earphones are placed over the ears. A series of different tones in varying degrees of loudness are played through the earphones and the patient indicates by hand signs which or both ears heard the sound.

A *tympanogram* is a way of recording the movement of the ear drum. A rubber plug is inserted in one ear and mild pressure is applied which is similar to the pressure experienced when flying in a plane. The tympanogram reveals if the eardrum is thickened due to infection, perforated, or if there is an obstruction in the middle ear.

Patients who experience dizziness may have an *electronystagmogram*, which measures and records the abnormal movements of the eye that can indicate a problem with the balance mechanism (vestibular system). Contacts or glasses are removed and the technician tapes a small metal disk under each eye and on the bridge of the nose. These sensors are attached by lead wires to a graph machine. Small lights are flashed on the wall, which the patient is asked to look at. The patient then lies down, closes his eyes, and turns onto each side. Water is then put in the ears. The procedure often produces dizziness or nausea that persists for several hours.

Smears and cultures are the common lab tests for nose and throat complaints. X ray examinations may also be done. In some cases a biopsy may be necessary. For the nose, a needle aspiration is the common method, either through the nose or upper gum of the mouth. A local anesthetic is given first. An excisional biopsy may be necessary, in which case a small piece of tissue is removed. For the throat an excisional biopsy is commonly done, normally under general anesthesia, and an overnight stay in the hospital may be required. A laryngoscope is used to obtain the sample. The throat will be sore for several days afterwards.

The Eyes

The ophthalmologist specializes in eye disorders. The common eye exam involves several tests: visual acuity, refraction, color defectiveness, determination, muscle integrity, pupillary reflex response, slit-lamp exam, intraocular pressure determination, and retinal exam. The *visual acuity* test is the familiar wall chart. The patient covers each eye in turn and tries to read as many letters as he can see. In the *refraction* test a special device with various lenses is positioned in front of the patient. Different lenses are tried while the patient again tries to read the letters on the wall chart, telling the doctor which is better.

Color blindness is usually tested for with a series of cards covered with an array of colored dots which form a number. Those with no color defect will be able to read the number. The doctor performs the *muscle integrity* exam simply by asking the patient to look in different directions and observing that the patient is able to. The *pupillary reflex response* is tested when the doctor directs the patient to look straight ahead while he shines a small light at each eye and watches what happens to the size of the pupil.

The slit-lamp examination is done in two parts and involves a special instrument called a biomicroscope. The patient's eyes may be stained with a special dye (a fine strip of paper is quickly touched to the side of each eye) and the chin and forehead are positioned on their respective rests. The ophthalmologist sits in front and looks into the eyes, viewing the sclera, iris, conjunctiva, cornea, and the lens. Next drops are put into the eyes to dilate the pupils, which takes about 20 to 30 minutes. With the pupils dilated, the doctor can then see the retina.

Focusing

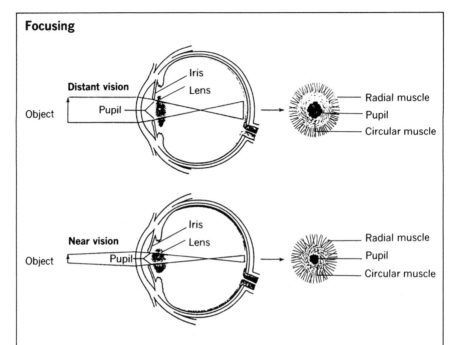

When viewing a distant object (more than 20 feet away), the lens flattens and the pupil dilates, allowing more light to enter the eye. The pupil is dilated by the action of the outer radial muscles of the iris, which contract and thus stretch the previously contracted circular muscles. When viewing a near object, the lens becomes more oval and the pupil contracts as more light enters the eye. This prevents overstimulation of the retina. The pupil is reduced in size by the contraction of the inner circular muscles, which serve to stretch the previously contracted radial muscles.

Glaucoma is a condition of increased pressure within the eyes that, if discovered too late, can cause blindness. The *intraocular pressure determination,* or *tonometry,* is the test for this problem. First, a drop of local anesthetic is put into each eye. Then the ophthalmologist uses a *tonometer,* a penlike tube with a small retractable tip, to touch the front of each eye. It is recommended that this painless procedure be done for those 40 and over every 2 to 3 years, or annually if there is a family history of glaucoma.

The final test in the general eye exam is the *retinal exam.* The room is darkened, and the doctor uses an ophthalmoscope to look through the pupil into the back of the eye.

Diagnostic Tests and the Patient's Rights

As medical costs continue to rise, questions about the necessity of various diagnostic tests will continue to be raised. For the healthy individual, it makes little sense to undergo more than the few routine screening tests necessary for his particular age group; there is always the chance of an error that may lead to additional tests at even greater expense, not to mention the emotional trauma that a false positive could cause.

For the patient experiencing particular symptoms, or those in high risk categories, the number and kind of diagnostic tests are a concern. *Batteries,* or sets, of tests are a particular cause for concern. The batteries can be complex, and the physician may not take the time to explain each one in detail so that the patient thoroughly understands what they mean in terms of discomfort, risk, and cost. The value of a particular test must also be weighed against its results. Expensive CT and MRI tests are the "study of choice" for many problems, but for others, the less expensive X ray might do just as well or better. When approaching diagnostic tests, then, the patient should make sure that he is as informed as possible about what is necessary. As already mentioned, having a physician with whom you can converse easily and understand is an important factor in the quality of the medical care you receive.

27

Nutrition and Weight Control

Just as it was for our earliest ancestors, food is an integral part of our daily lives. Not only is food essential for survival, but oftentimes the way in which we structure our lives—our work habits, our recreational activities—revolves around how, when, and where we get food and eat it.

Ironically, however, because most of us live a much faster-paced lifestyle than we did even twenty years ago, we spend less time choosing, preparing, and eating food. We grab breakfast on the run (if we eat it at all), hurry through lunch, and rarely take time to plan and prepare a lei-surely, well-balanced dinner. Often everyone in the family is on a different schedule, with the result that all too often we rely on prepackaged microwave dinners or take out fast food. Consequently, many of us are not eating properly, spending money on expensive vitamins to make up for poor nutrition, starving ourselves to lose weight, or gaining extra pounds by filling up on empty calories.

Practicing good eating habits may take a little more time and planning than we think we can afford, but its benefits will pay off in the long run in a healthier, happier way of life.

Basic Nutritional Requirements

The process by which food is converted into useful energy is called *metabolism*. It begins with chemical processes in the gastrointestinal tract which change plant and animal food into less complex components so that they can be absorbed to fulfill their various functions in the body—growth, repair, and fuel. Different foods have different energy values, measured in calories. An ideal diet for the average healthy individual provides the highest nutritional benefits from the fewest number of calories. Information on the protein, fat, and carbohydrate content in specific foods, as well as the number of calories, may be obtained by consulting the table "Nutrients in Common Foods." The Metric Equivalents table converts spoon and cup measures into metric measures.

Protein

Of the several essential components of food, *protein* is in many ways the most important. This is so not only because it is one of the three principal sources of energy, but also because much of the body's structure is made up of proteins. For example, the typical 160-pound man is composed of about 100 pounds of water, 29 pounds of protein, 25 pounds of fat, 5 pounds of minerals, 1 pound of carbohydrate, and less than an ounce of vitamins. Because the muscles, heart, brain, lungs, and gastrointestinal organs are made up largely of protein, and since the protein in these organs is in constant need of replacement, its importance is obvious.

The recommended dietary allowance for protein is 0.8 g/Kg of body weight per day for persons aged 15 and up and 1 g/Kg of body weight for children under 15. (To convert your weight from pounds to kilograms, divide by 2.2. Thus a woman weighing 130 pounds weighs about 59 kilograms and needs about 47 grams of protein a day. A man weighing 175 pounds needs about 64 grams of protein a day.) Most Americans, however, eat about twice the amount they need, and while more may sound better, too much is too much. Your body uses only what it needs. Some excess protein is excreted as urine; the rest is converted to fat.

Chemically, proteins are varying mixtures of amino acids that contain various elements, including nitrogen. There are 22 different amino acids that are essential for the body's protein needs. Nine of these must be provided in the diet and are thus called *essential* amino acids; the rest can be synthesized by the body itself.

Meat, fish, poultry, eggs, and milk or milk products are the primary protein foods and contain all of the necessary amino acids; they are therefore called *complete* proteins. Grains and vegetables are partly made up of protein, but more often than not, they do not provide the whole range of amino acids required for proper nourishment. When properly combined, however, vegetable proteins, too, can be complete. For example, mixing rice and dried beans provides the same quality of protein as a steak (with a lot less fat).

One gram of protein provides four calories of energy.

Carbohydrates

Carbohydrates are another essential energy source. Called *starches* or *sugars,* they are present in large quantities in grains, fruits, and nuts. As

complex carbohydrates, or polysaccha-
rides, they are found in the foods
named and particularly in breads,
breakfast cereals, flours, pastas, barley, legumes, rice, and starchy vegetables. Simple carbohydrates, or
mono- or disaccharides, are found in
such foods as table sugars, candy,
pastries, and soft drinks.

Complex carbohydrates are primary sources of calories, nutrients,
and fiber—for such purposes as muscle contraction, weight reduction, and
control of sodium and cholesterol.
Simple carbohydrates, on the other
hand, are pure sources of calories and
contain little nutritional value. It is for
this reason that they are often termed

"empty" calories. Lack of adequate
carbohydrates means the body will
begin to convert body fat or protein
into sugar.

Although there is no absolute dietary requirement for carbohydrates,
it is generally recommended that
more than half the energy requirement beyond infancy be provided by
complex carbohydrates. One gram of
carbohydrate provides four calories of
energy. Thus the average man consuming about 2,900 calories per day
should consume about 360 grams of
carbohydrate. The average woman
consuming about 2,200 calories per
day should consume about 275 grams
of carbohydrate.

Fats

Fats are a chemically complex food
component composed of glycerol (a
sweet, oily alcohol) and fatty acids.
Fats exist in several forms and come
from a variety of sources. One way to
think of them is to group them as visible fats, such as butter, salad oil, or
the fat seen in meat, and as invisible

fats, which are mingled, blended, or
absorbed into food, either naturally,
as in nuts, meat, or fish, or during
cooking. Another way is to think of
them as solid at room temperature
(fats), or as liquid at room temperature (oils).

Saturated and Unsaturated

Fats are also classified as saturated or
unsaturated. This is a chemical distinction based on the differences in
molecular structure of different kinds
of fat. If the carbon atoms in a fat
molecule are surrounded or boxed in
by hydrogen atoms, they are said to
be saturated. This type of fat tends to
be solid at room temperature, and
high consumption of it increases the
cholesterol content of the blood,
which can lead to heart disease. Un-

saturated fats, such as those found in
fish and vegetable oils, contain the
least number of hydrogen atoms and
do not add to the blood cholesterol
content. They are either monounsat-
urated or polyunsaturated. In general,
fats in foods of plant origin are more
unsaturated than in those of animal
origin (except for coconut and palm
oils, which are highly saturated). It is
recommended that you consume no
more than 30 percent of your daily

calories from fats; 10 percent of each of the three types, or, for our average man, about 32 grams total; for our average woman, about 24 grams total.

Fats play several essential roles in the metabolic process. First of all, they provide more than twice the number of calories on a comparative weight basis than do proteins and carbohydrates (one gram of fat contains nine calories). They also can be stored in the body in large quantities (in adipose tissue) and used as a later energy source. They serve as carriers of the fat-soluble vitamins A, D, E, and K, and—of no little importance—they add to the tastiness of food.

Vitamins

Vitamins, which are present in minute quantities in foods in their natural state, are essential for normal metabolism and for the development and maintenance of tissue structure and function. In addition to the fat-soluble vitamins noted above, there are a number of B vitamins, as well as vitamin C, also called *ascorbic acid.* If any particular vitamin is missing from the diet over a sufficiently long time, a specific disease will result.

Vitamin A

Vitamin A is essential for vision, growth, cell growth and development, reproduction, a strong immune system, and healthy hair, skin, and mucous membranes.

Vitamin A is fat soluble and is therefore stored by the body (in the liver). It comes in two forms: retinol, found only in animal foods (chiefly liver), and beta-carotene, found in fruits and vegetables (chiefly deep green or orange ones like spinach and sweet potatoes). Retinol is instantly available for bodily use, while beta-carotene must be converted by the body into retinol before it can be used. (Because the body will not convert excess beta-carotene into retinol, there is no danger of overdosing on this form of vitamin A. Retinol, however, can be extremely toxic at high levels.)

Symptoms of vitamin A deficiency include dry rough skin, slow growth, night blindness, thickening of bone, and increased susceptibility to infection. Vitamin A deficiency is rare in the United States.

Formerly measured in International Units (IU), vitamin A content is now expressed retinol equivalents (RE). One RE equals 10 IU of beta-carotene and 3.33 IU of retinol. The Recommended Daily Allowance (RDA) for vitamin A for adult males is 1000 RE and for adult women, 800 RE.

Vitamin D

Vitamin D is essential for proper metabolism of calcium, which is primarily responsible for the healthy growth of bones and teeth.

Low Calorie Diet

Sample Menus

	800 calories		1,200 calories		1,600 calories	
	Weight (grams)	Household measure	Weight (grams)	Household measure	Weight (grams)	Household measure
Breakfast						
Orange, sliced	125	1 medium	125	1 medium	125	1 medium
Soft cooked egg	50	One	50	One	50	One
Toast	25	1 slice	25	1 slice	25	1 slice
Butter	5	1 teaspoon	5	1 teaspoon	5	1 teaspoon
Coffee or tea	—	As desired	—	As desired	—	As desired
Milk	240	1 cup skim	240	1 cup skim	240	1 cup whole
Luncheon						
Clear broth	—	As desired	—	As desired	—	As desired
Salad (cottage cheese, tomato, plain lettuce leaf)	90	½ cup	90	½ cup	90	½ cup
Egg			50	One	50	One
Green peas					100	½ cup
Baked apple, unsweetened	80	1 small	80	1 small	80	1 small
Bread			25	1 slice	25	1 slice
Butter			5	1 teaspoon	5	1 teaspoon
Milk	240	1 cup skim	240	1 cup skim	240	1 cup whole
Coffee or tea	—	As desired	—	As desired	—	As desired
Dinner						
Roast beef, lean	60	2 ounces	90	3 ounces	120	4 ounces
Carrots, plain	100	½ cup	100	½ cup	100	½ cup
Tossed vegetable salad with vinegar	50	¾ cup	50	¾ cup	50	¾ cup
Pineapple, unsweetened	80	½ cup	80	½ cup	80	½ cup
Bread			25	1 slice	25	1 slice
Butter			5	1 teaspoon	10	2 teaspoons
Coffee or tea	—	As desired	—	As desired	—	As desired
Nourishment						
Peach					100	1 medium

These diets contain approximately 800, 1,200, and 1,600 calories. The 800 calorie diet, even with variations in selections of food, will not meet the recommended daily allowances in iron and thiamine. The approximate composition is as follows:

	800 calories	1,200 calories	1,600 calories
Protein	60 gm.	75 gm.	85 gm.
Fat	30 gm.	50 gm.	80 gm.
Carbohydrate	75 gm.	110 gm.	130 gm.

From the *Clinical Center Diet Manual*, revised edition, prepared by the Nutrition Department. The Clinical Center, National Institutes of Health, Public Health Service, U.S. Department of Health, Education, and Welfare (Public Health Service Publication No. 989), pp. 67–68.

Vitamin D is fat soluble and therefore excessive intake can be toxic. It is consumed chiefly as an addition to milk and is also manufactured by the body by a reaction of sunlight on sterols present in the skin.

The major deficiency disease of vitamin D in children is rickets (deformation of the skeleton) and in adults excessive bone loss and fractures. The RDA for adults over 24 is 5 micrograms.

Vitamin E (tocopherol)

Vitamin E is essential for healthy nerve function and reproduction.

Vitamin E is found principally in plant oils, particularly wheat germ oil and nuts. It is fat soluble, but there is little danger of toxicity because absorption by the body is inefficient.

Vitamin E is measured in tocopherol equivalents (TE). The RDA for adult males is 10 TE and for adult women 8 TE. Deficiencies in a normal diet are rare.

Vitamin K

Vitamin K is essential for proper clotting of the blood.

Vitamin K is fat soluble and is found primarily in green leafy vegetables. Another form of the compound is synthesized by intestinal bacteria. Like vitamin E, there is little danger from ingesting too much vitamin K, and most diets provide an adequate supply.

The RDA for adult males over age 24 is 80 micrograms and for adult women 65 micrograms.

Vitamin C (ascorbic acid)

Vitamin C is essential for healthy skin, bones, teeth, and muscles, for producing and maintaining collagen, and for fighting infection.

Vitamin C is water soluble and therefore must be ingested every day. It is widely available in a variety of colorful fruits and vegetables, such as peppers, broccoli, cabbage, oranges, strawberries, and tomatoes. Unfortunately, vitamin C is also the most unstable of all vitamins and minerals: it is easily destroyed by heat and oxygen, and thus care should be taken in cooking and storing of fruits and vegetables.

The classic vitamin C deficiency disease is scurvy, typified by the wasting away of muscles, wounds and bruises that don't heal, and bleeding, deteriorating gums. Milder forms of vitamin C deficiency produce milder versions of these symptoms. Vitamin C deficiency has also been linked to such health problems as the common cold, anemia, atherosclerosis, asthma, cancer of the stomach and esophagus, infertility in males, rheumatoid arthritis, and cataracts.

Vitamin C is measured in milligrams (mg). The RDA for adults is 60 mg. Megadoses of vitamin C are often recommended to fight colds or as a general preventive measure against disease, although the body only uses as much as it needs; the rest is excreted in the urine. Toxicity is rarely a problem.

Average Daily Calorie Consumption

Men	Calories
Sedentary	2,500
Moderately active	3,000
Active	3,500
Very active	4,250
Women	**Calories**
Sedentary	2,100
Moderately active	2,500
Active	3,000
Very active	3,750

Guidelines for average daily calorie consumption by men and women. With increasing use of labor-saving devices, most Americans fall into the sedentary category.

Calorie Consumption for Some Activities

Type of Activity	Calories Per Hour
Sedentary: reading, sewing, typing, etc.	30–100
Light: cooking, slow walking, dressing, etc.	100–170
Moderate: sweeping, light gardening, making beds, etc.	170–250
Vigorous: fast walking, hanging out clothes, golfing, etc.	250–350
Strenuous: swimming, bicycling, dancing, etc.	350 and more

Table 1

Desirable Weights for Men and Women Aged 25 and Over[1]
(in pounds by height and frame, in indoor clothing)

	MEN (in shoes, 1-inch heels)				WOMEN (in shoes, 2-inch heels)		
Height	Small Frame	Medium Frame	Large Frame	Height	Small Frame	Medium Frame	Large Frame
5′ 2″	112–120	118–129	126–141	4′ 10″	92– 98	96–107	104–119
5′ 3″	115–123	121–133	129–144	4′ 11″	94–101	98–110	106–122
5′ 4″	118–126	124–136	132–148	5′ 0″	96–104	101–113	109–125
5′ 5″	121–129	127–139	135–152	5′ 1″	99–107	104–116	112–128
5′ 6″	124–133	130–143	138–156	5′ 2″	102–110	107–119	115–131
5′ 7″	128–137	134–147	142–161	5′ 3″	105–113	110–122	118–134
5′ 8″	132–141	138–152	147–166	5′ 4″	108–116	113–126	121–138
5′ 9″	136–145	142–156	151–170	5′ 5″	111–119	116–130	125–142
5′ 10″	140–150	146–160	155–174	5′ 6″	114–123	120–135	129–146
5′ 11″	144–154	150–165	159–179	5′ 7″	118–127	124–139	133–150
6′ 0″	148–158	154–170	164–184	5′ 8″	122–131	128–143	137–154
6′ 1″	152–162	158–175	168–189	5′ 9″	126–135	132–147	141–158
6′ 2″	156–167	162–180	173–194	5′ 10″	130–140	136–151	145–163
6′ 3″	160–171	167–185	178–199	5′ 11″	134–144	140–155	149–168
6′ 4″	164–175	172–190	182–204	6′ 0″	138–148	144–159	153–173

[1]Adapted from Metropolitan Life Insurance Co., New York. New weight standards for men and women. *Statistical Bulletin* 40:3.

Table 2

Average Weights for Men and Women[1]
(in pounds by age and height, in paper gown and slippers)

	MEN						
Height	18–24 Years	25–34 Years	35–44 Years	45–54 Years	55–64 Years	65–74 Years	75–79 Years
5' 2"	137	141	149	148	148	144	133
5' 3"	140	145	152	152	151	148	138
5' 4"	144	150	156	156	155	151	143
5' 5"	147	154	160	160	158	154	148
5' 6"	151	159	164	164	162	158	154
5' 7"	154	163	168	168	166	161	159
5' 8"	158	168	171	173	169	165	164
5' 9"	161	172	175	177	173	168	169
5' 10"	165	177	179	181	176	171	174
5' 11"	168	181	182	185	180	175	179
6' 0"	172	186	186	189	184	178	184
6' 1"	175	190	190	193	187	182	189
6' 2"	179	194	194	197	191	185	194
	WOMEN						
4' 9"	116	112	131	129	138	132	125
4' 10"	118	116	134	132	141	135	129
4' 11"	120	120	136	136	144	138	132
5' 0"	122	124	138	140	149	142	136
5' 1"	125	128	140	143	150	145	139
5' 2"	127	132	143	147	152	149	143
5' 3"	129	136	145	150	155	152	146
5' 4"	131	140	147	154	158	156	150
5' 5"	134	144	149	158	161	159	153
5' 6"	136	148	152	161	164	163	157
5' 7"	138	152	154	165	167	166	160
5' 8"	140	156	156	168	170	170	164

[1]Adapted from National Center for Health Statistics: Weight by Height and Age of Adults, United States. *Vital Health Statistics.* PHS Publication No. 1000—Series 11, No. 14.

Thiamin (vitamin B_1)

Thiamin is essential for the proper metabolism of carbohydrates and for a healthy nervous system.

Thiamin is water soluble and is found primarily in cereals, wheat germ, pork, and nuts. It is strongly susceptible to destruction during cooking. Deficiency is not common among the general population, but studies have shown heavy drinkers, pregnant women, and the elderly to be more deficient. Severe thiamin deficiency results in beriberi, a disease that weakens the body, disables the mind, and permanently damages the heart. Symptoms of deficiency include loss of appetite, nausea, vomiting, constipation, depression, fatigue, poor eye-hand coordination, irritability, headaches, and anxiety.

Thiamin is measured in milligrams. The RDA for adult males is 1.5 mg and for adult women 1.1 mg. Danger of toxicity is rare as excess thiamin is excreted in urine.

Riboflavin (vitamin B₂)

Riboflavin is essential for growth and repair of tissues and aids in DNA synthesis. It helps metabolize proteins, fats, and carbohydrates.

Most Americans get plenty of this water-soluble vitamin, which is readily found in liver, eggs, and milk products. Studies have found that children in low-income families, however, are less likely to get enough riboflavin. Signs of deficiency include a purplish-colored tongue; cracks at the corners of the mouth; sores and burning of the lips, mouth, and tongue; itchy inflamed eyelids; flaky skin around the nose, ears, eyebrows, or hairline; and light sensitivity of eyes. Deficiency in riboflavin often means deficiency in other B vitamins as well. Cataracts, birth defects, and anemia have been linked to riboflavin deficiency.

Unlike vitamin C and thiamin, riboflavin is not easily destroyed by cooking, although adding baking soda to vegetables when cooking creates an alkaline solution that destroys it. Risk of toxicity is very low, and excess riboflavin is excreted in the urine.

Riboflavin is measured in milligrams. The RDA for adult males is 1.7 mg and for adult women 1.3 mg.

Niacin (vitamin B₃)

Niacin is essential for the release of energy from carbohydrates, fats, and proteins and for the formation of DNA.

Most Americans get plenty of niacin from their diets; only heavy drinkers are at risk of deficiency. Severe deficiencies of niacin result in pellagra, a disease virtually wiped out in the United States since the 1930s with the advent of fortified flour and cereals with the vitamin.

Niacin is widely available in a variety of plant and animal foods, including fish, liver, turkey, cereals, and peanuts. The body is also able to convert the amino acid tryptophan into niacin, and thus proteins high in tryptophan also provide plenty of niacin.

Niacin is measured in milligrams (60 mg of tryptophan equal 1 mg of niacin). The RDA for adult males is 19 mg and for women 15 mg.

Vitamin B₆

Vitamin B₆ is essential for fat and carbohydrate metabolism and for the formation and breakdown of amino acids. It also helps regulate blood glucose levels and is needed to synthesize hemoglobin.

Vitamin B_6 occurs in three forms: pyridoxine, pyridoxal, and pyridoxamine, which are converted by the body into pyridoxal phosphate and pyridoxamine phosphate. It is most readily found in nuts, kidney, liver, eggs, pork, poultry, dried fruits, and fish.

Although few Americans get the full RDA of vitamin B_6, there is no evidence of corresponding overt deficiency symptoms. The following health problems, however, have been linked to B_6 deficiency: asthma, carpal tunnel syndrome, cancer (melanoma, breast, and bladder), diabetes, coronary heart disease, premenstrual syndrome, sickle-cell anemia, and aging and dementia.

In moderate doses B_6 is not toxic. Although excessive amounts of this water-soluble vitamin are to a great extent flushed out of the body in the urine, high doses have produced neurological disturbances such as numbness in the hands, feet, and mouth.

Vitamin B_6 is measured in milligrams. The RDA for adult men is 2 mg and for women 1.6 mg.

Vitamin B_{12}

Vitamin B_{12} is important for normal growth, healthy nerve tissue, and normal blood formation.

Most Americans get plenty of B_{12}. It is found chiefly in animal foods: meat, fish, eggs, and milk products. Only strict vegetarians (vegans), who eat none of these foods are in danger of deficiency. Problems for everyone arise with age, however; the stomach may become less able to absorb B_{12} and deficiency may result. Pernicious anemia is the classic B_{12} deficiency disease and may take years to appear. Other health problems that may be linked to B_{12} deficiency include infertility, nervous system disorders, and walking difficulties.

Cooking results in few losses of B_{12}, and toxicity is not a danger. The RDA for B_{12} for adults is 2 micrograms.

Folacin (folic acid, or folate)

Folacin is essential for many metabolic processes, especially cell growth and division.

Women, especially pregnant women, and alcoholics are most likely to be folacin deficient. Signs of deficiency include anemia, weakness, pallor, headaches, forgetfulness, sleeplessness, and irritability. Vitamin B_{12} deficiency can aggravate folacin deficiency because B_{12} is essential to release folacin from bodily storage. Other health problems that may be associated with folacin deficiency include depression, dementia, neuropsychological disorders, toxemia of pregnancy, infections, and fetal damage.

Folacin is widely distributed in fruits and vegetables, but it is easily destroyed during cooking and storage. The RDA for folacin for adult men is 200 micrograms and for women, 180 micrograms.

Biotin

Biotin is essential for overall growth and well-being. It is important in the metabolism of fats and in the utilization of carbon dioxide.

The best sources of biotin are liver, egg yolks, soy flour, cereals, and yeast. It is also produced by intestinal bacteria, although it is not known whether this form is readily absorbed by the body. Deficiencies are most often produced by the ingestion of large amounts of raw egg white, which contains a biotin-binding protein called avidin that prevents the absorption of biotin. Symptoms of deficiency include nausea, vomiting, swelling of the tongue, pallor, depression, hair loss, and dry scaly dermatitis.

The RDA for adults is a wide range: from 30 to 100 micrograms. Toxicity from a normal diet is not a concern.

Pantothenic acid

Pantothenic acid is essential for general growth and well-being. It is an important component in a number of metabolic reactions such as the release of energy from carbohydrates, fats, and proteins and the synthesis of sterols and steroid hormones.

Pantothenic acid is widely distributed among foods, chiefly animal tissues, cereals, and legumes. Evidence of dietary deficiency of pantothenic acid has not been clinically recognized in humans, and there is no specific disease associated with pantothenic acid deficiency.

Pantothenic acid is measured in milligrams. There is no RDA, but daily consumption by adults of between 4 and 7 mg is considered safe. Toxicity from a normal diet is not a concern.

Minerals

Minerals are another component of basic nutritional needs. All living things extract them from the soil, which is their ultimate source. Like vitamins, they are needed for normal metabolism and must be present in the diet in sufficient amounts for the maintenance of good health. The essential minerals include calcium, phosphorus, magnesium, iodine, iron, zinc, selenium, molybdenum, copper, manganese, fluoride, and chromium.

Calcium

Calcium is essential for bone growth, development, and retention as well as for proper nerve conduction, muscle contraction, blood clotting, and membrane permeability.

Dairy products are the primary sources of calcium, but the mineral is also found in green leafy vegetables and soft bones, such as those of sardines and salmon. Maximum calcium ingestion is extremely important during the years from birth to age 25, when the body reaches its peak bone mass. Deficiencies are most common

Recommended Dietary Allowances for Fat-Soluble Vitamins					
		Vit. A	Vit. D	Vit. E	Vit.K
	Age	(mcg RE)	(mcg)	(mgTE)	(mcg)
Infants	0 to .5	375	7.5	3	5
	.5 to 1	"	10	4	10
Children	1 to 3	400	"	6	15
	4 to 6	500	"	7	20
	7 to 10	700	"	"	30
Males	11 to 14	1,000	"	10	45
	15 to 18	"	"	"	65
	19 to 24	"	"	"	70
	25 to 50	"	5	"	80
	51 +	"	"	"	"
Females	11 to 14	800	10	8	45
	15 to 18	"	"	"	55
	19 to 24	"	"	"	60
	25 to 50	"	5	"	65
	51 +	"	"	"	"
Pregnant		"	10	10	"
Nursing	1st 6 months	1,300	"	12	"
	2nd 6 months	1,200	"	11	"

in women and have been linked to the development of osteoporosis in the later years.

The RDA for calcium for children between the ages of 11 and 24 is 1,200 mg. For adults over 24 the RDA is 800 mg. Ingestion of very large amounts of calcium may inhibit the absorption of iron, zinc, and other essential minerals.

Phosphorus

Phosphorus is a structural component of all cells. It is a part of DNA, and is therefore essential in the growth, maintenance, and repair of all body tissues. It is also critical for energy transfer and production.

Phosphorus is present in nearly all foods, principally cereals and pro-teins. Deficiency is a serious concern only for premature infants fed exclusively human milk.

The RDA for phosphorus is the same as that for calcium, 800 mg for adults over 24. Toxicity from a normal diet is not a concern.

Magnesium

Like phosphorus, magnesium is a structural component in soft tissue cells and is therefore important in the growth, maintenance, and repair of these tissues. It is also important in energy production, lipid and protein synthesis, the formation of urea, muscle relaxation, and in the prevention of tooth decay.

The best sources of magnesium are nuts, legumes, unmilled grains, and green vegetables. Deficiencies from a

Recommended Dietary Allowances for Water-Soluble Vitamins

	Age	Vit. C (mg)	Thiamin (mg)	Riboflav. (mg)	Niacin (mg)	Vit. B6 (mg)	Folate (mcg)	Vit. B12 (mcg)
Infants	0 to .5	30	0.3	0.4	5	0.3	25	0.3
	.5 to 1	35	0.4	0.5	6	0.6	35	0.5
Children	1 to 3	40	0.7	0.8	9	1	50	0.7
	4 to 6	45	0.9	1.1	12	1.1	75	1
	7 to 10	"	1	1.2	13	1.4	100	1.4
Males	11 to 14	50	1.3	1.5	17	1.7	150	2
	15 to 18	60	1.5	1.8	20	2	200	"
	19 to 24	"	"	1.7	19	"	"	"
	25 to 50	"	"	"	"	"	"	"
	51 +	"	1.2	1.4	15	"	150	"
Females	11 to 14	50	1.1	1.3	"	1.4	180	"
	15 to 18	60	"	"	"	1.5	"	"
	19 to 24	"	"	"	"	1.6	"	"
	25 to 50	"	1.1	"	"	"	"	"
51 +		"	1	1.2	13	"	"	"
Pregnant		70	1.5	1.6	17	2.2	400	2.2
Nursing	1st 6 months	95	1.6	1.8	20	2.1	280	2.6
	2nd 6 months	90	"	1.7	20	"	260	"

normal diet are rare and are related instead to various diseases such as those of the gastrointestinal tract, kidney dysfunction, and malnutrition and alcoholism. Symptoms of deficiency include weakness, confusion, personality changes, muscle tremor, nausea, lack of coordination, and gastrointestinal disorders.

The RDA for adult men is 350 mg and for adult women 280 mg.

Iodine

Iodine is an essential component of thyroid hormone, which is important in cellular reactions, metabolism, and growth and development.

Iodized salt and water are the most common sources, and most animal foods contain adequate supplies depending on the soil quality and the amount of iodine added to animal feeds. Iodine is also added in the processing of bread dough. Deficiencies in the United States are not common. The classic deficiency disease in adults is goiter. Iodine deficient fetuses are at a risk of developing cretinism.

The RDA for iodine for adults is 150 micrograms.

Iron

As an essential component of hemoglobin and myoglobin, iron is necessary for the proper transfer of oxygen to cells and muscles. It is also important for energy production and collagen synthesis.

Many Americans don't get enough iron. Women and very young children get the least, followed by the elderly. Iron deficiency leads to anemia: muscles become weak, and fatigue, listlessness, and a tendency to tire easily set in. Even mild iron deficiency, however, can affect a person's intellectual capabilities, especially children's. Symptoms of deficiency in children include irritability, hyperactivity, learning problems, shortened attention span, poor motivation, and poor intellectual performance.

There are two types of iron, heme and nonheme. Heme comes from animal foods and is much more readily absorbed than nonheme iron, which comes from vegetables. When eaten together, however, the rate of absorption for nonheme iron increases significantly. Also, iron eaten with just a little vitamin C dramatically increases its absorption. Tannins (in tea and red wine) block iron absorption. Iron-rich foods include liver and other organ meats, beef, dried fruits, pumpkin and sunflower seeds, legumes, dark green leafy vegetables, prune juice, and whole grain cereals.

The RDA for adult males is 10 mg and for adult women 15 mg. There is little danger of toxicity from a normal diet, although some people have an inherited defect in regulating iron absorption and can easily get too much.

Zinc

Zinc is essential for cell multiplication, tissue regeneration, sexual maturity, and proper growth. It is also important as a cofactor in more than 20 enzymatic reactions and serves as a binder in many others.

Severe zinc deficiency is not a problem in the United States, but the effects of mild deficiency—common especially in children, women, and the elderly—on overall health are feared to be widespread. Signs of deficiency include loss of appetite, stunted growth in children, skin changes, small sex glands in boys, delayed sexual maturation, impotence, loss of taste sensitivity, white spots on fingernails, delayed wound-healing, and dull hair color.

Animal foods are good sources of zinc as are oysters, milk, egg yolks, wheat germ, pumpkin and sunflower seeds, nuts, cheese, dry beans, lentils, and whole grains. Toxicity is rare. The RDA for adults is 12 mg.

Selenium

Selenium functions in a similar way to vitamin E, as an antioxidant helping to protect cells from destruction by toxic agents. Its consumption has also been associated with lower incidences of cancer and heart disease.

Good sources of selenium include whole grains, seafood, liver, kidney, meat, seeds, and nuts. Deficiency may be a problem in areas with selenium-poor soils. Selenium is toxic at higher than trace amounts. The RDA for adult males is 70 micrograms and for adult women 55 micrograms.

Molybdenum

Molybdenum is essential in the function of certain enzyme systems and is also necessary in iron metabolism.

Sources of molybdenum include meats, whole grains, legumes, leafy vegetables, and organ meats. The molybdenum content of vegetables varies widely depending on the content of the soil in which they were grown. Deficiency is not known in humans. Ingesting more than trace amounts is not recommended. The RDA for adults is between 75 and 250 micrograms.

Copper

Copper is important as a cofactor in several enzyme systems and as a catalyst in the synthesis of hemoglobin. It also aids in collagen formation and is involved in the synthesis of phospholipids, which maintain healthy nerve fibers.

Copper deficiency is believed to be more common than once thought, and it has been linked to heart disease, central nervous system disorders, anemia, and bone disorders. Good sources of copper include shellfish, liver, nuts and seeds, meats, and green leafy vegetables. Copper supplements are not recommended because they can interfere with other minerals, and copper is toxic at more than trace amounts. The RDA for copper is 1.5 to 3 mg.

Manganese

Manganese has a variety of functions, some that other minerals can perform in its place. It is known to play a role in such things as collagen formation, urea formation, synthesis of fatty acids and cholesterol, digestion of proteins, normal bone formation and development, and protein synthesis.

Manganese deficiency has not been observed in humans. Sources of manganese include liver, kidney, spinach, whole grain cereals and breads, dried peas and beans, and nuts. Excessive intake of manganese can interfere with iron absorption. More than trace amounts of manganese are not recommended. The RDA is 2 to 5 mg.

Fluoride

Fluoride is essential for the development of healthy teeth and bones and the prevention of tooth decay.

Fluoride deficiency shows up in increased incidences of tooth decay. Fluoridated water is the most common source of fluoride for many people. For those without access to such water fluoride tablets or toothpaste are helpful. Fish, tea, milk, and eggs are also sources of fluoride. The RDA for adults is between 1.5 and 4 mg.

Chromium

Chromium is important for maintaining normal glucose metabolism. It also acts as a cofactor for insulin.

Chromium deficiency can show up in the form of glucose intolerance in malnourished children and in some diabetics. Sources of chromium include whole grains, brewer's yeast, meats, and cheeses. Hard water also contains chromium. Chromium intake should not exceed trace amounts. The RDA for adults is between 50 and 200 micrograms.

Fiber

Fiber in the diet is important for proper elimination. It provides bulk, and its use has been linked to the prevention of many health problems: constipation, appendicitis, colon cancer, diverticular disease, spastic colon, hiatal hernia, varicose veins, hemorrhoids, coronary heart disease, high blood pressure, gallstones, diabetes, obesity, ulcerative colitis, and Crohn's disease.

Fiber is found almost exclusively in plant foods and comes in basically two types: water soluble or water insoluble. Soluble fiber is found primarily in fruits and vegetables and in oat bran in the form of gums and pectin and affects the way the body metabolizes sugars and fats. Insoluble fiber is primarily associated with whole grains, the traditional "bran," such as wheat bran and rice bran, and is the fiber we think of when we think of laxatives. Generally, the less processed the food, the higher it is in either kind of fiber.

Fiber in high doses can affect the absorption of other vitamins and minerals as well as cause flatulence, bloating, nausea, diarrhea, and impaction or rupture of the bowel. Daily consumption of 35 to 40 grams of fiber is recommended for optimum health and safety.

Water

Water is not really a food in the fuel sense, but it is in many ways a crucial component of nutrition: the body's need for water is second only to its need for oxygen. It makes up from 55 to 65 percent of the body's weight, and is constantly being eliminated in the form of urine, perspiration, and expired breath. It must be replaced regularly, for while a person can live for weeks without food, he can live for only a few days without water.

Normally, the best guide to how much water a person needs is his sense of thirst. The regulating mechanism of excretion sees to it that an excessive intake of water will be eliminated as urine. The usual water requirement is on the order of two quarts a day in addition to whatever amount is contained in the solids which make up the daily diet.

Recommended Dietary Allowances for Minerals

	Age	Calcium (mg)	Phospho. (mg)	Magnesium (mg)	Iron (mg)	Zinc (mg)	Iodine (mcg)	Selenium (mcg)
Infants	0 to .5	400	300	40	6	5	40	10
	.5 to 1	600	500	60	10	"	50	15
Children	1 to 3	800	800	80	"	10	70	20
	4 to 6	"	"	120	"	"	90	"
	7 to 10	"	"	170	"	"	120	30
Males	11 to 14	1,200	1,200	270	12	15	150	40
	15 to 18	"	"	400	"	"	"	50
	19 to 24	"	"	350	10	"	"	70
	25 to 50	800	800	"	"	"	"	"
	51 +	"	"	"	"	"	"	"
Females	11 to 14	1,200	1,200	280	15	12	"	45
	15 to 18	"	"	300	"	"	"	50
	19 to 24	"	"	280	"	"	"	55
	25 to 50	800	800	"	"	"	"	"
	51 +	"	"	"	10	"	"	"
Pregnant		1,200	1,200	320	30	15	175	65
Nursing	1st 6 months	"	"	355	15	19	200	75
	2nd 6 months	"	"	340	"	16	200	"

Basic Daily Diets

Everyone should have at least the minimal amount of basic nutrients for resting or basal metabolism. The specific needs of each individual are determined by whether he is still growing, and by how much energy is required for his normal activities. All those who are still growing—and growth continues up to about 25 years of age—have relatively high food needs.

For Infants

That food needs of an infant are especially acute should surprise no one. The newborn baby normally triples his birth weight during his first year and is very active in terms of calorie expenditure.

For his first six months, breast milk or formula, or a combination of both, fills his nutritional needs. The amount of milk he should get each day is about two and a half ounces per pound of his body weight. This provides 50 calories per pound, and in the early months is usually given in six feedings a day at four-hour intervals.

If his weight gain is adequate and he appears healthy, and if his stomach is not distended by swallowed air, his appetite is normally a satisfactory guide to how much he needs. The formula-fed baby should get a supplement of 35 milligrams of ascorbic acid each day and 400 international units of vitamin D if the latter has not been added to the milk during its processing.

Estimated Safe and Adequate Daily Dietary Intakes of Selected Vitamins and Minerals

		Biotin	Pant. acid	Copper	Manga-nese	Fluoride	Chro-mium	Molyb.
		(mcg)	(mg)	(mg)	(mg)	(mg)	(mcg)	(mcg)
Infants	0 to 0.5	10	2	0.4-.06	0.3-0.6	0.1-0.5	10-40	15-30
	0.5 to 1	15	3	0.6-0.7	0.6-1.0	0.2-1.0	20-60	20-40
Children/	1 to 3	20	"	0.7-1.0	1.0-1.5	0.5-1.5	20-80	25-50
Adoles-	4 to 6	25	3-4	1.0-1.5	1.5-2.0	1.0-2.5	30-120	30-75
cents	7 to 10	30	4-5	1.0-2.0	2.0-3.0	1.5-2.5	50-200	50-150
	11 +	30-100	4-7	1.5-2.5	2.0-5.0	"	"	75-250
Adults	30-100	"	1.5-3.0	"	1.5-4.0	"	"	

Solid Foods

Between two and six months of age, the baby should begin to eat solid foods such as cooked cereals, strained fruits and vegetables, egg yolk, and homogenized meat. With the introduction of these foods, it is not really necessary to calculate the baby's caloric intake. Satisfaction of appetite, proper weight gain, and a healthy appearance serve as the guides to a proper diet.

By one year of age, a baby should be getting three regular meals a day, and as his teeth appear, his food no longer needs to be strained. By 18 to 24 months, he should no longer need baby foods. For further information on the care and feeding of infants, see under "Birth, Infancy, and Maturation" in Ch. 2, *The First Dozen Years.*

Basic Food Groups

The recommended daily amounts of food for people over the age of two have been established with reasona-ble accuracy, but they always contain a fairly generous safety factor.

The Four Group Division

In general, foods are divided into four major groups:

- Meat, fish, eggs

- Dairy products

- Fruits and vegetables

- Breads and cereals

The Seven Group Division

For purposes of planning daily re-quirements, a more detailed way of considering food groupings is the fol-lowing:

- Leafy green and yellow vegetables

- Citrus fruits, tomatoes, and raw cabbage

- Potatoes and other vegetables and fruits

- Milk, cheese, and ice cream

- Meat, poultry, fish, eggs, dried peas, and beans

- Bread, flour, and cereals

- Butter and oils

The "Daily Food Guide" table can be used as a general guide to planning nutritionally balanced meals for pre-teens, teens, and adults of any age.

The Six Group Division

Very similar to the seven group division, the six group division puts all vegetables into one group. The pyramid chart is meant to convey three key points: eat less fat, eat a variety of foods, and eat the recommended number of servings from each group.

The Years of Growth

Even though a child will never again triple his weight in a single year as he did during his first, a proper diet is crucial during the years from 2 to 18, since this is a period of tremendous growth.

Other food goals that should be realized during the childhood and

**Fats, oils, sweets:
Use sparingly**

**Milk, yogurt, and cheese:
2–3 servings**

**Meat, poultry fish, dry beans, eggs, and nuts:
2–3 servings**

**Vegetables:
3–5 servings**

**Fruits:
2–4 servings**

Bread, cereal, rice, and pasta: 6–11 servings

Derived from the U.S. Department of Agriculture's "Eating Right Pyramid."

adolescent years are an awareness of what a balanced diet is, a reasonable tolerance for a variety of foods, decent manners at the table, and a sense of timing about when to eat and when not to eat.

These are also the years that a young person should begin to learn something about how to buy and prepare food, how to serve it attractively, and how to clean up after a meal.

Creating a Pleasant Atmosphere at Mealtime

Although a child's attitudes about food and eating can often be exasperating, it is up to the parent to make mealtime as pleasant as possible, and above all, to avoid any battles of will.

If a young child is too tired, too excited, or too hungry to cope with a meal without ending up in tears or a tantrum, he should not be forced to eat. There are several ways to help children develop a wholesome attitude toward food and eating; here are a few suggestions:

● Children should never be bribed with candy, money, or the promise of special surprises as a way of getting them to eat properly.

● They should not be given the idea that dessert is a reward for finishing the earlier part of the meal.

● Relatively small portions should be served and completely finished before anything else is offered.

● Between-meal snacks should be discouraged if they cut down on the appetite at mealtime.

● From time to time, the child should be allowed to choose the foods that he will eat at a meal.

Parents should keep in mind that the atmosphere in which a child eats and the attitudes instilled in him toward food can be altogether as basic as the nourishment for his body.

Teenage Diet

From the start of a child's growth spurt, which begins at age 10 or 11 for girls and between 13 and 15 for boys, and for several years thereafter, adolescent appetites are likely to be unbelievably large and somewhat outlandish. Special care, however, should be taken with the youngster who is putting on too much weight as well as with the one who is attracted by a bizarre starvation diet: both instances could indicate emotional problems.

Adult Nutrition

Adult nutrition is concerned with more than 50 years of an individual's life span. In typical cases, there is a slow but steady weight gain that may go unnoticed at first; for some, there is an obesity problem that begins at about age 40.

Because it is never easy to lose weight, it is especially important for adults to eat sensibly and avoid excess calories. See under "Weight," for a discussion of weight control and obesity.

For Older People

People over 60 tend to have changes in their digestive system that are related to less efficient and slower absorption. Incomplete chewing of food because of carelessness or impaired teeth can intensify this problem. Avoiding haste at mealtimes ought to be the rule.

In cases where a dental disorder makes proper chewing impossible, food should be chopped or pureed. Older people occasionally have difficulty swallowing; for example, they may choke on a large piece of unchewed meat.

Food for older people should be cooked simply, preferably baked, boiled, or broiled rather than fried, and menus excessively rich in fats should be avoided. A daily multivitamin capsule is strongly recommended for those over 60. A poor appetite can be stimulated by an ounce or two of sherry before a meal unless there are medical reasons for avoiding alcoholic beverages of any kind. See under "Aging and What To Do About It" in Ch. 6, *The Later Years,* for a discussion of diet and eating habits in the later years.

During Pregnancy

A pregnant woman needs special foods to maintain her own health as well as to safeguard the health of her baby. She should have additional vitamin D, folic acid, and iron, usually recommended as dietary supplements. More important for most women is the provision of adequate protein in the diet to prevent toxemia of pregnancy or underweight babies. Between 70 and 85 grams of protein a day should be eaten during pregnancy, even if this results in a weight gain of as much as 25 pounds. Adequate nutrition is more important than restricting weight gain to 20 pounds or less.

Nursing Mothers

A nursing mother has special dietary needs in addition to those satisfied by the normal adult diet. She should drink an extra quart of milk and eat two more servings of citrus fruit or tomatoes, one more serving of lean meat, fish, poultry, eggs, beans, or cheese, and one more serving of leafy green or yellow vegetables.

Eating for Life

The U.S. Department of Agriculture and the U.S. Department of Health and Human Services have recommended seven basic guidelines to follow to avoid excess weight and maintain optimum health:

- Eat a variety of foods
- Maintain a desirable weight
- Avoid too much fat, saturated fat, and cholesterol
- Eat foods with adequate starch and fiber
- Avoid too much sugar
- Avoid too much sodium
- If you drink alcoholic beverages, do so in moderation

The first two guidelines form the framework of a good diet: eat a variety of foods so that you get enough of the essential nutrients you need, and eat only enough calories to maintain desirable weight. The next five guidelines describe special characteristics of a good diet—getting adequate starch and fiber and avoiding too much fat, sugar, sodium, and alcohol. Although the guidelines are designed for healthy adult Americans, these suggestions are considered especially appropriate for people who may already have some of the risk factors for chronic diseases. These risk factors include a family history of obesity, premature heart disease, diabetes, high blood pressure, or high blood cholesterol levels.

As part of their *Dietary Guidelines for Americans,* the U.S.D.A. and the U.S.D.H.H.S. recommend the "Choose More Often" approach to healthful eating.

Choose More Often:

Low-fat meat, poultry, fish
Lean cuts of meat trimmed of fat (round tip roast, pork tenderloin, loin of lamb chop), poultry without skin, and fish, cooked without breading or fat added.

Low-fat dairy products
1 percent or skim milk, buttermilk; low-fat or nonfat yogurt; lower fat cheeses (part-skim ricotta, pot, and farmer); ice milk, sherbert.

Dry beans and peas
All beans, peas, and lentils—the dry forms are higher in protein.

Whole grain products
Breads, bagels, and English muffins made from whole wheat, rye, bran, and corn flour or meal; whole grain or bran cereals; whole wheat pasta; brown rice; bulgur.

Fruits and vegetables
All fruits and vegetables (except avocados, which are high in fat, but that fat is primarily unsaturated). For example, apples, pears, cantaloupe, oranges, grapefruit, pineapple, peaches, bananas, carrots, broccoli, Brussels sprouts, cabbage, kale, potatoes, tomatoes, sweet potatoes, spinach, cauliflower, and turnips, and others.

Fats and oils high in unsaturates
Unsaturated vegetable oils, such as canola oil, corn oil, cottonseed oil, olive oil, and soybean oil, and margarine; reduced-calorie mayonnaise and salad dressings.

To assure an adequate diet, choose a variety of foods daily including selections of vegetables; fruits; whole-grain breads and cereals; low-fat dairy products; poultry, fish, and lean meat, dry beans and peas. Here are some tips for following the Choose More Often approach in three important areas: grocery shopping, food preparation, and eating out.

Grocery Shopping

Focus on variety. Choose a wide selection of low-fat foods rich in fiber. Include whole grain breads and cereals, vegetables, fruits, low-fat dairy products, and poultry, fish, and lean meat. Although the goal is to reduce fat to 30 percent or less of calories, when choosing foods that do contain fat, try to choose ones that contain primarily unsaturated fats. For example, choose an unsaturated-rich margarine instead of butter; choose vegetable oils.

Read food labels. To help you find foods that are low in fat and cholesterol and high in fiber, get into the label-reading habit. Many nutritional labels on packaged foods show the amount of unsaturated and saturated fatty acids and the amount of cholesterol and fiber they contain. Check the type of fat on the ingredients list. Is it an animal fat, coconut or palm kernel oil high in saturated fat? Or, is it corn or soybean oil high in polyunsaturated fat? Choose a product with the lowest proportion of saturated fat. The label also tells you something else about a product. Ingredients are listed in order of amount from most to least by weight. So, when you buy a breakfast cereal, for example, choose one that has a whole grain listed first (such as whole wheat or oatmeal).

Pay attention to sodium. Many processed, canned, and frozen foods are high in sodium. Cured or processed meats, cheeses, and condiments (soy sauce, mustard, tartar sauce) are also high in sodium. Check for salt, onion or garlic salt, and any ingredient with "sodium" on the label. If the sodium content is given on the nutritional label, compare products and choose the ones with lower levels.

Food Preparation

Use small amounts of fat and fatty foods. There are lots of ways to use less fat. For example, when you saute or stir-fry, use only ½ teaspoon of fat per serving. When you use margarine, mayonnaise, or salad dressing, use half as much as usual. And, decrease portion sizes of other high fat foods—rich desserts, untrimmed and fatty types of meat, poultry with skin, and fried foods, especially breaded foods.

Use less saturated fat. While reducing your total fat intake, substitute unsaturated fat and oils for saturated fat in food preparation. For example, instead of butter, use margarine or vegetable oil. One teaspoon of butter can be replaced with equal portions (or less) of margarine or ¾ teaspoon of vegetable oil in many recipes without affecting the quality. Saturated fat may be reduced even more if you want to experiment with recipes. Poultry without skin and fish are good choices because they are often lower in fat and saturated fat than many meats.

Use low-fat alternatives. Substitute 1 percent, skim, or reconstituted nonfat dry milk for whole milk. Use low-fat yogurt, buttermilk, or evaporated skim milk in place of cream and sour cream. Try reduced-calorie mayonnaise and salad dressing in place of regular.

Choose lean meat. When you buy meat, choose lean cuts such as beef round, pork tenderloin, and loin lamb chops. Be sure to trim all visible fat from meat and poultry and remove poultry skin.

Use low-fat cooking methods. Bake, steam, broil, microwave, or boil foods rather than frying. Skim fat from soups and gravies.

Increase fiber. Choose whole grain breads and cereals. Substitute whole grain flour for white flour. Eat vegetables and fruits more often and have generous servings. Whenever possible, eat the edible fiber-rich skin as well as the rest of the vegetable or fruit.

Use herbs, spices, and other flavorings. For a different way to add flavor to meals, try lemon juice, basil, chives, allspice, onion, and garlic in place of fats and sodium. Try new recipes that use less fat or sodium-containing ingredients, and adjust favorite recipes to reduce fat and sodium.

Eating Out

Choose the restaurant carefully. Are there low-fat as well as high-fiber selections on the menu? Is there a salad bar? How are the meat, chicken, and fish dishes cooked? Can you have menu items broiled or baked without added fat instead of fried? These are important things to know before you enter a restaurant—fast food or otherwise. Seafood restaurants usually offer broiled, baked or poached fish, and you can often request butter and sauces on the side. Many steak houses offer small steaks and have salad bars.

Try ethnic cuisines. Italian and Asian restaurants often feature low-fat dishes—though you must be selective and alert to portion size. Try a small serving of pasta or fish in a tomato sauce at an Italian restaurant. Many Chinese, Japanese, and Thai dishes include plenty of steamed vegetables and a high proportion of vegetables to meat. Steamed rice, steamed noodle dishes and vegetarian dishes are good choices too. Ask that the chef cook you food without soy sauce or salt to decrease sodium. Some Latin American restaurants feature a variety of fish and chicken dishes that are low in fat.

Make sure you get what you want. Here are just a few things you can do to make sure that you're in control when you eat out. Ask how dishes are cooked. Don't hesitate to request that one food be substituted for another. Order a green salad or baked potato in place of french fries or order fruit, fruit ice, or sherbert instead of ice cream. Request sauces and salad dressings on the side and use only a small amount. Ask that butter not be sent to the table with your rolls. If you're not very hungry, order two low-fat appetizers rather than an entire meal, split a menu item with a friend, get a doggie-bag to take half of your meal home, or order a half-size portion. When you have finished eating, have the waiter clear the dishes away so that you can avoid postmeal nibbling.

Malnutrition

The classic diseases of nutritional deficiency, or malnutrition, such as scurvy and pellagra, are now rare, at least in the United States. The chief reason for their disappearance is the application of scientific knowledge gained in this century of the importance of vitamins and minerals in the diet. Thus most bread is fortified with vitamins and minerals, and in addition, commercial food processing has made it possible for balanced diets of an appealing variety to be eaten all year round.

Many people do not get an adequate diet, either through ignorance or because they simply cannot afford it. A number of food programs have been created to assist them, but unfortunately, the programs don't reach everyone who needs help.

Metric Equivalents of Traditional Food Measures	
1 teaspoon	= 5 milliliters
1 tablespoon	= 15 milliliters
¼ cup	= 60 milliliters
⅓ cup	= 80 milliliters
½ cup	= 120 milliliters
⅔ cup	= 160 milliliters
¾ cup	= 180 milliliters
1 cup	= 240 milliliters or 0.24 liter

Causes of Malnutrition

Some people, either because of ignorance or food faddism, do not eat a balanced diet even though they can afford to. There are also large numbers of people with nutritional deficiency diseases who can be described as abnormal, at least in regard to eating. Some are alcoholics; others live alone and are so depressed that they lack sufficient drive to feed themselves properly. Combination of any of these factors increase the likelihood of poor nutrition and often lead to health-damaging consequences.

Disease

People can also develop nutritional deficiencies because they have some disease that interferes with food absorption, storage, and utilization, or that causes an increased excretion, usually in the urine, of substances needed for nutrition. These are generally chronic diseases of the gastrointestinal tract including the liver, or of the kidneys or the endocrine glands.

Medications

Nutritional deficiencies can also result from loss of appetite caused by medications, especially when a number of different medications are taken simultaneously. This adverse affect on the appetite is a strong reason for not taking medicines unless told to do so by a physician for a specific purpose.

Most people are not aware of inadequacies in their diet until there are

Nutrients in Common Foods

Food	Food energy	Protein	Fat	Carbohydrate
	Calories	Grams	Grams	Grams
Milk and Milk Products				
Milk; 1 cup:				
Fluid, whole	165	9	10	12
Fluid, nonfat (skim)	90	9	trace	13
Buttermilk, cultured (from skim milk)	90	9	trace	13
Evaporated (undiluted)	345	18	20	24
Dry, nonfat (regular)	435	43	1	63
Yogurt (from partially skimmed milk); 1 cup	120	8	4	13
Cheese; 1 ounce:				
Cheddar or American	115	7	9	1
Cottage:				
From skim milk	25	5	trace	1
Creamed	30	4	1	1
Cream cheese	105	2	11	1
Swiss	105	7	8	1
Desserts (largely milk):				
Custard, baked; 1 cup, 8 fluid ounces	305	14	15	29
Ice cream, plain, factory packed: 1 slice or individual brick, ⅛ quart	130	3	7	14
1 container, 8 fluid ounces	255	6	14	28
Ice milk; 1 cup, 8 fluid ounces	200	6	7	29
Eggs				
Egg, raw, large:				
1 whole	80	6	6	trace
1 white	15	4	trace	trace
1 yolk	60	3	5	trace
Egg, cooked; 1 large:				
Boiled	80	6	6	trace
Scrambled (with milk and fat)	110	7	8	1
Meat, Poultry, Fish, Shellfish				
Bacon, broiled or fried, drained, 2 medium thick slices	85	4	8	trace
Beef, cooked without bone:				
Braised, simmered, or pot-roasted; 3 ounce portion:				
Entire portion, lean and fat	365	19	31	0
Lean only, approx. 2 ounces	140	17	4	0
Hamburger patties, made with Regular ground beef; 3-ounce patty	235	21	17	0
Lean ground round; 3-ounce patty	185	23	10	0
Roast; 3-ounce slice from cut having relatively small amount of fat:				
Entire portion, lean and fat	255	22	18	0
Lean only, approx. 2.3 ounces	115	19	4	0
Steak, broiled; 3-ounce portion:				
Entire portion, lean and fat	375	19	32	0
Lean only, approx. 1.8 ounces	105	17	4	0

Nutrients in Common Foods (continued)

Food	Food energy	Protein	Fat	Carbohydrate
	Calories	Grams	Grams	Grams
Beef, canned: corned beef hash; 3 ounces	155	8	10	9
Beef and vegetable stew; 1 cup	220	16	11	15
Chicken, without bone: broiled; 3 ounces	115	20	3	0
Lamb, cooked: Chops; 1 thick chop, with bone, 4.8 ounces: Lean and fat, approx. 3.4 ounces	340	21	28	0
Lean only, 2.3 ounces	120	18	5	0
Roast, without bone: Leg; 3-ounce slice: Entire slice, lean and fat	265	20	20	0
Lean only, approx. 2.3 ounces	120	19	5	0
Shoulder; 3-ounce portion, without bone: Entire portion, lean and fat	300	18	25	0
Lean only, approx. 2.2 ounces	125	16	6	0
Liver, beef, fried; 2 ounces	120	13	4	6
Pork, cured, cooked: Ham, smoked; 3-ounce portion, without bone	245	18	19	0
Luncheon meat: Boiled ham; 2 ounces	130	11	10	0
Canned, spiced; 2 ounces	165	8	14	1
Pork, fresh, cooked: Chops; 1 chop, with bone, 3.5 ounces: Lean and fat, approx. 2.4 ounces	295	15	25	0
Lean only, approx. 1.6 ounces	120	14	7	0
Roast; 3-ounce slice, without bone: Entire slice, lean and fat	340	19	29	0
Lean only, approx. 2.2 ounces	160	19	9	0
Sausage: Bologna; 8 slices (4.1 by 0.1 inches each), 8 ounces	690	27	62	2
Frankfurter; 1 cooked, 1.8 ounces	155	6	14	1
Tongue, beef, boiled; 3 ounces	205	18	14	trace
Veal, cutlet, broiled; 3-ounce portion, without bone	185	23	9	0
Fish and shellfish: Bluefish, baked or broiled; 3 ounces	135	22	4	0
Clams: raw, meat only; 3 ounces	70	11	1	3
Crabmeat, canned or cooked; 3 ounces	90	14	2	1
Fishsticks, breaded, cooked, frozen, 10 sticks (3.8 by 1.0 by 0.5 inches each), 8 ounces	400	38	20	15

Nutrients in Common Foods *(continued)*

Food	Food energy	Protein	Fat	Carbohydrate
	Calories	Grams	Grams	Grams
Haddock, fried; 3 ounces	135	16	5	6
Mackerel; broiled; 3 ounces	200	19	13	0
Oysters, raw, meat only; 1 cup (13-19 medium-size oysters, selects)	160	20	4	8
Oyster stew: 1 cup (6–8 oysters)	200	11	12	11
Salmon, canned (pink); 3 ounces	120	17	5	0
Sardines, canned in oil, drained solids; 3 ounces	180	22	9	1
Shrimp, canned, meat only; 3 ounces	110	23	1	—
Tuna, canned in oil, drained solids; 3 ounces	170	25	7	0
Mature Beans and Peas, Nuts Beans, dry seed: Common varieties, as Great Northern, navy, and others, canned; 1 cup:				
Red	230	15	1	42
White, with tomato or molassess:				
With pork	330	16	7	54
Without pork	315	16	1	60
Beans, dry seed: Lima, cooked; 1 cup	260	16	1	48
Cowpeas or black-eyed peas, dry, cooked; 1 cup	190	13	1	34
Peanuts, roasted, shelled; 1 cup	840	39	71	28
Peanut butter; 1 tablespoon	90	4	8	3
Peas, split, dry, cooked; 1 cup	290	20	1	52
Vegetables Asparagus: Cooked; 1 cup	35	4	trace	6
Canned, 6 medium-size spears	20	2	trace	3
Beans Lima, immature, cooked; 1 cup	150	8	1	29
Snap, green: Cooked; 1 cup	25	2	trace	6
Canned; solids and liquid; 1 cup	45	2	trace	10
Beets, cooked, diced; 1 cup	70	2	trace	16
Broccoli, cooked, flower stalks; 1 cup	45	5	trace	8
Brussels sprouts, cooked; 1 cup	60	6	1	12
Cabbage; 1 cup: Raw, coleslaw	100	2	7	9
Cooked	40	2	trace	9
Carrots: Raw: 1 carrot (5½ by 1 inch) or 25 thin strips	20	1	trace	5
Cooked, diced, 1 cup	45	1	1	9
Canned, strained or chopped; 1 ounce	5	trace	0	2
Cauliflower, cooked, flower buds; 1 cup	30	3	trace	6

some dramatic consequences. Nor is it easy to recognize the presence of a disorder that might be causing malnutrition. A physician should be consulted promptly when there is a persistent weight loss, especially when the diet is normal. He should also be informed of any changes in the skin, mucous membranes of the mouth or tongue, or nervous system function, because such symptoms can be a warning of dietary deficiency.

The family or friends of a person with a nutritional deficiency can often detect his condition because they become aware of changes in his eating patterns. They can also note early signs of a deficiency of some of the B vitamins, such as cracks in the mucous membranes at the corners of the mouth, or some slowing of intellectual function.

Correction of Nutritional Deficiencies

Nutritional deficiencies are among the most easily preventable causes of disease. It is important to realize that even mild deficiencies can cause irreparable damage, particularly protein deprivation in young children, which can result in some degree of mental retardation. Periodic medical checkups for everyone in the family are the best way to make sure that such deficiencies are corrected before they snowball into a chronic disease. In most cases, all that is required is a change of eating habits.

Weight

Probably the most important dietary problem in the United States today is obesity. It is certainly the problem most talked about and written about, not only in terms of good looks, but more important, in terms of good health.

All studies indicate that people who are obese have a higher rate of disease and a shorter life expectancy than those of average weight. From a medical point of view, people who are too fat may actually suffer from a form of malnutrition, even though they look overnourished.

Being too fat and being overweight are not necessarily the same. Heavy bones and muscles can make a person overweight in terms of the charts, but only an excess amount of fat tissue can make someone obese. However, height and weight tables are generally used to determine obesity.

Table 1 lists standard desirable weights for people of various heights, calculated with indoor clothing and shoes on. Frame sizes are estimated in a general way. This table applies to anyone over the age of 25, indicating that weight gain for the rest of the life span is unnecessary for biological normalcy.

Table 2 gives average weights of American men and women, according to height and age. These measurements are made without clothing or shoes. Note that the weights are considerably higher than the corresponding ones of Table 1. There is a modest weight gain until the middle years and then a gradual loss.

To determine whether a person is obese according to the tables, the percent that he is overweight has to be calculated. An individual is usually considered obese in the clinical sense if he weighs 20 percent more than the standard tables indicate for his size and age.

The Pinch Test

Another method of determining obesity is to use the "pinch" test. In most adults under 50 years of age, about half of the body fat is located directly under the skin. There are various parts of the body, such as the side of the lower torso, the back of the upper arm, or directly under the shoulder blade, where the thumb and forefinger can pinch a fold of skin and fat away from the underlying bone structure.

If the fold between the fingers—which is, of course, double thickness when it is pinched—is thicker than one inch in any of these areas, the likelihood is that the person is obese.

The Problem of Overweight

The percentage of overweight people in this country has been increasing steadily, chiefly because people eat more and use less physical energy than they used to. Americans do very little walking because of the availability of cars; they do very little manual labor because of the increasing use of machines. They may eat good wholesome meals, but they have the time for nibbling at all hours, especially when sitting in front of the television screen.

These patterns usually begin in childhood. Youngsters rarely walk to school any more; they get there by bus or car. They often have extra money for snacks and soft drinks, and frequently parents encourage them to overeat without realizing that such habits do them more harm than good.

Most overweight children remain overweight as adults. They also have greater difficulty losing fat, and if they do lose it, tend to regain it more easily than overweight adults who were thin as children. Many adults become overweight between the ages of 20 and 30. Thus, by age 30, about 12 percent of American men and women are 20 percent or more overweight, and by age 60, about 30 percent of the male population and 50 percent of the female are at least 20 percent overweight. As indicated above, the phenomenon of weight gain while aging does not represent biological normalcy.

Why People Put On Weight

Why does weight gain happen? Excess weight is the result of the imbalance between caloric intake as food and caloric expenditure as energy, either in maintaining the basic metabolic processes necessary to sustain life or in performing physical activity. Calories not spent in either of these ways become converted to fat and accumulate in the body as fat, or *adipose* tissue.

A *calorie* is the unit of measurement that describes the amount of energy potentially available in a given food. It is also used to describe the amount of energy the body must use up to perform a given function.

Counting Calories

If an adult gets the average 3,000 calories a day in his food from the age of 20 to 70, he will have consumed about 55 million calories. About 60 percent of these calories will have been used for his basic metabolic processes. The rest—22 million calories—might have resulted in a gain of about 6,000 pounds of fat, since each group of 3,500 extra calories could have produced one pound of fat.

In some ways, it's a miracle that people don't become more obese than they do. The reason, of course, is

that most or all of these extra calories are normally used to provide energy for physical activity. Elsewhere in this chapter are some examples of calorie expenditure during various activities.

A reasonably good way for an adult to figure his daily caloric needs for moderate activities is to multiply his desirable weight (as noted in Table 1) by 18 for men and 16 for women. If the typical day includes vigorous or strenuous activities, extra calories will, of course, be required.

Parental Influences and Hereditary Factors

Although there are exceptions, almost all obese people consume more calories than they expend. The reasons for this imbalance are complex. One has to do with parental weight. If the weight of both parents is normal, there is only a 10 percent likelihood that the children will be obese. If one parent is obese, there is a 50 percent probability that the children will be too, and if both are, the probability of obese offspring is 80 percent.

No one knows for certain why this is so. It is probably a combination of diet habits acquired in youth, conditioning during early years to react to emotional stress by eating, the absence of appropriate exercise patterns, and genetic inheritance.

Some obese people seem to have an impairment in the regulatory mechanism of the area of the central nervous system that governs food intake. Simply put, they do not know when to stop eating. Others, particularly girls, may eat less than their nonobese counterparts, but they are considerably less active. Some researchers think that obese people have an inherent muscle rhythm deficiency. In rare cases, a few people appear to have an abnormality in the metabolic process which results in the accumulation of fat even when the balance between calories taken in and expended is negative and should lead to weight loss.

Nutrients in Common Foods *(continued)*

Food	Food energy	Protein	Fat	Carbohydrate
	Calories	Grams	Grams	Grams
Celery, raw: large stalk, 8 inches long	5	1	trace	1
Collards, cooked; 1 cup	75	7	1	14
Corn, sweet:				
Cooked; 1 ear 5 inches long	65	2	1	16
Canned, solids and liquid; 1 cup	170	5	1	41
Cucumbers, raw, pared; 6 slices (⅛-inch thick, center section)	5	trace	trace	1
Lettuce, head, raw:				
2 large or 4 small leaves	5	1	trace	1
1 compact head (4¾-inch diameter)	70	5	1	13
Mushrooms, canned, solids and liquid; 1 cup	30	3	trace	9
Okra, cooked; 8 pods (3 inches long, ⅝-inch diameter)	30	2	trace	6
Onions: mature raw; 1 onion (2½-inch diameter)	50	2	trace	11
Peas, green; 1 cup:				
Cooked	110	8	1	19
Canned, solids and liquid	170	8	1	32
Peppers, sweet:				
Green, raw; 1 medium	15	1	trace	3
Red, raw; 1 medium	20	1	trace	4
Potatoes:				
Baked or boiled; 1 medium, 2½-inch diameter (weight raw, about 5 ounce):				
Baked in jacket	90	3	trace	21
Boiled; peeled before boiling	90	3	trace	21
Chips; 10 medium (2-inch diameter)	110	1	7	10
French fried:				
Frozen, ready to be heated for serving; 10 pieces (2 by ½ by ½ inch)	95	2	4	15
Ready-to-eat, deep fat for entire process; 10 pieces (2 by ½ by ½ inch)	155	2	7	20
Mashed; 1 cup:				
Milk added	145	4	1	30
Milk and butter added	230	4	12	28
Radishes, raw; 4 small	10	trace	trace	2
Spinach:				
Cooked; 1 cup	45	6	1	6
Canned, creamed, strained; 1 ounce	10	1	trace	2
Squash:				
Cooked, 1 cup:				
Summer, diced	35	1	trace	8
Winter, baked, mashed	95	4	1	23
Canned, strained or chopped; 1 ounce	10	trace	trace	2

Nutrients in Common Foods (continued)

Food	Food energy Calories	Protein Grams	Fat Grams	Carbohydrate Grams
Sweet potatoes:				
Baked or boiled; 1 medium, 5 by 2 inches (weight raw, about 6 ounces):				
Baked in jacket	155	2	1	36
Boiled in jacket	170	2	1	39
Candied, 1 small, 3½ by 2 inches	295	2	6	60
Canned, vacuum or solid pack; 1 cup	235	4	trace	54
Tomatoes:				
Raw; 1 medium (2 by 2½ inches), about ⅓ pound	30	2	trace	6
Canned or cooked; 1 cup	45	2	trace	9
Tomato juice, canned; 1 cup	50	2	trace	10
Tomato catsup; 1 tablespoon	15	trace	trace	4
Turnips, cooked, diced; 1 cup	40	1	trace	9
Turnip greens, cooked; 1 cup	45	4	1	8
Fruits				
Apples, raw; 1 medium (2½ inch diameter), about ⅓ pound	70	trace	trace	18
Apple juice, fresh or canned; 1 cup	125	trace	0	34
Apple sauce, canned:				
Sweetened; 1 cup	185	trace	trace	50
Unsweetened; 1 cup	100	trace	trace	26
Apricots, raw; 3 apricots (about ¼ pound)	55	1	trace	14
Apricots, canned in heavy syrup; 1 cup	200	1	trace	54
Apricots, dried; uncooked; 1 cup (40 halves, small)	390	8	1	100
Avocados, raw, California varieties: ½ of a 10-ounce avocado (3½ by 3¼ inches)	185	2	18	6
Avocados, raw, Florida varieties: ½ of a 13-ounce avocado (4 by 3 inches)	160	2	14	11
Bananas, raw; 1 medium (6 by 1½ inches), about ⅓ pound	85	1	trace	23
Blueberries, raw; 1 cup	85	1	1	21
Cantaloupes, raw, ½ melon (5-inch diameter)	40	1	trace	9
Cherries, sour, sweet, and hybrid, raw; 1 cup	65	1	1	15
Cranberry sauce, sweetened; 1 cup	550	trace	1	142
Dates, "fresh" and dried, pitted and cut; 1 cup	505	4	1	134
Figs:				
Raw; 3 small (1½-inch (diameter), about ¼ pound	90	2	trace	22
Dried; 1 large (2 by 1 inch)	60	1	trace	15
Fruit cocktail, canned in heavy syrup, solids and liquid; 1 cup	175	1	trace	47
Grapefruit:				
Raw; ½ medium (4¼-inch diameter, No. 64's)	50	1	trace	14
Canned in syrup; 1 cup	165	1	trace	44

Nutrients in Common Foods *(continued)*

Food	Food energy	Protein	Fat	Carbohydrate
	Calories	Grams	Grams	Grams
Grapefruit juice:				
Raw; 1 cup	85	1	trace	23
Canned:				
Unsweetened; 1 cup	95	1	trace	24
Sweetened; 1 cup	120	1	trace	32
Frozen concentrate, unsweetened:				
Undiluted; 1 can (6 fluid				
ounces:	280	4	1	72
Diluted, ready-to-serve; 1 cup	95	1	trace	24
Frozen concentrate, sweetened:				
Undiluted; 1 can (6 fluid				
ounces)	320	3	1	85
Diluted, ready-to-serve; 1 cup	105	1	trace	28
Grapes, raw; 1 cup:				
American type (slip skin)	70	1	1	16
European type (adherent skin)	100	1	trace	26
Grape juice, bottled; 1 cup	165	1	1	42
Lemonade concentrate, frozen,				
sweetened:				
Undiluted; 1 can (6 fluid ounces) ...	305	1	trace	113
Diluted, ready-to-serve; 1 cup	75	trace	trace	28
Oranges, raw; 1 large orange				
(3-inch diameter)	70	1	trace	18
Orange juice:				
Raw; 1 cup:				
California (Valencias)	105	2	trace	26
Florida varieties:				
Early and midseason	90	1	trace	23
Late season (Valencias)	105	1	trace	26
Canned, unsweetened; 1 cup	110	2	trace	28
Frozen concentrate:				
Undiluted; 1 can 6 fluid				
ounces)	305	5	trace	80
Diluted, ready-to-serve; 1 cup	105	2	trace	27
Peaches:				
Raw:				
1 medium (2½-inch diameter),				
about ¼ pound	35	1	trace	10
1 cup, sliced	65	1	trace	16
Canned (yellow-fleshed) in heavy				
syrup; 1 cup	185	1	trace	49
Dried: uncooked; 1 cup	420	5	1	109
Pears:				
Raw; 1 pear (3 by 2½-inch				
diameter)	100	1	1	25
Canned in heavy syrup; 1 cup	175	1	trace	47
Pineapple juice; canned; 1 cup	120	1	trace	32
Plums				
Raw; 1 plum (2-inch diameter,				
about 2 ounces	30	trace	trace	7
Canned (Italian prunes, in syrup;				
1 cup	185	1	trace	50

Nutrients in Common Foods (continued)

Food	Food energy	Protein	Fat	Carbohydrate
	Calories	Grams	Grams	Grams
Prunes, dried:				
Uncooked; 4 medium prunes	70	1	trace	19
Cooked, unsweetened; 1 cup (17–18 prunes and ⅓ cup liquid	295	3	1	78
Prune juice, canned; 1 cup	170	1	trace	45
Raisins, dried; 1 cup	460	4	trace	124
Raspberries, red:				
Raw; 1 cup	70	1	trace	17
Frozen; 10-ounce carton	280	2	1	70
Strawberries:				
Raw; 1 cup	55	1	1	12
Frozen; 10-ounce carton	300	2	1	75
Tangerines; 1 medium (2½-inch diameter), about ¼ pound	40	1	trace	10
Watermelon; 1 wedge (4 by 8 inches), about 2 pounds (weighed with rind	120	2	1	29
Grain Products				
Biscuits, baking powder, enriched flour; 1 biscuit (2½-inch diameter)	130	2	4	20
Bran flakes (40 percent bran) with added thiamine; 1 ounce	85	3	1	22
Breads:				
Cracked wheat:				
1 pound (20 slices)	1,190	39	10	236
1 slice (½-inch thick)	60	2	1	12
Italian; 1 pound	1,250	41	4	256
Rye:				
American (light):				
1 pound (20 slices)	1,100	41	5	236
1 slice (½-inch thick)	55	2	trace	12
Pumpernickel; 1 pound	1,115	41	5	241
White:				
1–2 percent nonfat dry milk:				
1 pound (20 slices)	1,225	39	15	229
1 slice (½-inch thick)	60	2	1	12
3–4 percent nonfat dry milk:				
1 pound (20 slices)	1,225	39	15	229
1 slice (½-inch thick)	60	2	1	12
5–6 percent nonfat dry milk:				
1 pound (20 slices)	1,245	41	17	228
1 slice (½-inch thick)	65	2	1	12
Whole wheat, graham, or entire wheat:				
1 pound (20 slices)	1,105	48	14	216
1 slice (½-inch thick)	55	2	1	11
Cakes:				
Angel food: 2-inch sector (¹⁄₁₂ of cake, 8-inch diameter)	160	4	trace	36
Butter cakes:				
Plain cake and cupcakes without icing:				
1 square (3 by 3 by 2 inches)	315	4	12	48

Nutrients in Common Foods *(continued)*

Food	Food energy	Protein	Fat	Carbohydrate
	Calories	Grams	Grams	Grams
1 cupcake (2¾-inch diameter)	120	2	5	18
Plain cake with icing: 2-inch sector of iced layer cake (¹⁄₁₆ of cake, 10-inch diameter)	320	5	6	62
Rich cake: 2-inch sector layer cake, iced (¹⁄₁₆ of cake, 10-inch diameter)	490	6	19	76
Fruit cake, dark; 1 piece (2 by 1½ by ¼ inches)	60	1	2	9
Sponge; 2-inch sector (¹⁄₁₂ of cake, 8-inch diameter	115	3	2	22
Cookies, plain and assorted; 1 cookie (3-inch diameter)	110	2	3	19
Cornbread or muffins made with enriched, degermed cornmeal; 1 muffin 2¾-inch diameter)	105	3	2	18
Cornflakes; 1 ounce	110	2	trace	24
Corn grits, degermed, cooked; 1 cup	120	3	trace	27
Crackers: Graham; 4 small or 2 medium	55	1	1	10
Saltines; 2 crackers (2-inch square	35	1	1	6
Soda, plain: 2 crackers (2½-inch square	45	1	1	8
Doughnuts, cake type; 1 doughnut	135	2	7	17
Farina, cooked; 1 cup	105	3	trace	22
Macaroni, cooked; 1 cup: Cooked 8–10 minutes (undergoes additional cooking as ingredient of a food mixture)	190	6	1	39
Cooked until tender	155	5	1	32
Noodles (egg noodles), cooked; 1 cup	200	7	2	37
Oat cereal (mixture, mainly oat flour), ready-to-eat; 1 ounce	115	4	2	21
Oatmeal or rolled oats, regular or quick cooking, cooked; 1 cup	150	5	3	26
Pancakes; baked; 1 cake (4-inch diameter): Wheat (home recipe)	60	2	2	7
Buckwheat (with buckwheat pancake mix)	45	2	2	6
Pies; 3½-inch sector (⅛ of 9-inch diameter pie): Apple	300	3	13	45
Cherry	310	3	13	45
Custard	250	7	13	27
Lemon meringue	270	4	11	40
Minced	320	3	14	49
Pumpkin	240	5	13	28
Pretzels; 5 small sticks	20	trace	trace	4

Nutrients in Common Foods (continued)

Food	Food energy	Protein	Fat	Carbohydrate
	Calories	Grams	Grams	Grams
Rice, cooked; 1 cup:				
Converted	205	4	trace	45
White	200	4	trace	44
Rice, puffed or flakes; 1 ounce	110	2	trace	25
Rolls:				
Plain, pan (16 ounces per dozen); 1 roll	115	3	2	20
Hard, round (22 ounces per dozen); 1 roll	160	5	2	31
Sweet, pan (18 ounces per dozen); 1 roll	135	4	4	21
Spaghetti, cooked until tender; 1 cup	155	5	1	32
Waffles, baked, with enriched flour: 1 waffle (4½ by 5½ by ½ inches)	215	7	8	28
Wheat, puffed; 1 ounce	100	4	trace	22
Wheat, rolled, cooked; 1 cup	175	5	1	40
Wheat flakes; 1 ounce	100	3	trace	23
Wheat flours:				
Whole wheat; 1 cup, sifted	400	16	2	85
All purpose or family flour: 1 cup, sifted	400	12	1	84
Wheat germ; 1 cup, stirred	245	17	7	34
Fats, Oils, Related Products				
Butter; 1 tablespoon	100	trace	11	trace
Fats, cooking:				
Vegetable fats:				
1 cup	1,770	0	200	0
1 tablespoon	110	0	12	0
Lard:				
1 cup	1,985	0	220	0
1 tablespoon	125	0	14	0
Margarine; 1 tablespoon	100	trace	11	trace
Oils, salad or cooking; 1 tablespoon	125	0	14	0
Salad dressings; 1 tablespoon:				
Blue cheese	90	1	10	1
Commercial, plain (mayonnaise type)	60	trace	6	2
French	60	trace	6	2
Mayonnaise	110	trace	12	trace
Thousand Island	75	trace	8	1
Sugars, Sweets				
Candy; 1 ounce:				
Caramels	120	1	3	22
Chocolate, sweetened, milk	145	2	9	16
Fudge, plain	115	trace	3	23
Hard	110	0	0	28
Marshmallow	90	1	0	23
Jams, marmalades, preserves; 1 tablespoon	55	trace	trace	14
Jellies; 1 tablespoon	50	0	0	13
Sugar; 1 tablespoon	50	0	0	12
Syrup, table blends; 1 tablespoon	55	0	0	15

Nutrients in Common Foods *(continued)*				
Food	**Food energy**	**Protein**	**Fat**	**Carbohydrate**
	Calories	**Grams**	**Grams**	**Grams**
Miscellaneous				
Beverages, carbonated, cola types; 1 cup	105	—	—	28
Bouillon cubes; 1 cube	2	trace	trace	0
Chocolate, unsweetened; 1 ounce	145	2	15	8
Gelatin dessert, plain, ready-to-serve; 1 cup	155	4	0	36
Sherbet, factory packed; 1 cup (8-fluid-ounce container)	235	3	trace	58
Soups, canned, prepared with equal amount of water; 1 cup:				
Bean with pork	168	8	6	22
Beef noodle	140	8	5	14
Bouillon, broth, and consomme	30	5	0	3
Chicken consomme	44	7	trace	4
Clam chowder, Manhattan style	80	2	3	12
Tomato	90	2	3	16
Vegetable beef	80	5	2	10
Vinegar; 1 tablespoon	2	0	—	1

Adapted from *Nutritive Value of American Foods* by Catherine F. Adams. Agriculture Handbook No. 456. U.S. Department of Agriculture, issued November 1975. The cup measure used in the following table refers to the standard 8-ounce measuring cup of 8 fluid ounces or one-half liquid pint. When a measure is indicated by ounce, it is understood to be by weight—1/16 of a pound avoirdupois—unless a fluid ounce is indicated. All weights and measures in the table are in U.S. System units.

Obesity and Health

There are many reasons why obesity is a health hazard. The annual death rate for obese people between the ages of 20 and 64 is half again as high as that for people whose weight is close to normal. This statistical difference is due primarily to the increased likelihood that the obese person will suffer from diabetes mellitus and from diseases of the digestive and circulatory systems, especially of the heart.

One possible reason for the increased possibility of heart disease is that there are about two-thirds of a mile of blood vessels in each pound of adipose tissue. Thus 20 or more pounds of excess weight are likely to impose a great additional work load on the heart.

Obese people are also poorer surgical risks than the nonobese, and it is often more difficult to diagnose and therefore to treat their illnesses correctly.

Permanent loss of excess weight makes the formerly obese person come closer to matching the life expectancy of the nonobese. However, losing and regaining weight as a repeated pattern is even more hazardous in terms of health than consistent obesity.

Psychological Consequences of Obesity

In ways that are both obvious and subtle, obesity often has damaging psychological consequences. This is particularly true for obese children, who tend to feel isolated and rejected by their peers. They may consider themselves victims of prejudice and blame their obesity for everything that goes wrong in their lives. In many cases, the destructive relationship between obesity and self-pity keeps perpetuating itself.

Obese adults are likely to experience the same feelings, but to a somewhat lesser degree. For some, obesity is an escape which consciously or unconsciously helps them to avoid situations in which they feel uncomfortable—those that involve active competition or relationships with the opposite sex.

Avoiding Excess Weight

Clearly, obesity is a condition that most people would like to avoid. Not putting on extra pounds does seem to be easier, in theory at least, than taking them off. One possible explanation for this is that additional adipose tissue consists of a proliferation of fat cells. Shrinking these cells is one thing, eliminating them is another. Our present lack of fundamental knowledge about the regulatory and metabolic mechanisms relating to obesity limits the technique of preventing overweight to recommending a balance between caloric intake and expenditure.

The real responsibility for preventing the onset of obesity in childhood rests with parents. It is important for the parents to set a good example and to instill early on all of the fundamentals of good nutrition and healthy eating habits; these are of the utmost importance in this connection. Caloric expenditure in the form of regular exercise is equally important.

Exercising by Habit

This does not necessarily mean that exercise should be encouraged for its own sake. What it does mean is making a habit of choosing an active way of approaching a situation rather than a lazy way: walking upstairs rather than taking the elevator; walking to school rather than riding; walking while playing golf rather than riding in a cart; running to get the ball that has rolled away rather than ambling toward it. These choices should be made consistently and not just occasionally if obesity is to be avoided. Those people who naturally enjoy the more active way of doing things are lucky. Those who don't should make an effort to develop new patterns, especially if obesity is a family problem.

Anyone with the type of physical handicap that makes a normal amount of exercise impossible should be especially careful about caloric intake.

Weight Reduction

The treatment of obesity is a complicated problem. In the first place, there is the question of who wants or needs to be treated and how much weight should be lost. Except in unusual situations, anyone who wants to lose weight should be encouraged to do so. Possible exceptions are teenagers who are not overweight but who want to be as thin as they can possibly be—the boy who is involved in an athletic event such as wrestling, or the girl who has decided she wants to look like a fashion model.

Crash dieting is usually unwise if the goal is to lose too much weight too rapidly and should be undertaken only after consulting a doctor about its advisability. As for adolescents who have become slightly overweight during puberty, they may be ill-advised to try to take off the extra pounds that probably relate to a temporary growth pattern.

Losing Weight Must Be Self-Motivated

Unless there are compelling medical reasons for not doing so, anyone weighing 20 percent or more over the normal limit for his age and body build should be helped to slim down. It is extremely important, however, for the motivation to come from the person himself rather than from outside pressure.

Unless an overweight person really wants to reduce, he will not succeed in doing so, certainly not permanently, even though he appears to be trying. He must have convinced himself—intellectually and emotionally—that the goal of weight loss is truly worth the effort.

It is very difficult not only for his friends and family but for the person himself to be absolutely sure about the depth of his motivation. A physician treating an overweight patient has to assume that the desire to re-

duce is genuine and will try to reinforce it whenever he can. However, if a patient has made a number of attempts to lose weight over a period of years and has either been unable to reduce to any significant degree, or has become overweight again after reducing, it is probably safe to assume that the emotional desire is absent, or that there are emotional conflicts that stand in the way.

It is very possible that such a person could be harmed psychologically by losing weight, since he might need to be overweight for some deep-seated reason. This can be true for both children and adults. Occasionally it is possible for a psychiatrist or psychologist to help the patient remove a psychological block against losing weight, after which weight reduction can occur if the caloric balance is straightened out.

Effective Planning for Weight Loss

The ultimate key to successful weight reduction is proper eating combined with proper physical activity. This

balance is extremely difficult for many people to achieve because it involves a marked change in attitudes and be-

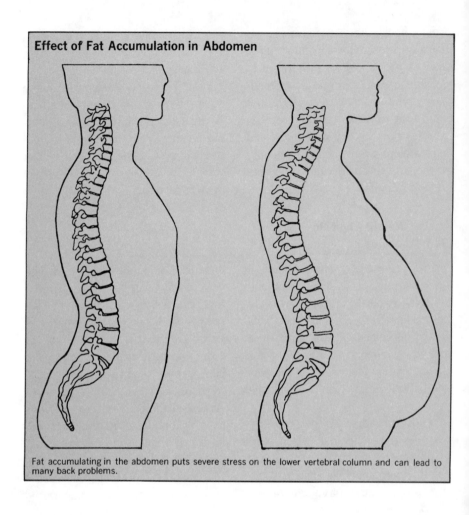

Effect of Fat Accumulation in Abdomen

Fat accumulating in the abdomen puts severe stress on the lower vertebral column and can lead to many back problems.

havior patterns that are generally solidly established and of long duration. Furthermore, once the changes are made, they will have to endure for a lifetime if the weight that has been lost is not to be regained.

It is therefore important that the reducing diet should be somewhat similar to the person's usual eating pattern in terms of style and quality. Intake of fat and calories should be reduced and that of fiber increased, and probably the word "dieting"

should not be used to describe the process, since most people don't find the idea of permanent dieting congenial.

Similarly, the increased physical activity that must accompany the new eating style should be of a type that the person enjoys. It is virtually impossible for an overeating person to reduce merely by restricting his caloric intake, or merely by increasing his caloric expenditure. The two must go together.

Cutting Down Step by Step

The first thing to determine when planning to lose weight is the number of pounds that have to go. A realistic goal to set is the loss of about one pound a week. This may seem too slow, but remember that at this rate, fifty pounds can be lost in a year.

Getting Started

Start by weighing yourself on arising, and then for two weeks try to eat in your customary manner, but keep a careful record of everything that you eat, the time it is eaten, and the number of calories it contains. During this period, continue to do your usual amount of physical activity.

When the two weeks are over, weigh yourself again at the same time of day as before. If you haven't gained any weight, you are in a basal caloric state. Then check over your food list to see what might be eliminated each day without causing discomfort.

Try to think in terms of eliminating fats and simple carbohydrates first, because it is essential that you continue to get sufficient vitamins and minerals which are largely found in proteins and complex carbohydrates. The foods described in the "Daily Food Guide" chart should all continue to be included in your daily food consumption. If you are in the habit of having an occasional drink, remember that there are calories in alcohol but no nutrients, and that most alcoholic beverages stimulate the appetite.

Planning Meals

When you replan your meals, keep in mind that the items you cut down on must add up to between 300 and 400 calories a day if you are going to lose one pound a week.

Your total daily food intake should be divided among at least three meals a day, more if you wish. If you need to eat more food or to eat more often, try snacking on low calorie foods such as cabbage, carrots, celery, cucumber, and cauliflower. All of these can be eaten raw between meals.

There is definitely something to be said in favor of having breakfast every morning, or at least most mornings. This may be psychologically difficult, but try to do it, because it will be easier to control your urge to eat too much later in the day.

Increasing Exercise

At the same time that you begin to cut down on your food intake, start to increase your daily exercise in whatever way you find congenial so that the number of calories expended in increased exercise plus the number of calories eliminated from your diet comes to 500 or more. This is your daily caloric loss compared with your so-called basal caloric state.

Daily Food Guide

	Child	Preteen and Teen	Adult	Aging Adult
Milk or milk products *(cups)*	2–3	3–4 or more	2 or more	2 or more
Meat, fish, poultry, and eggs *(servings)*	1–2	3 or more	2 or more	2 or more
Green and yellow vegetables *(servings)*	1–2	2	2	at least 1
Citrus fruits and tomatoes *(servings)*	1	1–2	1	1–2
Potatoes, other fruits, vegetables *(servings)*	1	1	1	0–1
Bread, flour, and cereal *(servings)*	3–4	4 or more	3–4	2–3
Butter or margarine *(tablespoons)*	2	2–4	2–3	1–2

1. The need for the nutirents in 1 or 2 cups of milk daily can be satisfied by cheeses or ice cream. (1 cup of milk is approximately equivalent to 1½ cups of cottage cheese or 2–3 large scoops of ice cream.)
2. It is important to drink enough fluid. The equivalent of 3–5 cups daily is recommended.
3. The recommended daily serving of meat, fish, and poultry (3 oz.) may be alternated with eggs or cheese, dried peas, beans, or lentils.
4. Iron-rich foods should be selected as frequently as possible by teenage and adult females to help meet their high requirement for this mineral (liver, heart, lean meats, shellfish, egg yolks, legumes, green leafy vegetables, and whole grain and enriched cereal products).

From *Your Age and Your Diet* (1971), reprinted with permission from the American Medical Association.

Achieving Your Goal

You may wish to double your daily caloric loss so that you lose two pounds a week. Do not try to lose any more than that unless you are under close medical supervision.

If you gained weight during your two-week experimental period, you will have to increase your daily caloric loss by 500 for every pound gained per week. Thus, if you gained one pound during the two weeks, you will have to step up your daily caloric loss to 750 to lose a pound a week.

You'll have to keep plugging away to achieve your goal. It will be trying and difficult in many ways. You may get moody and discouraged and be tempted to quit. Don't. You'll probably go on periodic food binges. All this is natural and understandable, so try not to brood about it. Just do the best you can each day. Don't worry about yesterday, and let tomorrow take care of itself.

In many ways it can help, and in some cases it's essential, to have the support and encouragement of family and friends, particularly of those with whom you share meals. You may find it helpful to join a group that has been formed to help its members lose weight and maintain their weight loss. This is a good psychological support.

Maintaining Your Weight Loss

Once you have achieved your desired weight, you can test yourself to see what happens if you increase your caloric intake. Clearly, anyone who can lose weight in the manner described can't stay in a state of negative caloric imbalance indefinitely. But you will have to be careful, or you'll become overweight again. It's a challenge, but people who stick to a disciplined program can be rewarded by success.

Special Problems

If you do not succeed in losing weight in spite of carrying out the program described above, you may need professional help because of some special problem. A qualified physician may try some special diets, or he may even suggest putting you into a hospital so that he can see to it that you have no caloric food at all for as long as three weeks.

Perhaps the situation is complicated by a metabolic abnormality that can be corrected or helped by medication. Although such conditions are rare, they are not unheard of.

Obesity is almost never caused by a "glandular" problem—which usually means an underactive thyroid. Do not take thyroid pills to reduce unless your thyroid has been found to be underactive on the basis of a specific laboratory test.

The indiscriminate use of pills to reduce, even when prescribed, is never helpful in the long run, although it may appear to be at first. The unsupervised use of amphetamines, for example, can be extremely dangerous. See Ch. 29, *Substance Abuse,* for further information about the dangers of amphetamine abuse.

Because so many people are eager to reduce, and because losing weight isn't easy, there are many unethical professionals who specialize in the problem. Avoid them. All they are likely to do for you is take your money and make your situation no better—and often worse—than it was to begin with.

Underweight

Weighing too little is a problem that is considerably less common than weighing too much. In fact, in many cases, it isn't accurate to call it a problem at all, at least not a medical one.

There are some times, however, when underweight may indicate the presence of a disease, especially when a person rather suddenly begins and continues to lose weight, even though there has been no change in his eating habits. This is a situation that calls for prompt medical evaluation. Fortunately, such a person may already be under a physician's care at the time the weight loss is first noticed.

More often, however, underweight is a chronic condition that is of concern to the person who feels his looks would improve if he could only add some extra pounds. This is especially true in the case of adolescent girls and young women.

What To Do About
Weighing Too Little

Chronic underweight is rarely a reflection of underlying disease. It is rather an expression of individual heredity or eating patterns, or a combination of both. Treatment for the condition is the opposite of the treatment for overweight. The achievement of a positive caloric balance comes first; more calories have to be consumed each day than are expended. An underweight person should record his food history over a two-week period in the manner described for an overweight one. Once this has been done, various adjustments can be made.

First of all, he should see that he eats at least three meals a day and that they are eaten in a leisurely way and in a relaxed frame of mind. All of the basic foods should be represented in the daily food intake, with special emphasis on protein and complex carbohydrates. The daily caloric intake should then be gradually increased at each meal and snacks added, so long as the snacks don't reduce the appetite at mealtimes.

Carbohydrate foods are the best ones to emphasize in adding calories. Since the extra food intake may cause a certain amount of discomfort, encouragement and support from family and friends can be extremely helpful. Just as there may be psychological blocks against losing weight, there may well be a complicated underlying resistance to adding it.

Anyone trying to gain weight should remain or become reasonably active physically. Adding a pound or two a month for an adult—and a little more than that for a growing youngster—is an achievable goal until the desired weight is reached. There will probably have to be some adjustments in eating and exercise patterns so that a state of caloric balance is achieved.

How Food Relates
to Disease

Just as proper food is essential in the prevention of some diseases, it is helpful in the treatment of others. It also plays an important role in protecting and fortifying the general health of a patient while a specific illness is being treated.

The components of therapeutic diets are usually prescribed by the physician in charge, but some general principles will be presented here. Remember that diets designed to treat a given disease must supply the patient's basic nutritional requirements.

Ulcers

Special diet is a major treatment consideration in the case of peptic ulcer, whether located in the stomach (gastric) or in the small intestine (duodenal). A major aim of such a diet is the neutralizing of the acidity of gastric juices by the frequent intake of high protein foods such as milk and eggs. Foods which irritate an ulcer chemically, such as excessive sweets, spices, or salt, or mechanically, such as foods with sharp seeds or tough skins, and foods that are too hot or too cold, should be avoided. It is also advisable to eliminate gravies, coffee, strong tea, carbonated beverages, and alcohol, since all of these stimulate gastric secretion. Such a diet is called a *bland* diet. A soft diet is recommended for some forms of gastrointestinal distress and for those people who have difficulty chewing. It is often combined with the bland diet recommended for peptic ulcer patients to reduce the likelihood of irritation. See Ch. 11, *Diseases of the Digestive System,* for further information about ulcers.

Diabetes

As the section on diabetes mellitus indicates (see Ch. 15), the major objectives of the special diet are weight control, control of the abnormal carbohydrate metabolism, and as far as possible, psychological adjustment by the patient to his individual circumstances. To some extent, he must calculate his diet mathematically. First, his daily caloric needs have to be determined in terms of his activities:

If he is overweight or underweight, the total calories per pound of body weight will have to be adjusted downward or upward by about five calories per pound.

After his total daily caloric needs have been figured out, he can calculate the number of grams of carbohydrate, protein, and fat he should have each day: 58 percent of the calories should come from carbohydrates, 12 percent from protein, and 30 percent from fat. One-fifth of the total should be obtained at breakfast and the rest split between lunch and dinner. Snacks that are taken during the day should be subtracted equally from lunch and dinner.

It is important that meals and planned snacks be eaten regularly and that no food servings be added or omitted. Growing children from 1 to 20 years of age who have diabetes will require considerably more daily calories. A rough estimate is 1,000 calories for a one-year-old child and 100 additional calories for each year of age.

Salt-Free Diets

There are a number of chronic diseases which are treated in part by restricting the amount of sodium in the diet. These diseases, which are associated with fluid retention in the body, include congestive heart failure, certain types of kidney and liver diseases, and hypertension or high blood pressure.

The restriction of sodium intake helps to reduce or avoid the problem of fluid retention. The normal daily diet contains about seven or more grams of sodium, most of it in the form of sodium chloride or table salt. This amount is either inherent in the food or added during processing, cooking, or at mealtime. Half the weight of salt is sodium.

For people whose physical condition requires only a small restriction of the normal sodium intake, simply not salting food at the table is a sufficient reduction. They may decide to use a salt substitute, but before doing so should discuss the question with their physician.

A greater sodium restriction, for example, to no more than 5 grams a day, requires the avoidance of such high salt content foods as ham, bacon, crackers, catsup, and potato chips, as well as almost entirely eliminating salt in the preparation and serving of meals. Severe restriction—1 gram or less a day—involves special food selection and cooking procedures, as well as the use of distilled water if the local water has more than 20 milligrams of sodium per quart. In restricting sodium to this extent, it is important to make sure that protein and vitamins are not reduced below the minimum daily requirements. See "Sodium Restricted Diets."

Sodium Restricted Diets

Diets Moderately Restricted in Sodium

If only a moderate sodium restriction is necessary, a normal diet *without added salt* may be ordered. Such an order is interpreted to mean that the patient will be offered the regular salted food on the general selective menu with the following exceptions:

1. No salt will be served on the tray.
2. Soups that are salted will be omitted.
3. Cured meats (ham, bacon, sausage, corned beef) and all salted cheeses will be omitted.
4. Catsup, chili sauce, mustard, and other salted sauces will be omitted.
5. Salt-free gravies, sauces, and salad dressings will be substituted for the regular salted items.
6. Salted crackers, potato chips, nuts, pickles, olives, popcorn, and pretzels will be omitted.

This diet contains approximately 3 grams of sodium or 7.5 grams of sodium chloride, depending on the type and quantity of the food chosen.

Other Diseases Requiring Special Diets

There are several other disorders in which diet is an important consideration: all chronic gastrointestinal disorders, such as gallbladder stones, ulcerative colitis, enteritis, and diverticulitis; a variety of hereditary disorders such as phenylketonuria and galactosemia; atherosclerosis, especially when it is associated with elevated blood levels of cholesterol or triglycerides or both; liver disease such as cirrhosis; many of the endocrine diseases; kidney stones; and sometimes certain neurological diseases such as epilepsy. Diet also plays a special role in convalescence from most illnesses and in post-surgical care. A modified fat diet and low fat diet are recommended for some diseases of the liver and gall-bladder. A minimal residue diet is recommended for some digestive troubles and before and after gastrointestinal surgery.

Diet and Individual Differences

Most discussions about food and eating tend to suggest that all normal people have identical gastrointestinal and metabolic systems. This is simply not true. There are many individual differences that explain why one man's meat is another man's poison. A person's intolerance for a given food may be caused by a disorder, such as an allergy or an ulcer, and it is possible that many of these intolerances will ultimately be related to enzyme deficiencies or some other biochemical factor.

More subtle are the negative physical reactions to particular foods as a result of psychological conditioning. In most such cases, the choice is between avoiding the food that causes the discomfort or eating it and suffering the consequences. Of course, compulsive overeating can also cause or contribute to discomfort. Practically no one can eat unlimited quantities of anything without having gastrointestinal discomfort or *dyspepsia.*

The establishment of so-called daily minimum food requirements suggests that every day's intake should be carefully balanced. Although this is beneficial, it is by no means necessary. Freedom from such regimentation can certainly be enjoyed during a holiday, or a trip to another country, or on a prolonged visit to relatives with casual food habits.

Sometimes a change in diet is dictated by a cold or an upset stomach or diarrhea. Liquids containing carbohydrates, such as tea with sugar and light soups, should be emphasized in treating a cold, while at the same time solid food intake should be somewhat reduced. In the case of an upset stomach or diarrhea, the discomfort may be eased by not eating or drinking anything at all for a whole day. This form of treatment may be helpful for an adult, but since children with diarrhea can become dehydrated in a day or so, professional advice is indicated when cutting down liquid intake.

Diet and Disease Prevention

More and more, medical specialists agree that diet can be helpful in preventing various diseases. Consensus has become general that a diet low in cholesterol and saturated fats can help prevent cardiovascular disease caused by atherosclerosis. Among the foods that reduce total cholesterol levels are rice bran and oat bran. Other sources of the soluble fiber that decreases blood cholesterol include peas, lentils, barley, and pectin fruits like apples, oranges, pears, and prunes. Also recommended are skin-less poultry and fish, lean meat, and low-fat dairy products.

Food-Borne Diseases

There are several ways in which food can be the *cause* of disease, most commonly when it becomes contaminated with a sufficient amount of harmful bacteria, bacterial toxin, viruses, or other poisonous substances. The gastrointestinal diseases typically accompanied by nausea, vomiting, diarrhea, or stomach cramps that are produced in this way are not, strictly speaking, caused by the foods themselves, and are therefore called food-borne diseases.

Most food-borne illnesses are caused by a toxin in food contaminated by staphylococcal or salmonella bacteria. In general, milk, milk products, raw shellfish, and meats are the foods most apt to be contaminated. This is most likely to happen when such foods are left standing at room temperature for too long between the time they are prepared and the time they are eaten. However, food can also become contaminated at many different points in time and at various stages of processing. Standards enforced by federal and local government agencies provide protection for the consumer for foods bought for the home as well as for use in restaurants, although whether the protection is adequate is a matter of dispute.

Food Storage

Food is best protected from contamination when it is stored below 40 degrees Fahrenheit or heated to 145 degrees or more. Cold slows bacterial growth; cooking kills it. Bacteria present in food can double in number every 15 minutes at room temperature.

All food stored in the refrigerator should be covered except ripe fruits and vegetables. Leftover foods cannot be kept indefinitely, nor can frozen foods be stored beyond a certain length of time. Specific information about these time periods for individual items is available from the Agricultural Extension Service in each state.

Commercially processed foods sold in the United States are under government control and generally are safe. However, any food can spoil or become contaminated at any point in time, and the consumer should not buy or serve food whose container (package or can) has been broken, cracked, or appears unusual.

Food Additives

From time to time, concern is expressed about one or another food additive as a hazard to health. Most of these additives are put into foods during processing in order to increase their nutritional value, or to improve their chemical or physical characteristics, such as taste and color. Perhaps as many as 2,000 different substances are used in this way in the United States. Some are natural products such as vanilla, others are chemicals derived from other foods, and a few, like artificial sweeteners, are synthetic. Other additives are referred to as indirect, since they are residues in the food from some stage of growing, processing, or packaging. Although additives are controlled and approved by agencies such as the federal Food and Drug Administration, they continue to be a cause of concern to many people.

Pesticides

The pesticides and fertilizers used in growing fruits and vegetables and the additives given to livestock may pose additional health hazards to humans. The National Academy of Sciences, for example, in 1988 estimated the national risk of cancer from pesticide use alone at as many as 20,000 cases a year.

Although it is not known how much is too much, it only makes sense to try and eliminate as much of the risk as possible. This is fairly easy to do. First of all, eat a wide variety of foods to help minimize your exposure to any one pesticide. Eat what's in season and what's grown locally or domestically. (The right season and less transportation mean less chemicals to ripen and preserve food; food and animals from abroad are subject to different health standards that are hard to regulate and check.) Wash all meat and produce carefully; many toxins are easily removed with soap and wa-

ter. Peel any fruit or vegetable with a wax coating. (Although it is generally advisable to retain as much of the skin of produce as possible for higher vitamin content, wax coatings hold in toxic residues.) Trim produce.

You may also want to go further in reducing your chances of consumption of added toxins by buying organically grown and raised produce and meat. These foods are not widely available in all areas of the country, and they often cost quite a bit more than foods raised with chemicals, but many people not only feel safer eating these foods, but find them tastier as well. Home gardening without the use of chemical fertilizers and pesticides is another healthful option. Be sure to wash and trim carefully all organic or home-grown vegetables, however, to guard against ingestion of naturally occurring toxins such as fungus.

Psychological Aspects of Food and Meals

Food and meals play an important role in emotional well-being and interpersonal relationships as well as in physical health and appearance.

During Infancy

The infant whose needs are attended to by a loving family develops a general sense of trust and security. The major contribution to his emotional contentment is probably made at mealtimes, and perhaps in a special way if he is breast-fed.

For most infants, food comes to be identified with love, pleasure, protection, and the satisfaction of basic needs. If there is an atmosphere of tension accompanying his feeding times, his digestion can be impaired in such a way as to cause vomiting, fretting, or signs of colic. If the tension and the baby's reaction to it—and inevitably the mother's increasing tension as a consequence—become a chronic condition, the result may be a failure to gain weight normally, and in extreme cases, some degree of mental retardation. Throughout life, good nutrition depends not only on eating properly balanced meals that satisfy the body's physiological requirements, but also on a reasonable degree of contentment and relaxation while eating.

Everybody develops individual emotional reactions and attitudes about food and its role as a result of conditioning during the years of infancy and childhood. These attitudes relate not only to food itself and to mealtimes in general, but also to other aspects of eating, including the muscle activities of sucking, chewing, and swallowing.

If food symbolized contentment during the early years, it probably will have the same role later on. If it was associated with conflict, then it may be associated throughout life with strife and neurotic eating patterns.

During Childhood

For the preschool child, mealtimes should provide the occasion for the development of interpersonal relationships, because they are a daily opportunity for both verbal and nonverbal self-expression. The child who eats with enthusiasm and obvious enjoyment is conveying one message; the one who dawdles, picks at food, and challenges his mother with every mouthful is conveying quite a different one.

Meals can become either positive or negative experiences depending in large part on how the adults in the family set the stage. Communication can be encouraged by relaxed conversation and a reasonably leisurely schedule. It can be discouraged by watching television or reading while eating, by not eating together, or by eating and running.

Reasonably firm attitudes about eating a variety of foods in proper quantities at proper times and avoiding excessive catering to individual whims can also help in the development of wholesome eating patterns.

Those who select and prepare the food can transmit special messages of love and affection by serving favorite dishes, by setting the table attractively, and by creating an atmosphere of grace and good humor. Or they can show displeasure and generate hostility by complaining about all the work involved in feeding everyone, or by constant criticism of table manners, or by bringing up touchy subjects likely to cause arguments at the table.

Diet Fads

There are many fads and fallacies about losing weight. Everyone wants an easy solution; cosmetic and food product manufacturers know this and develop products that play to this desire. Thus we have pills that are supposed to burn fat while we sleep; machines that are supposed to give us a "workout" while we're lying down by electrically stimulating our muscles; plastic suits that we wear while exercising that are supposed to produce dramatic weight loss; and special creams and body scrubbers that are supposed to take away unsightly cellulite.

The truth is that a pill will not burn calories for you, a machine will not do your exercise for you, a plastic suit will only make you lose water, not fat, and the idea that there is a special kind of fat called cellulite is a myth.

Cellulite, in fact, is fat, plain and simple; there are no special varieties. Much of the body's fat is stored directly beneath the skin where there is also a sheath of connective tissue, which tends to compartmentalize the fat cells. The more fat the more this tissue is stretched and the more the fat bulges around and through it, producing cellulite's characteristic dimpled effect. Women tend to have thinner skin and less flexible connective tissue, making them more "prone" to cellulite than men. There is no point in spending money on special creams or brushes; you cannot scrub away excess fat. You have to reduce your intake and burn it through exercise.

Similarly, most diet programs that consist of pills, powders, or foolish eating habits are ineffective and usually harmful. Many of them are addictive and those who benefit from the diet programs often gain back the weight lost once they return to their "normal" eating habits.

One controversial drug that appears frequently in pills is phenylpropanolamine hydrochloride (PPA). Producers of PPA claim that it acts as an appetite suppressant, though its effectiveness is questionable.

Taken in large doses, its effects resemble those of amphetamines. It can produce such side effects as anxiety, sleeplessness, headaches, irregular heart rhythm, and even lead to strokes or seizures.

Another diet drug, benzocaine, is present in chewing gum and candy. It deadens taste receptors, which supposedly suppresses one's appetite. It does not, however, stop the habit of munching, which is a great cause of weight gain.

Guar gum is another diet substance that gives the dieter a sense of fullness. It is a vegetable gum that swells when it absorbs moisture. When

FOODS TO AVOID	FOODS TO EAT
High saturated fat percentages	Low or no saturated fat
Avocado 15-20%	Apples 0%
Biscuits 23%	Apricots 0%
Bread stuffing 25%	Cherries 0%
Sweet rolls 27 + %	Cranberry sauce 0%
Fried chicken 27%	Fruit 0%
Bran muffins 30%	Fruit juices 0%
Veal 30-50%	Herbs 0%
Chicken livers 33%	Peaches 0%
Ham 33%	Plums 0%
Lunch meats 35 + %	Rice, plain 0%
Duck 35%	Split peas 0%
Pancakes 35%	Vegetables, raw or steamed 0%
Pork 35%	Squid 1%
Beef brisket 40%	Cornmeal 10%
Ground beef 40%	Popcorn, plain 12%
Hotdogs 40%	Sweet and sour sauce 12%
Lamb 40-50%	Teriyaki sauce 14%
Rib roast 42%	Spaghetti, no egg 15%
Gravy 50 + %	Halibut 17%
Custard 50%	Chestnuts 19%
Cheese 50-80%	Salmon 19%
Cream 60%	Carp 20%
Ice cream 60 + %	Perch 20%
Beef heart 80%	Abalone 21%
Coconut 88%	Clams 21%
Cream substitute 90 + %	Trout 22%
Sour cream 91%	Octopus 27%

NOTE: The same percentage number may appear in both columns; the determining factor is then the grams of fat in each item. The left column has more grams of fat, even if the percentage is the same for an item in the right column.

taken improperly, it can swell in the throat and cause an obstruction, resulting in suffocation. At least 1 death and 50 injuries have been reported as a result of ingesting guar gum diet products.

Anybody interested in losing a substantial amount of weight should consult with his or her physician. The physician will know of a nutritionist who can provide a healthy program for weight reduction. If a person chooses to try one of the over-the-counter diet programs, read the directions carefully.

Weight loss involves a complete change in one's lifestyle. The solution includes eating balanced meals, reducing the intake of fat, increasing proportionately the consumption of carbohydrates, and exercising three or four times a week. It is a slow process that does not offer the quick yet temporary loss offered by over-the-counter diet programs. Rather, it is a permanent commitment to a healthy way of life. Only then, can a person maintain an optimal weight.

28

Mental and Emotional Disorders

The ability to adapt is central to being emotionally fit, healthy, and mature. An emotionally fit person is one who can adapt to changing circumstances with constructive reactions and who can enjoy living, loving others, and working productively. In everyone's life there are bound to be experiences that are anxious or deeply disturbing, such as the sad-ness of losing a loved one or the disappointment of failure. The emotionally fit person is stable enough not to be overwhelmed by the anxiety, grief, or guilt that such experiences frequently produce. His sense of his own worth is not lost easily by a setback in life; rather, he can learn from his own mistakes.

Communication and Tolerance

Even the most unpleasant experiences can add to one's understanding of life. Emerging from a crisis with new wisdom can give a sense of pride and mastery. The emotionally fit person can listen attentively to the opinions of others, yet if his decision differs from that being urged by friends and relatives, he will abide by it and can stand alone if necessary, without guilt and anger at those who disagree.

Communicating well with others is an important part of emotional fitness. Sharing experiences, both good and bad, is one of the joys of living. Although the capacity to enjoy is often increased by such sharing, independence is also essential, for one person's pleasure may leave others indifferent. It is just as important to appreciate and respect the individuality of others as it is to value our own individual preferences, as long as these are reasonable and do not give pain to others.

Ways of Expressing Disagreement

Communication should be kept open at all times. Anger toward those who disagree may be an immediate response, but it should not lead to cutting off communication, as it so frequently does, particularly between husbands and wives, parents and children.

Emotional maturity enables us to disagree with what another says, feels, or does, yet make the distinction between that person and how we feel about his thoughts and actions. To tell someone, "I don't like what you are doing," is more likely to keep the lines of communication open than telling him "I don't like you." This is particularly important between parents and children.

It is unfortunately common for parents to launch personal attacks when children do something that displeases them. The child, or any person to whom this is done, then feels unworthy or rejected, which often makes him angry and defiant. Revenge becomes uppermost, and communication is lost; each party feels misunderstood and lonely, perhaps even wounded, and is not likely to want to reopen communication. The joy in a human relationship is gone, and one's pleasure in living is by that much diminished.

Function of Guilt

The same principles used in dealing with others can be applied to ourselves. Everyone makes mistakes, has angry or even murderous thoughts that can produce excessive guilt. Sometimes there is a realistic reason for feeling guilty, which should be a spur to take corrective action.

Differentiate clearly between thoughts, feelings, and actions. Only actions need cause guilt. In the privacy of one's own mind, anything may be thought as long as it is not acted out; an emotionally fit person can accept this difference.

Role of the Subconscious

Emotional disorders are similar to other medical diseases and can be treated by physicians or other professionals just as any other disease can be treated. Fortunately, this truth is widely accepted today, but as recently as 200 years ago it was believed that the emotionally ill were evil, possessed by the devil. Their illness was punished rather than treated. The strange and sometimes bizarre actions of the mentally ill were feared and misunderstood.

Freud and Psychoanalysis

Although we have penetrated many of the mysteries of the mind, much remains to be discovered. Significant steps toward understanding mental functioning came about through the work of Sigmund Freud. Building upon the work of others before him and making his own detailed observations, Freud demonstrated that there is a subconscious part of the mind which functions without our awareness.

He taught that mental illness resulting from subconscious memories could be cured by *psychoanalysis,* which brings the memories out into consciousness. He believed that dreams are a major key to the subconscious mind and that thoughts, dreams, fantasies, and abnormal fears follow the rules of cause and effect and are not random. This is called *psychic determinism,* meaning that emotional disorders can be understood by exploring the subconscious. *Psychiatrists* help the patient understand how his mind works and why it works that way—often the first step toward a cure.

Does psychic determinism rule out will power as a function of the mind? No, because the subconscious is only one part of the mind. Although it has an important influence, there are other forces influencing behavior and thought: the *id,* or instinctive force, the *superego,* or conscience, and the *ego,* or decision-maker. The more we know about how our minds work, what underlies our wishes and thoughts, the more control we can exercise in choosing how to behave in order to achieve our goals.

Role of Sexuality

Freud discovered that young children and even babies are aware of the sensations, pleasurable and painful, that can be experienced from all parts of the body. The sexual organs have a rich supply of nerves; the baby receives pleasure when these organs are touched, for example, during a bath or a diaper change. The child learns that when he touches these organs he obtains a pleasant feeling; therefore he repeatedly touches and rubs them (*infantile masturbation*).

This concept, that the child derives pleasure from his body and sex organs, is called *infantile sexuality.* It does not mean that the baby has adult sexual ideas or wishes. These do not develop until puberty. It does mean that parents have the responsibility to see to it that children learn early that sex is associated with tenderness and love between man and woman. Even young children are aware of what their parents do and how they treat each other.

Types of Mental Illness

Although there is considerable disagreement about the classification of mental disorders, a convenient system used by many doctors divides mental illnesses into two general categories, organic and functional.

Some types of mental illness show little or no evidence of changes in brain tissue: these are called *functional* disorders. Another group of mental illnesses does involve some definable impairment of brain tissue resulting from disease, injury, the introduction of poisonous substances, malfunction of the body's metabolic processes, nutritional problems, or inherited defects. These are *organic* disorders. Organic brain damage may be *congenital*—that is, existing at or prior to birth—or *acquired.* Examples of congenital defects are *hydrocephalus,* an accumulation of fluid within the skull of a newborn infant that destroys brain tissue; *phenylketonuria* (PKU), a type of mental retardation associated with an inability of the child's body to metabolize a protein substance; and *Down's syndrome* (also called *Mongolism*), a form of retardation that occurs more frequently in children of older mothers and which is marked by certain physical features such as eyes that resemble those of Oriental people. Some examples of acquired defects are cerebrovascular accidents such as stroke; injuries to the brain, as from a fall or from the introduction of poisonous substances such as lead, arsenic, or mercury; and arteriosclerosis, resulting in senile psychosis in aged people.

This chapter will deal only with functional illness. Organic disorders are treated in the chapters on diseases of particular systems of the body and often in other sections as well. If you are in doubt about where to find information about a particular disorder, consult the index.

Who Is Mentally Ill?

Most people occasionally experience spells of anxiety, blue moods, or temper tantrums, but unless the psychological suffering they endure or inflict upon others begins to interfere with their job or marriage, they seldom seek professional guidance. There is no exacting scientific standard for determining when an eccentric pattern of behavior becomes a mental illness. Norms vary from culture to culture and within each culture, and, as every student of history and every parent know, norms also change from generation to generation.

Just how can a determination be made as to who is mentally ill? No temperature reading, no acute pain, no abnormal growth can be looked for as evidence of a serious problem. Yet there are warning signs, and among the common ones are these:

- Anxiety that is severe, prolonged, and unrelated to any identifiable reason or cause

- Depression, especially when it is followed by withdrawal from loved ones, from friends, or from the usual occupations or hobbies that ordinarily afford one pleasure

- Loss of confidence in oneself

- Undue pessimism

- A feeling of constant helplessness

- Uncalled for or unexplainable mood changes—for example, an abrupt switch from happiness to unhappiness when nothing has happened to warrant it

- Rudeness or aggression that is without apparent cause or which is occasioned by some trivial incident

- An unreasonable demand for perfectionism, not only in oneself but in one's loved ones, friends, busi-ness associates, and even from things or situations

- Habitual underachievement, especially if one is adequately equipped to do the work one is called upon to perform

- The inability to accept responsibility, often manifested by a recurrent loss of employment

- Phobias

- Unreasonable feelings of persecution

- Self-destructive acts

- Sexual deviation

- A sudden and dramatic change in sleeping habits

- Physical ailments and complaints for which there are no organic causes

If one or more of these warning signs occur frequently or in severe form, a mental illness may be present, and professional help should be sought to evaluate the underlying problem.

Types of Functional Mental Illness

Functional mental disorders may be broken down into four general categories: neuroses; psychophysiologi-cal (or psychosomatic) disorders; personality or character disorders; and psychoses.

Neurosis

A *neurosis* (or *psychoneurosis*) is characterized primarily by emotional rather than physical symptoms—although physical symptoms may be present. The neuroses are usually categorized according to the type of reaction that the patient exhibits in his attempt to resolve the underlying emotional conflict. All of them involve anxiety as a prominent symptom.

Anxiety Reaction

The *anxiety reaction* is probably the most widespread of all the neurotic response patterns. Although, as noted above, all the neuroses share anxiety as a symptom, the most common and outstanding characteristic of the anxiety reaction is a feeling of dread or apprehension that is not related to any apparent cause. The anxiety is caused by conflicts of which the patient himself is unaware but which may be stimulated by thoughts or events in his present life. For example, the junior executive who is constantly apprehensive that his employer will ridicule his work and dismiss his ideas may be expressing an anxiety reaction to a childhood fear that equated ridicule with abandonment or mutilation.

While anxiety reaction symptoms are primarily mental or emotional—the patient feels inadequate or ineffectual, or behaves irrationally—anxiety is always accompanied by physiological changes such as sweating and heart palpitations. Fatigue and feelings of panic are also common symptoms.

Conversion Reaction

The *conversion reaction* (or *conversion hysteria*) describes a type of neurotic behavior in which the patient, instead of coming to grips with his underlying psychic conflict, manages to convert it into physical symptoms involving functions over which he ordinarily exerts complete control. Sometimes the physical symptoms are unimportant, but often they are markedly dramatic. For example, the soldier who becomes deaf to the sound of explosions even though there is no organic defect that would account for a loss of hearing has effectively obliterated a sensation that evokes associations too painful to acknowledge.

Obsessive-Compulsive Reaction

A person beset by persistent, unwanted ideas or feelings (*obsessions*), who is impelled to carry out certain acts (*compulsions*) ritualistically, no matter how irrational they are, is reacting to a psychic conflict in an *ob-

sessive-compulsive manner. The obsession may involve a feeling of violence or sexuality directed toward a member of his own family. Usually the feeling will never lead to any overt action of the type imagined, but the idea is nevertheless persistent and painful.

Obsessive-compulsive patients are typically exceptionally meticulous and conscientious, often intelligent and gifted in their work. But they expend an enormous amount of energy and time in observing compulsive acts. For example, they may take a dozen or more showers every day because they are obsessed with the idea that they are dirty or carrying a contagious disease. By performing an apparently harmless compulsive act, the patient is temporarily relieved of the obsession.

Depressive Reaction

Most people have blue moods from time to time in their lives. Indeed, when faced with a personal tragedy like the death of a loved one, a normal healthy individual may well undergo a period of depression. A person suffering from the *depressive reaction,* however, has persistent feelings of worthlessness and pessimism unrelated to events that might depress a normal person. An inability to cope with problem situations is gradually magnified into an inability to cope with anything at all. Attempts to mask the crisis by putting on a "front"—feigning cheerfulness and optimism—give way to episodes of total hopelessness. Suicide is often considered and sometimes attempted. Threats of suicide from a depressed person should always be regarded seriously.

Common physical symptoms accompanying depression are fatigue, loss of appetite, and insomnia.

Phobic Reaction

A *phobic reaction* is the result of an individual's attempt to deal with an anxiety-producing conflict, not by facing up to the actual source of that conflict but by avoiding something else. The substitute—whether it be an animal, closed places, or whatever—is responded to with the intense anxiety that is really felt for the true source of anxiety. This process is known as *displacement,* and the irrational fears or dreads are known as *phobias.*

Thus, a person who had been regularly punished as a child by having been forcibly confined in a closet might be unable to deal with the anxiety of the experience consciously. The anxiety might be displaced and emerge later in life in the form of terror of crowded or confined places—*claustrophobia.*

Phobias can involve almost anything one encounters in life—including things that go on in one's body and one's mind. Some of the most common phobias have to do with disease—*bacteriophobia*, for example, the fear of germs.

Scores of phobias exist, ranging alphabetically from *acrophobia*, the fear of heights, to *xenophobia*, the fear of strangers. Other well-known examples are *ailurophobia*, the fear of cats; *cynophobia*, the fear of dogs; *algophobia*, the fear of pain; *agoraphobia*, the fear of open spaces; *erythrophobia*, the fear of blushing; *mysophobia*, the fear of dirt and contamination; *nyctophobia*, the fear of the dark; and *lyssophobia*, the fear of rabies.

Dissociative Reaction

The *dissociative reaction* involves a basic disruption of the patient's personality. The dissociative reaction permits a person to escape from a part of his personality associated with intolerable anxiety. The escape is made in various ways: by forgetfulness or absent-mindedness, dream states (including sleepwalking), amnesia, and—most seriously—the adoption of multiple personalities, in which the patient behaves like one person at certain times and like an altogether different person at other times.

Psychophysiological Disorders

It has been estimated that one-half or more of the patients of a general practitioner either do not have any organic illness or do not have any organic disease that could account for the severity or extent of the symptoms described. These patients are obviously not inventing their symptoms. The symptoms—whether they be itching, constipation, asthma, or heart palpitations—are real enough. But in many cases they are either wholly or partly of psychological origin—*psychogenic* is the medical term.

The psychological and physiological aspects of humans are so closely interwoven that the problem of *psychophysiological* (or *psychosomatic*) disorders must be considered with attention to both aspects. Consider how many physiological changes in normal people can be induced by psychological states: sweating, blushing, gooseflesh, sexual arousal, weeping, the feeling of "a lump in the throat," etc. It should hardly be surprising, then, that when someone has a physical illness there are profound concomitant psychological factors that can materially affect the physiological disease.

In many cases, however, as noted above, there is no detectable organic disease. Anxiety and other disturbing emotions such as rage are sometimes dealt with by the individual by constructing a pattern of defense that involves physiological reactions. Confronted with an emotional conflict that cannot be handled consciously, the individual may channel his feelings inward and deal with it by the formation of troublesome physical symptoms. It must be stressed that this strategy is not consciously engineered by the patient and that the symptoms are genuinely experienced.

Psychophysiological disorders affect many parts of the body, but certain organs and tissues seem more vulnerable than others. The digestive tract, for example, is frequently beset by disorders that are psychophysiological, including diarrhea, constipation, regional enteritis (inflammation of the intestine), ulcerative colitis (ulcers and inflammation of the colon), and peptic ulcers. Hypertension is frequently associated with psychogenic causes. Muscle cramps, recurrent stiff necks, arthritis, backaches, and tension headaches are other common complaints. Many skin conditions such as hives and eczema can be triggered by or are aggravated by psychological factors.

The symptoms of a psychophysiological illness appear to have no logical relation to the conflict that is responsible for them, nor do they relieve the underlying anxiety.

Personality or Character Disorders

Another group of mental illnesses is the *personality* or *character disorders,* so called because they appear to stem from a kind of defect in or arrested development of the personality. Unlike neurotic patients, individuals with personality disorders do not especially suffer from anxiety, nor is their behavior markedly eccentric. But when observed over a period of time, the personality problem becomes evident.

Personality disorders fall into various categories including:

● The *passive-dependent* individual needs excessive emotional support and reassurance from an authority figure.

● The *schizoid* individual is withdrawn from and indifferent to other people.

● The *paranoid* individual is exqui-sitely sensitive to praise or criticism and often suspicious of expressed or implied attitudes toward him, and often is subject to feelings of persecution.

● The *cyclothymic* (or *cycloid*) individual is subject to sharply defined moods of elation or depression, seemingly without relation to external circumstances.

● The *sociopathic* individual is characteristically lacking in a sense of personal responsibility or of morality. Formerly called the *psychopathic* personality, the sociopath may be disposed to aggressive, hostile, sometimes violent behavior and frequently engages in self-destructive behavior such as alcoholism or addiction to drugs. Sociopathic behavior also includes sexual deviation.

Psychosis

The chief distinction between *psychosis* and neurosis is that a psychosis represents a more complete disintegration of personality and a loss of contact with the outside world. The psychotic is therefore unable to form relationships with people. Most people who suffer from nonpsychotic mental disorders are seldom, if ever, hospitalized, and then usually for very brief periods. But many psychotics are so crippled by their illness that they are hospitalized repeatedly or for protracted periods of time.

Schizophrenic Reaction

Schizophrenia, the most common and destructive of the psychotic reactions, is characterized by withdrawal from external reality, inability to think clearly, disturbances in affective reaction (capacity to feel and express emotion), and a retreat into a fantasy life—all of these resulting in a progressive deterioration of the patient's ordinary behavioral patterns.

Simple Schizophrenia

The patient with *simple schizophrenia* experiences a gradual loss of concern and contact with other people, and a lessening of the motivation needed to perform the routine activities of everyday life. There may be some personality deterioration, but the presence of hallucinations and delusions is rare.

Hebephrenic Schizophrenia

This form of schizophrenia is marked by delusions, hallucinations, and regressed behavior. Hebephrenics babble and giggle, and often react in inappropriately childish ways. Their silly manner can make them seem happier than other schizophrenics, but this disorder often results in severe personality disintegration— more severe, in fact, than in other types of schizophrenia.

Catatonic Schizophrenia

In *catatonic schizophrenia* there are dramatic disturbances of the motor functions. Patients may remain in a fixed position for hours, days, or even weeks. During this time their muscles may be rigid, their limbs held in awkward positions. They may have to be fed, and their urinary and bowel functions may be abnormal. This stuporous state may be varied by an occasional period of frenzied but purposeless excitement.

Paranoid Schizophrenia

The *paranoid schizophrenic* is preoccupied with variable delusions of persecution or grandeur. Men working with pneumatic drills on the street, for example, are really sending out supersonic beams designed to destroy his brain cells; the water supply is being poisoned by visitors from other planets; any mechanical malfunction, as of a telephone or an elevator, is part of a deliberate plot of harassment or intimidation.

Paranoid schizophrenia is often marked by the presence of hallucinations, by disturbances in mental processes, and by behavioral deterioration. The disorder is regarded as particularly serious—hard to deal with and likely to become permanent.

Paranoid Reaction

The patient with this disorder suffers from delusions, usually of persecution, sometimes of grandeur. In this respect, *paranoia* is very similar to paranoid schizophrenia. However, in paranoid schizophrenia the delusions are often variable, and usually there is a breakdown of the patient's behavioral patterns.

A case of true paranoia, by contrast, is characterized by an invariable delusion around which the patient constructs and adheres to a highly systematized pattern of behavior. When the delusion is of such a nature that its persistence does not engender a conflict between the patient and his surrounding social structure, the patient may never be suspected of mental illness, perhaps merely of eccentricity. If, however, the delusion does provoke conflict, the patient may react with destructive hostility, and hospitalization or some other kind of professional treatment will be necessary.

Manic-Depressive Reaction

This disorder, also called an *affective reaction,* is characterized by two phases—*mania* and *depression.* Patients are governed by one phase or another or by the alternation of both.

The manic phase may be mild and bring elation and a general stepping up of all kinds of activity. The patient tends to talk endlessly and in an associative rather than a logical way. If the disorder is more severe, he may act or dress bizarrely; he may be a whirlwind of activity and become so excited and agitated that he foregoes food and sleep and ends in a state of total collapse.

In a mild depressive phase, the individual feels dull and melancholy, his confidence begins to drain away, and he becomes easily fatigued by daily routines. When the depressive phase is more severe, the patient starts to retreat from reality, gradually entering into a state of withdrawal that is very much like a stupor. At this point he hardly moves or speaks. He may be unable to sleep. Eventually he begins to question his value as a human being and is crushed by feelings of guilt. He may refuse to eat. Symptoms may progress to the point where an attempt at suicide is a real possibility.

Although the manic-depressive psychosis may alternate from one of its phases to the other, one or the other phase is usually dominant for a prolonged period of time. Depression is more often dominant than mania. Manic-depressive patients often recover spontaneously for periods of time, but relapses are fairly common.

Depressive Reaction

The *depressive reaction* is a disorder connected with aging and its attendant changes in sexual functioning; it usually occurs at the time of the menopause in women, in the middle or late 40s, and somewhat later in men. Formerly called *involutional melancholia,* it is characterized, as that name suggests, by a sense of hopeless melancholy and despair.

Patients begin to feel that life has passed them by. They experience real physical symptoms such as loss of vigor, and develop various hypochondriacal complaints. Their interests become narrower, and they begin to retreat from the world.

As the melancholy deepens, there are periods of senseless weeping, bouts of intense anxiety, feelings of worthlessness, and growing concern—coupled with delusions—about dying and death. The depth of the depression is overwhelming, and the danger of suicide greater than in any other psychosis.

Treatment of Emotional Problems and Mental Disorders

When should help be sought for an emotional problem? Sometimes individuals themselves realize that they need help and seek it without urging. They may have symptoms such as anxiety, depression, or troublesome thoughts that they cannot put out of their mind. But many others who need help do not know it or do not want to know that they need it. They usually have symptoms that disturb others rather than themselves, such as irritability, impulsive behavior, or excessive use of drugs or alcohol that interferes with their family relationships and work responsibilities.

Other people in need of psychological guidance are those who have a physical disease that is based on psychological factors. They react to stress internally rather than externally. Instead of displaying anger, they feel it inside. We are all familiar with headaches or heartburn caused by tension; more serious diseases clearly associated with emotional factors are asthma, certain skin disorders, ulcerative colitis, essential hypertension, hyperthyroidism, and peptic ulcer. Other physical symptoms that may be related to psychological factors are some types of paralysis, blindness, and loss of memory.

In all these situations the patient's enjoyment of life is curtailed. He has no feeling of control over what he does and little or no tolerance for himself and others. Such an existence is completely unnecessary today, with the many agencies and specialists capable of effectively treating these problems.

Mental Health Professionals

Who can help those with emotional problems? Confusion about the different professions in the mental health field is understandable. To add to the muddle, self-appointed counselors without professional training and experience have set themselves up in this field, so it is necessary to know whom to consult to obtain the best help possible.

Psychiatrists

Psychiatrists are medical doctors; that is, they have graduated from a medical school, served internships and afterwards residencies specializing in emotional disorders. They are specialists in the same way that a surgeon or an eye doctor is a specialist. Most are members of the American Psychiatric Association. They are experienced in treating medical illnesses, having done so for many years before being certified as specialists in emotional disorders. Generally they can be relied upon to adhere to the ethical and professional standards of the medical field.

The American Psychiatric Association, 1400 K St., N.W., Washington, D.C. 20005, can supply the names of members. The American Board of Psychiatry and Neurology, One American Plaza, Suite 800, Evanston, Illinois 60201, examines and certifies psychiatrists who pass its tests, so that the term "board certified" means that the psychiatrist has passed its tests. If a family physician is consulted about an emotional problem, he will often refer the patient to a psychiatrist, just as he would to any other specialist.

Psychologists

Psychologists have gone to college, majored in psychology, and most often have advanced degrees, for example, a doctorate in psychology. They are not medical doctors and may get a degree in psychology without ever working with a human being, e.g., by working in animal behavior, experimental psychology, or other fields. They may or may not have clinical training, but many acquire this training and experience with human beings. There is no guarantee that a psychologist has this background, however, without looking into the qualifications of each individual.

Psychotherapists

Psychotherapy is the general term for any treatment that tries to effect a cure by psychological rather than physical means. A psychotherapist may be a psychiatrist, or he may be a psychologist, or may have no training at all. Anyone can set up an office and call himself a psychotherapist, psychoanalyst, marriage counselor, family therapist, or anything else he desires. It is up to the patient to check on the training and background of a therapist. Any reputable therapist should be pleased to tell patients his credentials and qualifications for helping them. A psychoanalyst, for example, may be a psychiatrist with several years of additional training in psychoanalysis, or may be someone whose qualifications consist of a few college psychology courses.

Social Workers

Social workers are another group of trained persons who may also counsel those with emotional problems. They may work either with individuals, families, or groups after meeting the educational requirements for the profession, which include a bachelor's degree and two years of professional training leading to a master's degree in social work.

Professionals should be associated with recognized groups of their peers, or perhaps with a medical center or hospital. Generally a person with emotional problems should consult a psychiatrist first, who will then either treat the problem or be in a good position to advise what is necessary and who can best be available for treatment.

Types of Therapy

Functional mental illnesses are treated by a variety of tools, among them psychotherapy and chemotherapy (treatment with drugs).

Psychotherapy

As noted above, psychotherapy applies to various forms of treatment that employ psychological methods designed to help patients understand themselves. With this knowledge, or insight, the patient learns how to handle his life—with all its relationships and conflicts—in a happier and more socially responsible manner.

The best known form of psychotherapy is psychoanalysis, developed by Freud but modified by many others, which seeks to lift to the level of awareness the patient's repressed subconscious feelings. The information about subconscious conflicts is explored and interpreted to explain the causes of the patient's emotional upsets.

The technique employs a series of steps beginning with *free association,* in which the patient is encouraged to discuss anything that comes to mind, including things that the patient might be reluctant to discuss with anyone else but the analyst. Other steps include dream analysis and *transference,* which is the redirection to the analyst of repressed childhood emotions.

Group therapy is a form of therapeutic treatment in which a group of approximately six to ten patients, usually under the guidance of a therapist, participate in discussions of their mental and emotional problems.

The therapist may establish the direction of the discussion or may remain mostly silent, allowing the patients' interaction to bring about the special cathartic benefits of this technique.

Family therapy is much like group therapy, with an individual family functioning as a group. It is felt that the family members may be better able to discuss the problems of relating to each other within the context of a group than they would be on an individual basis with a therapist.

Psychodrama is a therapeutic technique in which a patient or a group of patients act out situations centered about their personal conflicts. The psychodrama is "performed" in the presence of a therapist and, sometimes, other people.

Children are sometimes enrolled in programs of *play therapy* in which dolls, doll houses, and other appropriate toys are made available so that they can express their frustrations, hostilities, and other feelings through play. This activity, carried on under the observation of a therapist, is considered a form of catharsis in that it often prevents the repression of hostile emotions. In the case of a maladjusted child, it can also act as a helpful diagnostic tool—revealing the source of the child's emotional problem.

Chemotherapy

The relationship between body chemistry and mental illness has been studied for over half a century. The result of this study is the therapeutic technique known as *chemotherapy,* the treatment of disease with drugs or chemicals.

Early Uses of Chemical Agents

Sedatives to provide treatment of mental diseases were used during World War I for soldiers suffering from shell shock. *Sodium amytal,* one of the early chemicals used, offered a prolonged restful sleep, after which the army patients could tolerate some form of psychotherapeutic treatment.

In the 1930s, physicians introduced *insulin shock therapy* as a method for treating psychotic patients. The patients received injections of insulin in doses large enough to produce a deep coma, after which they were revived by doses of sugar. As with the use of sodium amytal, the insulin treatment was accompanied by psychotherapy for most effective results.

Present-Day Uses of Chemical Agents

More recently, the control of mental illness has taken a giant step forward with the development of *tranquilizers* and *antidepressants.* Tranquilizers counteract anxiety, tension, and overexcitement; they are used to calm patients whose behavior is dangerously confused or disturbed. Antidepressants help to stimulate the physiological activity of depressed patients, thereby tending to relieve the sluggishness that attends depression.

The treatment of the manic-depressive psychosis has been facilitated with the use of salts derived from lithium, a metal. Lithium salts seem to control the disease without producing the undesirable emotional and intellectual effects that resulted from the previous treatment with tranquilizers and antidepressants. The medication has been found to be particularly effective in treating patients with frequent manic episodes; it is also said to be effective as a preventive measure against future manifestations of mania or depression. Lithium may have adverse side effects and must be administered carefully.

Chemotherapy does not usually cure mental illness. It does, however, improve the patient's mental state, thereby enabling him to cope more effectively with the problems of everyday life.

Electroshock Treatment

Electroshock is a form of therapy in which a carefully regulated electric current is passed through a patient's head, thereby producing convulsions and unconsciousness.

Electroshock is primarily a treatment for the manic-depressive psychosis; to a lesser extent the therapy is used on schizophrenic patients. It often shortens depressed periods, and sometimes the patient seems totally free of the symptoms of his disorder. Unfortunately, the remission may be temporary; electroshock does not prevent further attacks. Also, transitory memory impairment often occurs.

Because of the recent advances in the techniques of chemotherapy, electroshock is used much less frequently than it was in the past.

Facilities Available for the Mentally Ill

The last decade has seen a number of hopeful changes in the facilities for treatment of mental disorders in the United States. The great majority of severely ill mental patients used to be cared for in county or state mental hospitals, many of which were crowded and able to offer custodial care but very little in the way of therapeutic programs. The picture has changed, however, and the extent and quality of care in these hospitals is expanding and improving.

Patients with mental illnesses are also being treated in greater numbers at general hospitals. As a matter of fact, more patients who need hospitalization for such illnesses are being admitted to general hospitals than to public mental hospitals.

Treatment for the mentally or emotionally disturbed is also provided in other facilities, including private mental hospitals, mental health clinics, and various social agencies.

Among the new facilities for treating mental illness is one which permits many patients who would formerly have been hospitalized, perhaps for the rest of their lives, to be served by community mental health centers. These centers offer both inpatient and outpatient care. The services they provide go beyond diagnosis and treatment to include rehabilitation, thus making it possible for more and more of today's mental patients to live at home, function in a job situation, and be a part of their own community.

Results of Treatment

What can be expected from treatment? Does a person who has been through treatment emerge bland, uncaring about others, with absolutely no problems, and without guilt for his misdeeds? Absolutely not. What treatment can do, said Freud, is to change neurotic misery into common unhappiness. There will always be things in life that are disappointing or otherwise upsetting. No treatment can eliminate such problems. After successful treatment, however, one should be better able to handle these stresses with flexible and constructive responses and to see his own difficulties in relation to the problems of others.

To feel emotionally fit is to have a capacity for enjoying life, working well, and loving others. Fear, shame, and guilt about undergoing needed treatment should not prevent anyone from reaching that potential.

29

Substance Abuse

"Drug-Related Deaths up 59%." "Driving-and-Drinking Accident Claims 5 Lives." "Teen Drug Abuse—The News Is Bad."

The headlines tell a story with a moral, or lesson. The lesson is that the United States has a major health and social problem. Once called by a number of names, including *alcoholism, drug addiction,* and *drug abuse,* the problem today goes by the designation *substance abuse.* In this usage, the phrase applies to all forms of addiction or abuse, whether the substance is alcohol or such vegetation-derived drugs as marijuana, cocaine, and heroin.

In a broad sense, substances include any material aside from food that can be imbibed, injected, or taken into the body in any way and that changes or affects the body or mind. This definition covers aspirin,

many medications, tobacco, and a broad range of other substances. But *substance abuse* refers to unhealthy or excessive use of any material, alcohol, or addictive drugs at an individual's discretion and not according to a physician's prescription.

The dimensions of the substance-abuse problem are almost incalculable. Americans in 1986 spent an estimated $110 billion on addictive drugs alone. At least 40 percent of all Americans between the ages of 18 and 25 had experimented with one or more illegal substances. As one authority wrote,

Not only the poor, the uneducated, the deprived, or the shadow types are being destroyed. We're dealing with the privileged, the successful, the professional.

Alcohol Abuse

Alcohol abuse is not unique to the United States or to the twentieth century. Alcoholic beverages, and their use or abuse, have an ancient history.

Long before humans began to keep records of any kind, these beverages were valued as food, medicine, and ceremonial drinks. When people today have a beer with dinner, or toast newlyweds with champagne, or share wine at a religious ritual or festival, they are continuing traditions that have deep roots in the past.

The consumption of alcoholic beverages has always been a fact of life. So has, in a sense, alcohol abuse. The immigrants who came to the United States brought their ethnic ceremonies and drinking habits with them. The frontiersmen who moved continually west found liquor to be a source of release and comfort. Inevitably, alcohol use and abuse occurred.

Most drinkers have been, and are, able to control what they are doing and are none the worse for the habit. However, of the estimated 100 million drinkers in the United States, about 10 million have some kind of problem with alcohol: they are *alcohol abusers.* The 10 million alcoholics cost the economy some $60 billion annually. Drunken drivers are implicated in about half of the nearly 50,000 traffic deaths occurring yearly.

Scientists have come to believe that habitual alcohol abuse is a disease and should be treated as such. In 1956, the American Medical Association officially termed alcoholism an illness and a medical responsibility.

Kinds of Alcohol

The alcohol in beverages is chemically known as *ethyl alcohol.* It is often called *grain alcohol.* It is produced by the natural process of *fermentation:* When certain foods such as honey, fruits, grains, or their juices remain in a warm place, airborne yeast organisms begin to change the sugars and starches in these foods into alcohol. Ethyl alcohol is in itself a food in the sense that its caloric content produces energy in the body, but it contains practically no essential nutriments.

Methyl alcohol, also called *wood alcohol,* because it is obtained by the dry distillation of maple, birch, and beech, is useful as a fuel and solvent. It is poisonous if taken internally and can cause blindness and death. Other members of the same family of chemicals, such as *isopropyl alcohol,* are also used as rubbing alcohols—as cooling agents and skin disinfectants—and are also poisonous if taken internally.

Present-Day Drinking Trends

On a per capita basis, Americans drink twice as much wine and beer as they did a century ago, and half as much distilled spirits. Where the drinking takes place has also changed. There is less hard drinking in saloons and more social drinking at home and in clubs. The acceptance of drinking in mixed company has made it more a part of social situations than it used to be.

Here are some facts about the current consumption of alcoholic beverages in the United States:

- Drinking is more common among men than among women, but the gap is closing.

- It is more common among people who are under 40.

- It is more common among the well-to-do than among the poor.

- Beyond the age of 45, the number of drinkers steadily declines.

Teenagers and Alcohol

One fact emerges clearly and consistently from all the surveys of teenage drinking in all parts of the country: the drinking behavior of parents is more related to what children do about drinking than any other factor. It is more influential than children's friends, their neighborhoods, their religion, their social or economic status, or their local laws.

Statistics on teenage (and adult) drinking vary from one ethnic group or one part of the country to another. But overall, the statistics show that about two-thirds of all Americans 18 and older consume alcoholic beverages. Some three-quarters of all students in the tenth to twelfth grade range also drink.

In general, drinking is an activity that is associated with growing up. For boys, it represents manhood; for girls, sophistication.

Kinds of Alcoholic Beverages

The way any alcoholic drink affects the body depends chiefly on how much alcohol it contains. The portion of alcohol can range from less than 1/20th of the total volume, in the case of beer, to more than one-half in the case of rum. As a general rule, distilled drinks have a higher alcohol content than fermented ones.

The five basic types of beverages are beers, table wines, dessert or cocktail wines, cordials and liqueurs, and distilled spirits such as brandy and whisky. The labels of beers and wines usually indicate the percentage of alcohol by volume. The labels of distilled spirits indicate *proof*.

Proof

The proof number is twice the percentage of alcohol by volume. Thus a rye whisky that is 90-proof contains 45 percent alcohol, 80-proof bourbon is 40 percent alcohol, and so on. The word *proof* used in this way comes from an old English test to determine the strength of distilled spirits. If gunpowder soaked with whisky would still ignite when lighted, that fact was "proof" that the whisky contained the right amount of alcohol. The amount, approximately 57 percent, is still the standard in Canada and Great Britain.

How Alcohol Affects the Body

The overall effects of alcohol on the body and on behavior vary a great deal depending on many factors. One factor should be noted at once: if the blood reaching the brain contains a certain percentage of alcohol, there are marked changes in reaction. As the percentage increases, the functioning of the brain and central nervous system is increasingly affected. As the alcohol is gradually metabolized and eliminated, the process reverses itself.

If at any given time the blood contains a concentration of about 3/100 of one percent (0.03 percent), no effects are observable. This amount will make its way into the bloodstream after you have had a highball or cocktail made with one and one-half ounces of whisky, or two small glasses of table wine, or two bottles of beer. It takes about two hours for this amount of alcohol to leave the body completely.

Twice that number of drinks produces twice the concentration of alcohol in the bloodstream (0.06 percent) with an accompanying feeling of warmth and relaxation.

If the concentration of alcohol in the bloodstream reaches 0.1 percent — when one part of every thousand parts of blood is pure alcohol — the person is legally drunk in most states. The motor areas of the brain are affected; there is a noticeable lack of coordination in standing or walking. If the percentage goes up to 0.15 percent, the physical signs of intoxication are obvious, and they are accompanied by an impairment of mental faculties as well.

A concentration of as much as 0.4 percent can cause a coma. At the level of 0.5 to 0.7 percent there may be paralysis of the brain centers that control the activities of the lungs and heart, a condition that can be fatal.

Alcohol affects the brain and nervous system in this way because it is a depressant and an anesthetic.

How Alcohol Moves through the Body

Although it is negligible as nourishment, alcohol is an energy-producing food like sugar. Unlike most foods, however, it is quickly absorbed into the bloodstream through the stomach and small intestine without first having to undergo complicated digestive processes. It is then carried to the liver, where most of it is converted into heat and energy. From the liver, the remainder is carried by the blood-stream to the heart and pumped to the lungs. Some is expelled in the breath and some is eventually eliminated in sweat and urine. From the lungs, the alcohol is circulated to the brain.

People who use good judgment when drinking rarely, if ever, get drunk. The safe and pleasurable use of alcoholic beverages depends on the drinker's weight and his or her physical condition and emotional state. Other factors include the following:

1.*The Concentration of Alcohol in the Beverage* The higher the alcohol content in terms of total volume, the faster it is absorbed. Three ounces of straight whisky—two shot glasses—contain the same amount of alcohol as 48 ounces (or four cans) of beer.

2.*Sipping or Gulping* Two shots of straight whisky can be downed in seconds or, more normally, in a few minutes. The same amount diluted in two highballs can be sipped through an entire evening. In the latter case, the body has a chance to get rid of much of the alcohol.

3. *Additional Components of the Drink* The carbohydrates in beer and wine slow down the absorption of alcohol in the blood. Vodka mixed with orange juice travels much more slowly than a vodka martini.

4.*Food in the Stomach* The alcohol concentration in two cocktails consumed at the peak of the hunger before dinner can have a nasty effect. Several glasses of wine with a meal or a brandy sipped after dinner get to the bloodstream much more slowly and at a lower concentration. The sensible drinker doesn't drink on an empty stomach.

The Hangover

The feeling of discomfort that sometimes sets in the morning after excessive drinking is known as a hangover. It is caused by the disruptive effect of too much alcohol on the central nervous system. The symptoms of nausea, headache, dry mouth, diarrhea, fatigue, dizziness, heartburn, and a feeling of apprehension are usually most acute several hours after drinking and not while there is still any appreciable amount of alcohol in the system.

Although many people believe that "mixing" drinks, such as switching from whisky drinks to wine, is the main cause of hangovers, a hangover can just as easily be induced by too much of one type of drink or by pure alcohol. Nor is it always the result of drinking too much because emotional

stress or allergy may well be contributing factors.

Some aspects of a hangover may be caused by substances called *congeners*. These are the natural products of fermentation found in small amounts in all alcoholic beverages, among them tannic acid and fusel oil. Some congeners have toxic properties that produce nausea by irritating certain nerve centers.

In spite of accumulated lore about hangover remedies, there is no certain cure for the symptoms. Neither raw eggs, oysters, alkalizers, sugar, black coffee, nor another drink has any therapeutic value. A throbbing head and aching joints can sometimes be relieved by aspirin and bed rest. Stomach irritation can be eased by bland foods such as skim milk, cooked cereal, or a poached egg. Persons seeking relief may also try analgesics such as aspirin or acetaminophen for the headache, antacids if the problem is upset stomach, or over-the-counter medications for the diarrhea.

Alcohol and General Health

As a result of new studies of the effect of alcohol on the body, many myths have been laid to rest. In general, it is known that in moderate quantities, alcohol causes the following reactions: the heartbeat quickens slightly, appetite increases, and gastric juices are stimulated. In other words, a drink makes people "feel good." But drinking does have harmful effects when consumed in large quantities.

Tissue Impairment

Habitual drinking of straight whisky can irritate the membranes that line the mouth and throat. The hoarse voice of some heavy drinkers is the result of a thickening of vocal cord tissue. As for the effect on the stomach, alcohol doesn't cause ulcers, but it does aggravate them.

There is no evidence to support the belief that port wine or any other alcoholic beverage taken in moderation will cause gout. Studies have shown that as many as 60 percent of all patients with this disease had never drunk any wine at all.

Brain Damage

Alcohol abuse continued over many years has been found to contribute to cognitive defects. These may, in turn, indicate brain impairment. Researchers do not know what the defects represent—whether greater susceptibility to the problems of aging or an actual, alcohol-caused "premature aging" effect. Whatever the case, long-term chronic alcohol abuse leads to more rapid aging of the brain. Neuropsychologically, the alcoholic's brain resembles that of an older nonalcoholic.

Long-term abuse can have many other effects. These include withdrawal symptoms beginning 12 to 48 hours after a person stops drinking, sometimes followed by *delirium tremens* (DTs), which brings hallucinations and can be fatal; the Werner-Korsakoff syndrome, a type of beriberi characterized by a lack of the B vitamins; alcoholic peripheral neuropathy, involving damage to the nerve tissue outside the brain and spinal cord; and liver damage, including alcoholic hepatitis and cirrhosis. In the latter the liver becomes hard and yellowed.

Alcohol and Immunity to Infection

Moderate drinkers who maintain proper health habits are no more likely to catch viral or bacterial diseases than nondrinkers. But heavy drinkers, who often suffer from malnutrition, have conspicuously lower resistance to infection. Even well-nourished heavy drinkers have a generally lower immunity to infection than normal. When the blood-alcohol level is 0.15 percent or higher, the alcohol appears to weaken the disease-fighting white blood cells.

Alcohol and Stroke

Studies have shown that heavy drinkers face nearly three times the teetotaler's risk of hemorrhagic stroke. Light drinkers face twice the risk. About one stroke in four occurring in the United States is hemorrhagic, but these strokes are more likely to be fatal than those caused by blood clots.

Alcohol and Life Expectancy

It is difficult to isolate drinking in itself as a factor in longevity. One study reported the shortest life span for heavy drinkers, a somewhat longer one for those who don't drink at all, and the longest for moderate drinkers. But other factors, such as general health and heredity, play important roles.

Alcohol and Sex Activity

Alcohol in sufficient quantity depresses the part of the brain that controls inhibitions. This liberating effect has led some people to believe that alcohol is an aphrodisiac, in men. This is a conclusion that is far from the truth. At the same time that alcohol increases the sexual appetite, it reduces the ability to perform.

Alcohol as an Irritant

Many otherwise healthy people cannot tolerate alcoholic beverages of any kind, or of a particular kind, without getting sick. In some cases, the negative reaction may be psychological in origin—connected with a disastrous experience with drunkenness in the early years or with an early hatred for a drinker in the family. Some people can drink one type of beverage but not another because of a particular congener, or because of an allergy to a specific grain or fruit. People suffering from such diseases as peptic ulcers, kidney and liver infections, and epilepsy should never drink any alcoholic beverages unless allowed to do so by a physician.

Uses and Hazards

At practically all times and in many parts of the world today, alcoholic beverages of various kinds have been and are still used for medicinal purposes. This should not be taken to mean that Aunt Sally is right about the curative powers of her elderberry wine, or that grandpa knows best when he says brandy is the best cure for hiccups. Today an American physician may recommend a particular alcoholic beverage as a tranquilizer, a sleep-inducer, or an appetite stimulant.

Use of Alcohol with Other Drugs

Alcoholic beverages should be avoided by anyone taking barbiturates or other sedatives. See "Drug Use and Abuse" later in this chapter for a discussion of barbiturates.

Alcohol and Driving

For many people, coordination, alertness, and general driving skills are impaired at blood-alcohol levels below the legal limit (0.1 percent). There are some people who become dangerous drivers after only one drink. Attempts are constantly being made, but so far with less than perfect success, to educate the public about the very real dangers of drunken driving.

Possible Causes of Alcohol Abuse

A popular myth holds that alcohol causes alcohol abuse. It doesn't—any more than sugar causes diabetes. Various theories have been evolved to explain what does cause alcohol abuse.

Physiological Causes

Although several physiological factors seem to be involved in the progression of alcohol abuse, no single one can be pinpointed as the cause of the disease. Among the theories that have come under investigation are the following: abnormal sugar metabolism, disorders of the endocrine glands, and dietary deficiencies.

Psychological Causes

Recent studies have pointed to a possible relationship between personality and alcohol abuse. Researchers indicate that one definable segment of the alcoholic population has the character disorder known as *antisocial personality*. Once called a *sociopath,* the person with an antisocial personality is usually charming in a social sense, manipulative, impulsive and rebellious, and egocentric. An estimated 25 percent of the alcoholic population falls in this category; in the general population the prevalence of antisocial personalities is about 3 percent.

Sociological Factors

Practically all studies of alcohol abuse in the United States indicate that ethnic groups vary dramatically in their rates of problem drinkers. A great deal of attention has therefore been focused on *learned attitudes* toward alcoholic beverages and how they are used or abused. Generally, in the low-incidence groups attitudes toward drinking are clearly defined and understood by all the members of the group. Drunkenness is consistently frowned upon. In the high-incidence groups, researchers have found extensive conflict over alcohol. The basic rules aren't clearly defined, and there are no clear-cut standards for acceptable and unacceptable drinking behavior.

Genetic Factors

Research into the genetics of alcohol abuse has led to a theory of "familial abuse." The theory holds that the person with a close relative who is alcoholic is at far greater risk of succumbing to the disease than are others without such connections. Familial abuse or "familial alcoholism" characterizes as many as three in four of all abusers. Therapy has thus begun to focus on the families of alcohol abusers—particularly young sons—as the ones most susceptible to the disease.

Recognizing the Danger Signals of Problem Drinking

The chronic alcohol abuser shows physical symptoms that a physician can recognize. Among them are hand tremors, deterioration of eye functions, reduced bladder control, liver disorders, anemia, memory lapses, and others. But there are many other symptoms that family members and friends can observe, among them these:

- Alcohol use as a way of handling problems or escaping from them

- Increased use of alcohol with repeated occasions of unintended intoxication

- Sneaking drinks or gulping them rapidly in quick succession

- Irritation, hostility, and lying when the subject of alcohol abuse is mentioned

- A noticeable deterioration in appearance, health, and social behavior

- Persistent drinking in spite of such symptoms as headaches, loss of appetite, sleeplessness, and stomach trouble

Treatment

Methods of treating alcohol abuse fall generally into three categories. Choice of any one form of treatment depends on the particular needs of a client, including the degree of dependency. The three categories include the hospital, the intermediate, and the outpatient settings. Other approaches to treatment may be geared to individual or group needs.

The family physician can in most cases provide guidance on what kind of treatment would most benefit a particular patient. The alcohol abuser may be referred first to a toxicologist for an interview and recommendations on treatment. A review of the patient's history is a typical first step in treatment. Family involvement during therapy may be critically important. More than 4,200 centers offer treatment programs; of these, many are nonprofit clinics while others are units owned by for-profit health care chains. Many centers and clinics specialize in team approaches to therapy.

The Hospital Setting

Whether undertaken voluntarily or involuntarily (for example, by court order) the treatment formats offered in a hospital can be individualized. Where some patients adjust best to inpatient care, others prefer partial hospitalization. In the latter case the patient is allowed to go home or to work at appropriate times, otherwise living in the hospital. In a hospital detoxification program, one designed to end physical addiction, the patient has a variable period, usually two weeks to a month, during which he or she undergoes a programmed regimen of activities. These may range from exercise classes to medications to bed rest and regulated diets.

The Intermediate Setting

The intermediate settings usually include at least halfway houses, quarterway houses, and residential care sites. The first of these offer not only living quarters but also job counseling, psychotherapy, and other services. In quarterway houses, the patient receives more attention in the form of counseling and psychotherapy. Residential care centers usually offer little beyond living quarters.

The Outpatient Setting

Again in the outpatient setting the patient has a range of treatment choices. Among them typically are individual counseling sessions held by a paraprofessional; individual therapy sessions with a professional who may have an advanced degree in social work, psychology, medicine, or a related specialty; and group therapy sessions supervised by either a paraprofessional or a professional.

Chemical Treatments

Some treatment programs utilize medications to help patients to "shake the habit." Tranquilizers may be used to reduce tensions and prepare the patient for a follow-up stage. In a program of *aversion therapy* a substance called emetine may be prescribed. Taken before an alcoholic drink, emetine causes nausea. The treatment should be undertaken only under medical supervision.

Where to Find Help

Volunteer organizations of various kinds offer the alcohol abuser and his or her family a wide range of services and programs. The best known is Alcoholics Anonymous (AA), which is supported by contributions from members. AA utilizes a group-support approach to treatment. Most larger communities have AA chapters as well as Al-Anon and Alateen units for family members, relatives, and friends of abusers. Alateen works with young people between 12 and 20 years of age. Counseling and referrals may be obtained from a local Alcoholic Treatment Center.

Information may also be obtained from the following national headquarters of organizations established to help alcohol abusers:

Alcoholics Anonymous World
 Services
P.O. Box 459
Grand Central Station
New York, NY 10163

National Association for Children of
 Alcoholics
31582 Coast Highway, Suite 201
South Laguna, CA 92677
(714/499-3889)

Al-Anon Family Group Headquarters
P.O. Box 862
Midtown Station
New York, NY 10018
(212/302-7240)

National Council on Alcoholism and
 Drug Dependence
12 W. 21 Street
New York, NY 10010
(212/206-6770)

Drug Abuse

Like alcohol abuse, drug abuse can wreck lives and break up families. But to many experts the problem of drug abuse is far more serious than alcohol abuse. The trade in addictive, harmful drugs is not only unlawful; it has grown year by year, to the point where many believe it is out of control. The U.S. government spent some $1.6 billion on efforts to combat illegal drug importation in 1986, calling on units of the military forces to join the campaign. Even so, heroin imports increased by about 10 percent and cocaine imports by about 4 percent.

The forms that drug abuse takes, and the numbers of drugs, are numerous and increasing. Many authorities believe we should examine our whole American society for the "pill-happy" context in which drug abuse occurs. Dr. Joel Fort, former consultant on drug abuse to the World Health Organization, called America

> "a drug-prone nation. . . . The average 'straight' adult consumes three to five mind-altering drugs a day, beginning with the stimulant caffeine in coffee, tea, and Coca Cola, going on to include alcohol and nicotine, often a tranquilizer, not uncommonly a sleeping pill at night and sometimes an amphetamine the next morning."

The social effects of drug abuse rank among the most alarming of all the symptoms of what has been called the drug crisis. By estimate, drugs are involved in one-third to one-half of all crimes committed in the United States in a typical year. In a single recent year, medical treatments for drug abusers cost the nation more than $2 billion. The costs of abuse to families, communities, and to abusers themselves cannot be calculated.

Making the problem of control of drug abuse unbelievably complex is the fact that literally thousands of drugs and drug combinations have basic roles in medical treatments. Legal and illicit uses may, because of the close connections, become confused. Physicians' instructions regarding use of such legal drugs as sleeping pills may be ignored or neglected. Legitimately prescribed drugs may, in some cases, unintentionally lead to abuse or dependency.

Other facts make it difficult to con-

trol drug abuse. More and more, for example, abusers are turning to multiple substance abuse. Cocaine "sniffers" may take alcohol in one form or another to soften the uncomfortable and even painful effects of cocaine withdrawal. Physicians report that "polydrug" abuse leads to progressive worsening of such medical symptoms as stomach ailments and liver problems.

Designer drugs add another complicating factor. Made in clandestine chemical laboratories, these drugs are imitations or analogs of such other drugs as cocaine, heroin, amphetamines, and many other basic substances. The new drugs are legal until declared illegal by the federal government's Drug Enforcement Administration because a chemist has altered their chemical compositions enough to take them out of the banned or controlled drug categories. Far more powerful than the basic drugs they imitate, the designer forms have been implicated in more than 200 deaths. Researchers indicate that there is no limit to the numbers of designer drugs that can be produced.

A designer drug called *new heroin* (*Ecstasy*) was, on analysis, found to contain the industrial chemical MPTP, a suspected causative element in cases of Parkinson's disease. A number of new-heroin abusers also had classic Parkinson's symptoms: rigidity, tremors in the arms, legs, and even the head, and slow or difficult movement. Thus new research has focused on MPTP as a possible clue to the degenerative brain processes that lead to Parkinson's.

Over-the-Counter Drugs

Americans consume over-the-counter (OTC) drugs in enormous quantities. Purchasable without a physician's prescription, these drugs have limited but real potential for abuse. They range from headache remedies to cold nostrums and from acne ointments to vitamins. In general, good practice is to use OTC drugs as seldom as possible, for short-term, minor illnesses. Medicines of proven effectiveness should be used exclusively: taking an aspirin for a headache is a good example. The U.S. Public Health Service offers these guidelines:

- Self-prescribed drugs should never be used continuously for long periods of time. . . . A physician is required for abdominal pain that is severe or recurs periodically; pains anywhere, if severe, disabling, persistent, or recurring; headache, if unusually severe or prolonged

more than one day; a prolonged cold with fever or cough; earache; unexplained loss of weight; unexplained and unusual symptoms; *malaise* lasting more than a week or two. . . .

The Food and Drug Administration (FDA), a branch of the U.S. Public Health Service, is responsible for establishing the safety and usefulness of all drugs marketed in the United States, both OTC and prescription. You can be assured that OTC drugs are safe provided you take them in strict accordance with the label instructions. These indicate the appropriate dosages, among other things, and carry warnings against prolonged or improper use, such as "discontinue if pain persists," or "do not take if abdominal pain is present." This labeling information is regulated by the FDA.

Drug Classifications

In addition to alcohol, the drugs of potential abuse fall into six categories: stimulants, depressants, and narcotic preparations, all of which can have legitimate medical uses; hallucinogens; cannabinoids such as marijuana; and inhalants (or volatile inhalants) such as aerosol sprays, glues, and fuels. See the accompanying table:

Drug abuse can lead to at least three kinds of addiction or dependency. *Physical addiction* results in unpleasant withdrawal symptoms, including, nausea, headache, or cold

Major Drug Classification	
Type	**Examples**
Stimulants	Amphetamines Cocaine derivatives
Depressants	Valium Seconal
Narcotics (opioids)	Morphine Codeine
Hallucinogens	LSD Mescaline Psilocybin

Marijuana	Marijuana
(cannabinoids)	Hashish
Inhalants	Gasoline
	Amyl nitrate

sweats when the abuser does not take the drug. Sudden withdrawal from some physically addictive drugs

can cause heart failure. *Psychological addiction,* more subtle, is a stage at which the abuser believes he or she cannot cope without the drug. In *functional addiction,* the abuser grows dependent on such drugs as decongestant nasal sprays to remain free of an annoying physical condition.

Definitions of Dependence and Addiction

Dependence and addiction is used to describe the compulsive and uncontrollable use of a substance. The use continues despite negative effects on health, lifestyle, work, or other aspects of one's life. Lack of the substance leads to craving, physical or psychological discomfort, and, at times, an overwhelming desire to obtain more of the substance to alleviate the negative sensations experienced from withdrawal.

Psychological dependence or addiction occurs when the user feels he or she cannot manage without the drug. This can occur for several reasons, with several types of drugs. The condition can be mild or can be extraordinarily severe.

Psychological addiction to painkillers—and this can include ibuprofen (Motrin), aspirin, and acetaminophen (Tylenol)—occurs when the user feels that pain may be too great without regular medication. As pain occurs without use, it fulfills the user's expectations. The pain may be real or may be psychosomatic (triggered by psychological expectations of pain), but it reassures the user that the drug is needed and does good. The prob-

lem is that with many types of drug, the effectiveness decreases as use increases.

Psychological addiction can accompany physical addiction, and it is usually difficult to distinguish where psychological needs leave off and physical needs begin. Many addictions are a combination of psychological and physical.

Physical dependence or addiction occurs when the body has developed a physical need for the drug. Physical dependence is usually recognized when the user stops taking the drug. Withdrawal symptoms occur when the body is denied the chemicals to which it has become habituated. Withdrawal symptoms can include dizziness, anxiety, restless sleep, dull ache, acute pain, heart tremors, seizures and convulsions, and heart attack. Sudden withdrawal from some physically addictive drugs can kill the user. Many of the street drugs, such as cocaine and heroin, and many of the prescription drugs, such as Xanax and codeine, can produce severe symptoms if withdrawal is sudden from quantities that were abusive.

Tolerance is the term used for the effect that occurs when the quantity of drug is progressively increased to achieve the desired result. For some chemicals, the body becomes habituated to one quantity and the dosage must be increased to maintain the same level of relief or pleasure experienced from the drug. Increased tolerance for some drugs is what frequently leads to levels that are physically addictive.

Three Classes of Prescription Drugs

Among the drugs that may be prescribed for you are some that have a tremendous potential for abuse. They include *stimulants,* such as amphetamines; *depressants,* such as sleeping pills; and *narcotic* painkillers, including morphine and codeine. When abused (that is, when taken in any way other than according to a physician's strict instructions) these drugs constitute a substantial part of America's burgeoning national drug problem.

Stimulant Drugs

The legitimate use of stimulant drugs and their great capacity for abuse stem from the same property: their ability to speed up the processes of the central nervous system. Physicians may prescribe amphetamines primarily to curb the appetites of patients who are dieting or to counteract mild depression. More rarely, they use stimulant drugs to treat *narcolepsy,* a disease in which the patient is subject to irresistible bouts of sleep, and to counteract the drowsiness caused by sedatives. Amphetamines and an amphetamine-like drug (Ritalin) may be used to treat some hyperactive children who are extremely excitable and easily distracted. For reasons that are imperfectly understood, the drug calms these children instead of stimulating them.

Amphetamines

The major forms of the amphetamines are: amphetamine (Benzedrine), the more powerful dextroamphetamine (Dexedrine), and methamphetamine (Methedrine, Desoxyn). The street name for these drugs is "speed."

The consumption of amphetamines is reportedly far greater than the prescription books indicate. Some 10 billion tablets are produced in the United States annually, enough for 50 doses for every man, woman, and child. Of this amount, probably half is diverted into illicit channels. Underground laboratories manufacture even more.

Abusers of amphetamines include students cramming for exams, housewives trying to get through the day without collapsing from exhaustion, and the businessman who has tossed and turned all night in a strange hotel bedroom and needs to be alert for a conference the next morning.

Used judiciously, amphetamines can improve performance, both mental and physical, over moderate periods of time. In effect, they delay the deterioration in performance that fatigue normally produces. Required to carry out routine duties under difficult circumstances and for extended periods, some astronauts have used amphetamines under long-range medical supervision.

Amphetamines give some persons feelings of self-confidence, well-being, alertness, and an increased ability to concentrate and perform. Others may experience an increase in tension ranging from the uncomfort-

able to an agonizing pitch of anxiety. High doses may produce dry mouth, sweating, palpitations, and raised blood pressure. Because amphetamines only defer the effects of fatigue, the letdown can be dangerous, especially for such users as long-distance truck drivers. In addition, the feelings of self-confidence about improved performance may be highly deceptive. Some college students who have crammed for exams while on speed have turned in blank examination books, or written a whole essay on one dense line.

Amphetamine abusers quickly develop a tolerance to the drug. They may have continually to increase dosages, and may undergo different kinds of drug experiences. Psychological dependence can build rapidly.

Amphetaminelike Stimulants

Several drugs that are chemically unrelated to the amphetamines produce very similar effects on the body. They are, also, equally amenable to abuse.

Among them are methylphenidate (Ritalin) and phenmetrazine (Preludin). The latter has been commonly used as a diet pill.

Cocaine

Ranked as powerful stimulants to the central nervous system, cocaine and its derivatives have become the trendy drugs of the late 20th century. An alkaloid found in the leaves of the coca bush, *Erythroxylon coca,* cocaine in its crystalline form is a white powder that looks like moth flakes. Cocaine can be sniffed, smoked, or taken intravenously. Abusers of cocaine may or may not develop a tolerance for the drug. But some evi-

dence indicates that the same dose repeated frequently will not produce similar effects over a period of time.

Very little street-purchased cocaine is pure. Usually, the drug is mixed, or cut, with other drugs or with substances that resemble it, such as talcum powder or sugar.

Physical dependence on cocaine is rare. Psychological dependence is much more common. When physical dependence occurs, the withdrawal symptoms may include hunger, irritability, extreme fatigue, depression, and restless sleep. With psychological dependence, abusers come to need the feeling of euphoria induced by cocaine. When a dose wears off, the abuser may go into a period of deep depression.

The use of cocaine as a legal anesthetic need not lead to addiction.It has been used particularly in surgical operations on the mouth, eyes, and throat because it can constrict blood vessels and because it is rapidly absorbed by the mucous membranes.

Cocaine's effects as a stimulant last only a short time. Generally, the effects depend on the size of the dose. A small dose may produce sensations of euphoria and illusions of increased strength and sensory awareness. A large dose may magnify these effects. The abuser may engage in irrational behavior, and may experience such physical side effects as sweating, dilation of the pupils, and rapid heartbeat.

In extreme cases abusers may have hallucinations and feelings of paranoia and depression. They may imagine that insects are crawling over their skins (formication) and may have chest pains. Injections by needle may produce skin abscesses. Both heavy and light users may develop runny noses, eczema around the nostrils, and deterioration of the nasal cartilage. The latter occurs because cocaine is usually "snorted" into the nostrils through a straw or a roll of paper, or from a spoon.

Death results, occasionally, from overdoses of cocaine, with respiratory arrest as a prime cause. The abuser may also have high fever, heart rhythm disturbances, or convulsions.

Crack Cocaine

By a simple process dealers in cocaine can convert cocaine in white powder form, cocaine hydrochloride, into cocaine alkaloid, called *freebase*. The process involves mixing powdered cocaine with baking soda and water to form a paste. Once the concoction hardens, it looks like lumpy, off-white granulated sugar. Unlike powdered cocaine, the drug in this form, called *crack* or *rock*, can be smoked, eliminating the need for needles.

However made, crack is a purified cocaine base that is usually smoked in a special pipe with wire screens, or sprinkled on a tobacco or marijuana cigarette. The drug produces a high that may start in eight seconds and last two minutes. By contrast, snorted cocaine takes effect after about five minutes.

Crack produces a very intense euphoria along with other physical symptoms. Because the drug in this form is far more potent than powdered cocaine, the heartbeat speeds up and the abuser's blood pressure may rise. Heart-lung problems may follow, and seizures can occur. Death may ensue. Because of the variations in the strength and purity of crack, and because of the variability of a body's response, death can occur on the first use or the thousandth. Abuse of crack may lead to physical addiction in weeks, with the victim needing continually larger doses to achieve a high.

Depressant Drugs

Making up a second class of medically useful drugs that are also widely abused, the depressants act as sedatives on the central nervous system (CNS). They may also act as hypnotic, or sleep-inducing, agents.

The depressants include mainly the barbiturates, which are both sedative and hypnotic, and the tranquilizers, which can calm without producing sleep. Though they are available as main or secondary constituents of more than 80 brand name preparations, the barbiturates are readily abused.

Tranquilizers act selectively on the brain and the central nervous system. Divided into major and minor tranquilizers, these drugs are similar to barbiturates in many ways, including their sedative or calming effect. The major tranquilizers, called *neuroleptics* because they are useful in the treatment of mental disorders, are *haloperidol* and *chlorpromazine*. These drugs lead to virtually no addiction or dependence even in long-term therapy.

The minor tranquilizers, among them *meprobamate* (Miltown), *chlordiazepoxide* (Librium), and *diazepam* (Valium), are, by contrast, highly addictive. Abusers take such drugs to achieve euphoric states as well as to offset the effects of alcohol, amphetamines, and other drugs.

Barbiturates

Barbiturates have many legitimate uses. For example, they may be prescribed to overcome insomnia, reduce high blood pressure, alleviate anxiety, treat mental disorders, and sedate patients both before and after surgery. Barbiturates may help to bring epileptic and other convulsions under control.

Barbiturates are metabolized, or broken down chemically, by the liver. They are then eliminated by the kidneys at different speeds depending on their types: slow- or long-acting, intermediate and short-acting, or ultra-short-acting. The first of these, primarily phenobarbital and barbital, take effect on the brain in one to two hours and last for six to 24 hours. The intermediate and short-acting barbiturates, including secobarbital and pentobarbital, take effect in 20 to 45 minutes and last five to six hours. The best known of the ultra-short-acting drugs, sodium pentothal or thiopental, can produce unconsciousness in a few minutes. Used mostly in hospitals as an anesthetic, pentothal is also injected by dentists to produce instant unconsciousness.

Abuse

Barbiturate abusers usually select the ultra-short-acting form of the drug because of the rapid action. Abusers as a group generally fall into four categories, with some overlap.

The "silent abuser" takes sleeping pills at first to get some sleep, probably with a physician's prescription. Progressively, the drug helps the abuser to deal with tension and anxiety. Indulging at home, he or she finds the barbiturates producing an alcohol-like high, with slurred speech, confusion, poor judgment and coordination, and sometimes wild emotional swings. Eventually the abuser is obtaining the drug through illicit channels. Some may end up spending most of their time in bed.

A second group, taking barbiturates for stimulation, has already developed a high tolerance that makes drug stimulation possible. Some other abusers find that the drug releases inhibitions.

Made up mostly of young people who are experimenting with various drugs, a third group uses barbiturates to "come down" from an amphetamine high. Members of this group may find themselves in a vicious cycle of stimulation and sedation. To obtain both effects at once, some abusers take the barbiturate-amphetamine combination in the same swallow—a so-called "set-up."

A fourth group, abusers of heroin and other narcotics, uses barbiturates as a substitute when drugs of choice are not available. They may also combine barbiturates with heroin to prolong its effect. In one hospital surveyed, 23 percent of the narcotics users said they were also dependent on barbiturates.

Effects and Dangers

Barbiturate abuse is generally considered to be far more dangerous than narcotic abuse. Every year brings some 3,000 deaths from barbiturate overdose, accidental or intentional. For such reasons many physicians believe barbiturates are the most dangerous of all drugs. Chronic abuse can lead to psychological dependence and increased tolerance, followed often by physical dependence of a particularly anguishing kind.

Abrupt withdrawal from barbiturates can be much more dangerous than withdrawal from heroin. Within a day the abuser withdrawing from barbiturates may experience headaches, muscle twitches, anxiety, weakness, nausea, and blood pressure drops. If the abuser stands up suddenly he or she may faint. Delirium and convulsions may come later. The latter can be fatal. Thus the withdrawal must always be undertaken under medical supervision. Even with supervision, a withdrawal from barbiturates may take two months.

Abuse of barbiturates presents other dangers. Unintentional overdosing frequently occurs when a person takes a regular dose to get to sleep and then remains awake or awakens soon afterward; tired and confused, the person may take another or repeated doses. Death may result. Mixing barbiturates and alcohol can produce the same outcome.

Other Barbiturate-Type Drugs

Some depressants are chemically unrelated to the barbiturates but have similar effects. These include *glutethimide, ethchlorvynol* (Placidyl), and *methyprylon* (Noludar). These too lead to tolerance when abused and sometimes to psychological and physical dependence.

Tranquilizers

The minor tranquilizers are manufactured as capsules and tablets in many sizes, shapes, and colors. They may also be purchased in liquid form for injection. Used legitimately to treat emotional tension and as muscle relaxants, these tranquilizers have high abuse potential because they produce both psychological and physical dependence. Tolerance develops with prolonged abuse.

Miltown, Librium, and Valium produce effects similar to those of barbiturates. But the minor tranquilizers act more slowly and have longer duration. Once considered completely harmless, these drugs came into such vogue that in the 1970s the federal government intervened. Both Valium and Librium as well as some other drugs were placed under federal control. From 1975 on anyone requiring a prescription for these drugs was limited to five prescription refills within a six-month period following the initial prescription. If more of the medication was required after that, a new prescription had to be written.

Withdrawal from the minor tranquilizers can be as dangerous and painful as withdrawal from barbiturates. Combining the tranquilizing drugs with others, including alcohol, is a highly dangerous form of abuse. Each drug reinforces the effects of the other. The result may be greater than the combined effects of the different drugs.

Narcotics (Opiates)

Narcotics are drugs that relieve pain and induce sleep by depressing the central nervous system. Under U.S. law, narcotics are addictive drugs that produce rapid and severe physical and psychological dependence; that category includes opium and such opium derivatives as heroin, morphine, and codeine. The narcotics, or *opioids,* also include the so-called synthetic opiates, among them *meperidine* and *methadone.*

Varieties of abused drugs

Name	Form	Drug
amphetamine methamphetamine	capsule, pill, liquid, powder, tablet, lozenge; swallowed	stimulant
barbiturate	sleeping pills, capsules, tablets; swallowed; injected	depressant, sedative
cocaine	white powder; sniffed, smoked, injected	stimulant, local anesthetic
hashish	resin; smoked	relaxant, euphoriant, hallucinogen (in large or strong doses)
heroin	powder; injected, or sniffed	narcotic
inhalants (for example, gasoline, paint, glue, aerosols, amyl nitrite)	aerosols, volatile substances, solvents; sniffed	
LSD (d-lysergic acid diethylamide)	tablet, capsule, liquid; swallowed	hallucinogen (psychedelic)
marijuana, marihuana	dried leaves; smoked	relaxant, euphoriant, hallucinogen (in large or strong doses)
mescaline	tablet, capsule; swallowed	hallucinogen
PCP	powder; smoked, swallowed	anesthetic (used only with animals)

Opium

The seedpods of the opium poppy, *Papaver somniferum,* produce a gummy resin that has narcotic effects when eaten or smoked. Opium has been used in many lands and many cultures since prehistoric times. It was used medicinally in ancient Egypt. But not until recently did its addictive properties become known. Of the more than two dozen active compounds, or *alkaloids,* that can be isolated from opium, the two most important are morphine and codeine.

Morphine

Morphine, named after Morpheus, the Roman god of dreams, is the chemical substance in opium that gives it sedative and analgesic properties. Isolated initially in the early 1800s, morphine was later synthesized in pure form. On the illicit drug market it appears usually as a white powder.

Morphine can relieve almost any kind of pain, particularly dull, continuous pain. It may also relieve the fear and anxiety that go with such suffering. In addition to drowsiness, euphoria, and impairment of mental and physical performance, morphine may have adverse effects including nausea, vomiting, and sweating. Intravenous injections of the drug may produce an orgasmic high sensation beginning in the upper abdomen and spreading throughout the body.

Taken in overdose, morphine can lead to respiratory depression that is sometimes severe enough to cause coma and death. Morphine is highly addictive and is used only short-term in hospitals because longer exposure easily leads to problems. Naloxone (Narcan) may be administered intravenously as an antidote for morphine overdose.

Codeine

Taking its name from the Greek word *kodeia,* meaning poppyhead, codeine is a mild pain-reliever that can be produced from gum opium or through conversion from morphine. The effects of codeine peak in 30 to 60 minutes; they disappear in three to four hours. Codeine is milder than either morphine or heroin in analgesic effect, and is the most effective cough medicine available. All forms can induce addiction problems with regular use.

Heroin

Originally thought to be nonaddictive, heroin was for a time used as a cure for opium and morphine addiction. It was then found to be more addictive than either of those drugs. It was prohibited in the United States in 1924 and became a staple on the drug black market. Heroin is several times as powerful as morphine.

All of the opiates, including heroin, produce feelings of well-being or euphoria. They also lead to dulled senses and to reduction or elimination of normal fears, tensions, and anxiety. The drug also produces sleepiness and lethargy; *nodding* is one of the characteristic symptoms of abuse. Possible side effects include nausea, flushing, constipation, slowed respiration rates, retention of urine, and, eventually, malnutrition resulting from loss of appetite. When first injecting heroin, nausea and vomiting can occur almost immediately.

The heroin abuser rapidly develops tolerance to the drug. Continually larger doses are then required to produce the same degree of euphoria. Used chronically, heroin leads to both psychological and physical dependence. The former is far more important, and is more difficult to break.

Caught in a cycle involving desperate efforts to obtain enough money, often by criminal means, and getting high, the heroin abuser is not necessarily driven by the search for escape. He or she may want, equally, to avoid withdrawal symptoms. For the chronic abuser these symptoms can be difficult and painful, and may include anxiety, sweating, muscle aches, vomiting, and diarrhea.

Heroin sold on the streets is cut with quinine, milk sugar, or baking soda. It may be cut several times before reaching the abuser. A bag may contain only 1 to 5 percent heroin. If the addict unknowingly buys a dose containing 30 percent or more pure heroin, the higher concentration can spell grave illness or death.

Because heroin can be taken in different ways, the drug's narcotic effects are variable. Sniffing is the mildest form of abuse, followed by skin-popping or subcutaneous injection anywhere on the body, and mainlining, injection directly into a vein, usually the large vein inside the elbow. Abscesses at the preferred site of injection are common, and the vein may become inflamed.

Heroin use does not necessarily lead to dependence. Many persons have experimented with the drug without becoming addicted. Others "joy-pop"—use the drug on weekends, usually for recreational purposes or "kicks."

Little agreement exists regarding treatments for heroin abuse. A promising yet controversial method is the substitution of controlled doses of *methadone* for heroin. Methadone is a synthetic opiate that does not produce the euphoria of heroin. The substitution can help the abuser to lead a normal life, but he or she may still be addicted—to methadone.

Other forms of treatment utilize group psychotherapy, often in live-in communities modeled after the West Coast's *Synanon*. Some experts believe that only multiple-approach treatment formats, combining chemical treatment, psychiatry, user communities, and rehabilitation, can be effective. But the five-year cure rate for heroin abusers is low—only about one-third of that for alcoholics.

Synthetic Opiates

Prescription pain-relievers such as Demerol, Dilaudid, Pantopon, and other synthetic opiates can become addicting if used indiscriminately. They occasionally appear on the illicit drug market. With the increased availability of methadone in treatment clinics, methadone itself is used illicitly, often in combination with alcohol or other drugs, and especially when heroin is in short supply.

The Hallucinogens: LSD and Others

LSD (lysergic acid diethylamide) is one of a class of drugs legally classed as *hallucinogens*—agents that cause the user to experience hallucinations, illusions, and distorted perceptions. Others include *mescaline, psilocybin* and *psilocin, PCP, DMT* (dimethyltryptamine), and *DOM* or *STP*.

A colorless, tasteless, odorless compound, LSD is a semisynthetic acid of immense potency. A single effective dose requires, on the average, only 100 millionths of a gram. A quantity of LSD equivalent to two aspirin tablets would furnish 6,500 such doses. When sold on the street, LSD is generally mixed with colored substances. It may be manufactured in capsule, tablet, or liquid form.

History of LSD

With names such as *California sunshine, acid, purple haze,* and others, LSD reached a peak of popularity in the 1960s. Today it cannot be made legally except for use in certain supervised experiments. Physicians may use it to treat alcoholism and some mental disease, but without uniformly convincing results. It may be sold illegally in sugar cubes, candy, cookies, on the surfaces of beads, even in the mucilage of stamps and envelopes. One dose may produce a 4- to 18-hour *trip*, a hallucinogenic experience.

In the 1960s this trip made LSD the drug of choice for many substance abusers. Among those who claimed that LSD and other psychedelic drugs were consciousness-expanding were well-known public figures. The drugs, in brief, were supposed to enhance the user's appreciation of everything in the environment, to increase creativity, open the gates of awareness to mind-bending mystical or religious experiences, and perhaps to bring about profound changes, hopefully for the better, in the user's personality.

While some users reported such results, various studies suggested that the improvements were illusory. Members of some groups nonetheless felt that it was "in" to be an *acidhead,* an LSD user. One authority estimates that less than 1 percent of the total population have experimented with LSD. Partly because knowledge of dangers in LSD use has become common, the drug has passed the peak of its popularity even though it can still be obtained illegally.

Addictive Aspects

Abuse of LSD is difficult; the drug produces such a spectacular high that daily ingestion is virtually out of the question. Thus LSD use does not lead to physical dependence. But the heavy user can develop a tolerance for the drug very quickly. The tolerance disappears after a few days of abstinence.

Effects

Taking LSD, the individual is usually prepared for minor physical discomforts: a rise in temperature, pulse, and blood pressure; the sensation of hair standing on end; and some nausea, dizziness, and headache. The trip begins about an hour after the drug is first taken. Vision is affected the most profoundly. Colors become more intense and more beautiful; those in a painting may seem to merge and stream. Flat objects become three-dimensional.

The LSD user's reactions are closely related to his or her expectations. Thus one trip may be mind-expanding, filled with brilliant sights and sensations as well as euphoric feelings of oneness with the universe. Another trip may bring anxiety, panic, fear, and depression verging on despair. The latter experience can be terrifying; some bad trips have ended in psychiatric wards, with the tripper suffering from a severe mental disorder, a *psychosis.* An individual's body image may be distorted; in the LSD-induced vision he or she may have no head, for example. Such psychotic episodes, or breaks, may clear up within a day or two. Others can last for months or years.

Some trips have ended in tragedy. Convinced that they could fly or float through the air, some trippers have walked through high windows to their deaths. Others have walked in front of trains or cars.

In effect, no one can predict what psychological changes LSD use will produce. One reason is that no one really knows how LSD works inside the body to affect the mind. What is known is that the drug moves quickly to the brain and throughout the body, acting on both the central and autonomic nervous systems. But all traces of the drug disappear from the brain in some 20 minutes. The effects, as noted, last many more hours.

As with all drugs, LSD should not be ingested by persons who have psychotic tendencies or who are unstable. A disquieting side effect, usually occurring after chronic or heavy use, appears in the flashback, a reexperiencing of the effects of the drug weeks or months after a trip. One theory holds that flashbacks are induced by stress or fatigue, or by resort to other drugs, but the theory remains a theory.

Studies have reported some statistical findings. One research project found that the children of LSD users are 18 times more likely to have birth defects than the children of non-users. Some research also suggests that the drug may have toxic effects on some cells of the human body. An unproved, and possibly unprovable, theory indicates that there may be a link between LSD use and breaks in chromosomes that could conceivably lead to leukemia or to birth defects in users' children.

Other Hallucinogens

Many other substances, both natural and synthetic, are used as hallucinogens. Most of them produce effects similar to those of LSD, but are far less potent.

Mescaline

Mescaline is the active ingredient of *peyote,* a Mexican cactus that has been used by American Indians for centuries to achieve mystical states in religious ceremonies. Users consume cactus "buttons" either ground up or whole. Mescaline itself may be obtained as a powder or a liquid. It can also be synthesized in a laboratory.

Psilocybin and Psilocin

Psilocybin and psilocin are the active hallucinogenic ingredients in the Aztec mushroom *Psilocybe mexicana.* The mushroom grows in southern Mexico and has been eaten raw by the natives since about 1500 B.C. Both derivatives can be made in the laboratory.

PCP (Phencyclidine Hydrochloride)

First developed in 1959 as an anesthetic, PCP in its pure form is a white crystalline powder that is readily soluble in water or alcohol. It appears on the drug black market as tablets, capsules, and colored powders. Abusers snort, smoke, or eat PCP. They can also inject the drug, but do not usually do so. PCP appears as an adulterant in many drug mixtures—in mescaline, psilocybin, or LSD, for example. PCP reportedly has as many or more undesirable effects as positive ones, among them forgetfulness, loss of behavior control, feelings of depersonalization, paranoid episodes, hallucinations, and suicidal impulses.

DMT (Dimethyltryptamine)

Called the "businessman's high" because its effects may last only 40 to 50 minutes, DMT is similar in structure to psilocin. DMT can be smoked or injected; in either case the effect is a powerful wave of exhilaration. An ingredient of various plants native to South America, DMT has long been used by Indian tribes in the form of intoxicating drinks or snuff, often very dangerous. In the United States, DMT is synthesized from tryptamine in the laboratory.

DOM or STP

DOM or STP is a synthetic compound originally developed by the Dow Chemical Company for possible use in the treatment of mental disorders. The drug was never released. Manufactured illicitly, it was allegedly given the name STP for Serenity, Tranquility, Peace. The drug is powerful, it produces vivid hallucinations, and it seems to last as long as LSD. It is also extremely poisonous, and can bring on fever, blurred vision, difficulty in swallowing, and occasionally death from convulsions. In some cases abusers suffer from manic psychoses lasting for days.

Marijuana (Cannabinoids)

Marijuana, or *marihuana,* is a Mexican-Spanish word originally used to refer to a poor grade of tobacco. Later it came to mean a smoking preparation made from the Indian hemp plant (*Cannabis sativa*). A tall, weedy plant related to the fig tree and the hop, cannabis grows freely in many parts of the world and in a variety of grades depending on climate and method of cultivation. The different grades produce drugs of varying strengths. Some 300 million people around the world obtain drug preparations of one kind or another from cannabis.

Drugs are obtained almost exclusively from the female hemp plants. The male plants produce the fiber for hemp. When the female plants are ripe, late in the summer, their top leaves and especially the clusters of flowers at their tops develop a minty, sticky, golden-yellow resin, which eventually blackens. This resin contains the highest concentrations of THC (tetrahydrocannabinol), the group of substances containing the active principles of the drug. The pure resin of carefully cultivated plants is the most potent form of cannabis. It is available in cakes, called *charas* in India, and as a brown powder called hashish in the Middle East.

An estimated 15,000 tons of marijuana are illegally smuggled into the United States annually. But cannabis cultivation has become a major underground business inside the United States. Most illegal shipments of the drug come from Colombia, Jamaica, and Mexico.

Abuse Potential

Marijuana has puzzling aspects. Scientists have not succeeded in establishing exactly what substances in the cannabis plant produce drug effects, or how. THC is, of course, believed to be the most important active element, but chemists believe it is not the only one.

Beyond that, marijuana seems to be in a special class as a drug. It is classed as a hallucinogen, but is less potent than the true hallucinogens. It is not a narcotic, and it resembles both stimulants and depressants in some of its effects. Its use does not lead to physical dependence, nor does the user or abuser develop tolerance. Some users, in fact, find that with regular use they need less marijuana to achieve the desired high.

Users do acquire a slight to moderate psychological dependence—less, in some experts' opinions, than do regular users of alcohol or tobacco. Thus much of the theorizing about marijuana is conjecture despite the fact that millions of persons use it regularly or occasionally.

Effects

Experimenters and newcomers to marijuana smoking may experience little at the beginning. A sense of panic may accompany early exposure to the drug. More serious reactions have been reported, however, including *toxic-psychosis* (psychosis caused by a toxic agent) with accompanying confusion and disorientation. But such reports are rare. Experimenters using large doses of marijuana, hashish, or THC have induced what they termed hallucinations and psychotic reactions.

The experienced smoker may feel halfway between elation and sleepiness. He or she may have some altered perceptions of sound or color, for example, and a greatly slowed-down sense of time. It is usually possible to control the extent of the high by stopping when a given point is reached. The smoker often experiences mild headache or nausea.

Medical Evidence

Research and medical use of marijuana have led to some relatively tentative findings. Some evidence indicates, for example, that the drug may produce genetic damage. More definitely, marijuana has been found to be effective for reducing the pressure of fluids in the eyes of patients suffering from glaucoma. In a 1976 case, the Food and Drug Administration (FDA) approved the use of marijuana for such treatment.

In 1985 the FDA licensed a small drug firm to manufacture THC for use in combating the nausea associated with cancer chemotherapy. Other studies indicated that the drug may also be useful in the treatment of such other diseases as multiple sclerosis.

The debate over full legalization of marijuana promises to continue. Few argue that all penalties for major suppliers should be dropped, at least as long as marijuana remains illegal. But many persons see a contradiction in sending a young person to prison for smoking a marijuana cigarette while his or her parents can drink three martinis every evening.

Inhalants

The inhalants as a class include solvents used in cleaning compounds, aerosol sprays, fuels, and glues. Abusers of these substances sniff or inhale the fumes for recreational and mind-altering purposes. But the substances, primarily chemical compounds, were never meant for human consumption. With some exceptions, they are available commercially and thus have appeal for persons who cannot afford or cannot obtain the more conventional drugs.

Strictly speaking, tobacco, cocaine, and marijuana could be considered inhalants. But the term more commonly refers to three categories of products: solvents, aerosols, and anesthetics. Among the solvents are commercial items such as gasoline, transmission fluid, paint thinner, and airplane cement. The aerosol products include shoeshine compounds, insecticides, spray paints, and hair spray. The type of inhalant used appears to vary according to geographic location, the ethnic backgrounds of abusers, and availability.

Anesthetics comprise a special group of inhalants. Some of them, including nitrous oxide, ether, and chloroform, were used recreationally before medical applications were found for them. Because they are not widely available, they are not abused as much as solvents and aerosols.

Abuse Patterns

Young teenagers are primary inhalant abusers. But some groups or classes of adults, such as prisoners in institutions, also use inhalants. Reasons for abuse vary; among teenagers they range from hostility and lack of affec- tion to peer pressure. Adults, say authorities, are attracted by the ready availability of many inhalants. Alcoholics may resort to inhalants while trying to forestall the symptoms of withdrawal from alcohol.

Effects

Among the active chemicals in many inhalants are toluene, naphtha, carbon tetrachloride, acetone, and others. The fumes from these chemicals enter the bloodstream quickly. They are then distributed to the brain and liver. Entering the central nervous system, the fumes depress such body functions as respiration and heartbeat.

Classed as depressants, inhalants are sometimes referred to as "deliriants." The reason is that they can produce illusions, hallucinations, and mental disturbances. These effects usually result in cases of overdose; in moderate doses, the abuser feels sedated, has changed perceptions and impaired judgment, and may experience fright or even panic. Depending on the dosage, the abuser may also feel intoxicated, and may have lowered inhibitions along with feelings of restlessness, uncoordination, confusion, and disorientation.

Prolonged abuse can lead to nausea, muscular weakness, fatigue, and weight loss. Other effects of such abuse can be extensive damage to the kidneys, bone marrow, liver, and brain. Inhalants have been implicated in some forms of cancer. A high can last from a few minutes to an hour or more. Repeated dosing can produce physical and psychological dependence; but inhalants are not considered as dangerously addictive as other depressants.

In the 1960s the many deaths resulting from glue-sniffing made inhalant abuse a matter of nationwide concern. Studies reported later that about two-thirds of these deaths came about because the abusers, usually children, put plastic bags over their heads to intensify the effect and suffocated.

More recently, deaths have occurred from children experimenting with all types of aerosol sprays and fumes and dying either from toxic poisoning or suffocating in their own vomit after they pass out.

Where to Find Help

Substance abuse has many disturbing aspects aside from the physical, psy- chological, and social damage that it can cause. With addictive medicines, the progression from a *therapeutic dose*—the amount prescribed by a physician—to a *toxic* dose may seem, to some persons, natural and even inevitable. Ingestion or injection of a *lethal* dose may follow as an unintended consequence.

Other factors are causes for concern. The proliferation of illicit street drugs, the rapidity with which dependence or addiction can develop, and the costs and complexity of treatment or detoxification programs all add to the dangers inherent in abuse as a spreading phenomenon. Researchers are discovering weapons that may help in some cases to make treatment more effective: *naloxone* (Narcan), for example, can be given intravenously to reduce the toxic effects of narcotics. But too often a drug has done irreversible harm in a human system before help arrives.

American society has begun to mobilize resources to aid those who need information, assistance, or counsel, for themselves or others, in cases of substance abuse. A National Partnership to Prevent Drug and Alcohol Abuse has established a network of community groups to inform teenagers about narcotics and their poten-

tially disastrous effects. Among helplines and hotlines is one operated by Fair Oaks Hospital in Summit, New Jersey, with the toll-free number 800-COCAINE. Counselors serving with 800-COCAINE are linked to a network of treatment centers and hospitals throughout the country. The addresses and telephone numbers of four national groups, including Fair Oaks Hospital and its program, are:

National Federation of Parents for
  Drug-Free Youth
1423 N. Jefferson
Springfield, MO 65802
417/836-3709

American Counsel for Drug Education
204 Monroe, Suite 110
Rockville, MD 20850
301/294-0600

National Parent Resource Institute for
  Drug Education (PRIDE)
50 Hurt Plaza, Suite 210
Atlanta, GA 30303
404/577-4500

Fair Oaks Hospital
19 Prospect Street
Summit, NJ 07901
800/COCAINE

30

The Environment and Health

How pure is the soil in which the food grows? How clean is the air? How unpolluted the water? How healthy the animals that provide substantial portions of our diets?

Americans were asking such questions with increasing frequency in the 1980s. Their concern had a basis in historic fact. Newspaper reports had for years told of the spread of toxic wastes, of the threat of radiation from nuclear power plants, of seepages of poisonous chemicals, and of polluted drinking water. The Environmental Protection Agency (EPA), established in 1970, had the task of monitoring the environment, but the agency could not prevent such accidents as Three-Mile Island, leaks of toxic gases and liquids in at least four states in 1983, and a toxic gas leak at a chemical plant in West Virginia in 1985. The latter accident raised new fears concerning health that had been generated by a 1984 accident that took 2,000 lives in Bhopal, India.

It became obvious that individual and public health depended on factors that were, in part, beyond governmental control. No one suggested that the American economy should shut down until every possible source of contamination had been removed or neutralized. But because the health fears were so real and so widespread, the environment—all of it, natural and manmade—became the focus of intense interest.

Today's Challenges

Can the health hazards in the environment be reduced or eliminated without hurting the American system and without changing Americans' lifestyles? Most experts believe it is possible.

Harmful ingredients in the environment may be the result of pollution, accidental or intentional. But some toxic substances enter the environment as a result of deliberate planning. Asbestos, for example, a mineral fiber that will not burn, has been widely used to insulate and fireproof buildings. The EPA called a halt to the use of asbestos in construction in the 1970s, when researchers proved that the fiber caused diseases such as *asbestosis,* a lung ailment, and several forms of cancer. Excluding such problems, the major health hazards fall in four main categories: Air, water, and noise pollution and food contamination. Some other hazards, including toxic wastes, nuclear radiation, and workplace dangers, received special attention.

Air Pollution

Air pollutants can damage health in a number of ways. Even where little scientific proof links these pollutants to specific maladies, much statistical or circumstantial evidence suggests that air pollution can lead to various forms of respiratory disease. Some cases of air pollution outside the workplace and exclusive of nuclear radiation hazards have been documented.

Inversions

An inversion is a freak weather condition in which a mass of warm air rests like a lid on top of cooler air. The warm air traps the lower air and prevents the pollutants in it from being ventilated. The results can be deadly.

Donora, Pennsylvania, experienced an inversion in 1948. Situated in a valley, at the center of an industrial complex, the town found its air becoming more and more polluted over a six-day period. Residents eventually had difficulty breathing; more than half of the valley's 14,000 inhabitants were coughing and gasping for breath. Thousands were hospitalized. Twenty-two persons died. Physicians used adrenalin to keep older people alive. Daytime visibility dwindled to a few yards. Some residents collapsed on the streets and in their homes.

What had happened? The temperature inversion, trapping the smoke and fumes from smoldering slag heaps, trash fires, coal-fueled home heating plants, and smokestacks, had filled the valley's air with soot, sulfur dioxide, and other pollutants.

Sulfur Dioxide

Sulfur dioxide enters the air from many sources. In the main, however, it is spewed into the atmosphere when heavy fuel oil and coal are burned to provide heat, generate electricity, and provide industrial power. Large cities are especially vulnerable because of their concentrations of heavy industry.

Sulfur dioxide apparently irritates the lungs and leads to a reduction of the lungs' oxygen-handling capacity. Persons who are particularly suscep-tible to carbon and sulfur dioxide-filled smogs are those suffering from bronchial asthma, chronic bronchitis, and emphysema. The respiratory systems of such persons are already defective. In emphysema, for example, the elasticity of the air sacs in the lungs has progressively broken down, usually after prolonged infection or repeated bronchial irritation. Cigarette smoking can produce such irritation; the sulfur dioxide only worsens the situation.

Lead

Substantial evidence indicates that lead in the air can cause neurological harm and impair body chemistry and bone growth. Most of the airborne lead comes from auto and smelter emissions. These are inhaled directly or they may "soak" food crops. Children are most immediately affected because they have fewer natural defenses against toxic absorption than adults. But adults too may feel the effects of such absorption. They may, for example, feel tired, cramped, or confused.

Because their bodies absorb and metabolize substances rapidly, children may have rates of lead absorption four times as high as those of adults. Workers in some industries, including the ceramic, glass, and lead industries, are also at risk. One study showed that 44 percent of the lead workers in two U.S. smelters suffered from clinical poisoning.

Specific effects of lead poisoning range across a broad spectrum. The formation of red blood cells may be inhibited even by low-level exposure to lead in the air. At higher levels, lead may cause anemia. In children, bone cell growth may be stunted; in pregnant women, lead may prevent the normal development of the fetal skeleton. But lead affects the brain primarily, in some cases interfering with motor skills, auditory development, memory, and the nervous system. Children with higher levels of lead absorption have been found to have serious learning disabilities. Fortunately, lead levels may fluctuate, and the lead in blood and soft tissue may pass out of the human system four to six weeks after exposure ends. But lead remains in bone for periods lasting as long as three decades.

Other Fuel Contaminants

Auto exhausts are major sources of other air pollutants besides lead. Exhaust emissions, for example, may include nitrogen oxides, carbon monoxide, hydrocarbons, and soot. The latter is made up of visible particles of carbon suspended in the air.

How can these substances affect your health? Nitrogen oxides irritate the eyes and the respiratory tract. When nitrogen oxide and hydrocarbons mix in sunlight, they form other noxious substances in the typical photochemical smog that has a yellowish cast. The new ingredients include *ozone,* a poisonous form of oxygen, and peroxyacetyl nitrate (PAN), which is intensely irritating to the eyes. Los Angeles was the first city to experience these smogs; they now occur in many other cities as well.

Worst of all, auto exhaust hydrocarbons include varieties that are possible *carcinogens,* causes of cancer in susceptible individuals. Carbon monoxide, another major hazard, is a colorless, odorless gas that is lethal even in small concentrations because it combines with hemoglobin and thus readily replaces oxygen in the blood. In concentrations that have been measured in heavy city traffic, carbon monoxide can make you tired, headachy, drowsy, and careless.

Acid Rain

While so-called *acid rain* has not been found to harm humans directly, scientists say it has begun to damage the natural food chain in certain regions. As industrial smokestacks emit pollutants, including sulfur and nitrogen oxides, these rise into the upper atmosphere. Mixed with water vapor and other substances, the airborne chemicals are changed by sunlight, becoming tiny acid droplets. The droplets fall to earth as rain or snow, raising the acid content of freshwater lakes and damaging trees and other plants. Under conditions of extreme acidity, fish populations have disappeared; where the food web is disrupted, aquatic animals, algae, and bacteria may dwindle in number. The effects of acid rain on crops and trees are less apparent but are thought to be harmful.

To some extent, acid rain is a geographic phenomenon in North America. Factories in the midwestern industrial belt throw off most of the pollutants, which are then carried east and north. Southeastern Canada and the northeastern and eastern regions of the United States are the areas primarily affected.

Indoor Air Pollution

Reports of illness associated with office and other nonresidential buildings have given rise to what has been termed the "sick building syndrome."

The causes of this syndrome, or complex of symptoms, have not been completely and precisely explained. Among the possible explanations are the following:

- Building ventilation has been reduced to conserve energy, with the result that ventilation is simply inadequate

- Indoor air has become contaminated by emissions from the building fabric and associated systems, furnishings, office equipment, or maintenance materials

- Entrainment or cross contamination has taken place, with contaminants generated in a different part of the building or in a separate building drawn in by an air-handling system

- Bioeffluents, or volatile human substances, spread throughout a building, polluting the air with pyruvic acid, lactic acid, acetaldehyde, butyric acid, carbon dioxide, and other body effluents

- Combustion byproducts from smoking tobacco have produced substances, smoke included, that contaminate indoor air

- Microorganisms or airborne particles from molds, dust mites, and other sources cause such illnesses as Legionnaires Disease

A common tendency has been to identify a public building's heating, ventilating, and air conditioning (HVAC) system as the cause of indoor air pollution. But that conclusion may be premature and overly nonspecific. The symptoms described by persons affected by the sick building syndrome should be studied closely. At least four separate illnesses have been isolated according to their symptoms and causes. Hypersensitivity Pneumonitis and Humidifier Fever usually produce such symptoms as coughing, wheezing, chest tightness, muscular aches, chills, headache, fever, and fatigue. While these conditions are rarely fatal, Legionnaires Disease, produced by the bacterium *Legionella pneumonophilae,* is notable because of its 15 to 20 percent mortality rate. Both Legionnaires Disease and the relatively less serious Pontiac Fever are identified by their pneumonialike symptoms.

Household Chemicals

Depending on its location, structural characteristics, and other factors, the typical home may have as many as 350 or more organic chemical pollutants in its interior air. Household chemical products like spray paints, insecticides, and furniture polish disperse tiny (and toxic) droplets into the air, adding the propellant to the chemicals in the basic product. Among the hazard-producing chemicals, some solvents in particular are known or suspected carcinogens. One of the worst is methylene chloride, found in paint sprays and paint strippers and in some hair sprays and insecticides. Product labels may identify methylene chloride as a "chlorinated solution" or as "aromatic hydrocarbons."

Radon

After cigarette smoking, say scientists, the second leading cause of lung cancer may be radon gas. Considered by many to be the most dangerous of all indoor air pollutants, radon, a naturally occurring radioactive gas, diffuses out of the ground into houses that happen to be built above subsurface sources.

Invading homes, according to the U.S. Environmental Protection Agency, radon causes between 5,000 and 20,000 lung cancer deaths annually. The gas breaks down into unstable elements called "radon daughters"; these become attached to particles of dust or other matter floating in the air. If breathed in, the radon daughters lodge in the linings of the lungs. Radioactive decay takes place almost at once, with the daughters emitting alpha particles that damage the adjacent lung cells, sometimes causing cancer.

Private homes can be tested for radon and, if hazardous levels are found, can be equipped with ventilation or other equipment to remove the health threat. A charcoal-based detector is available. Finally, many firms can conduct home radon checks for a fee.

Water Pollution

To an increasing extent, water pollution has prevented or limited use of many once-valuable sources of water. This progressive deterioration of the nation's water supply has resulted from years of abuse in which natural lakes and waterways were inundated with quantities of raw sewage, waste products of industrial plants and slaughterhouses, petroleum residues, poisonous herbicides and insecticides, and so on. But the pollutants generally fall into two categories: materials that change with time and contact with water, and materials that remain unchanged in form. Organic materials in sewage and such industrial wastes as pulp and paper effluents belong in the first group; inorganic salts like sodium sulfate and such inert inorganic materials as pesticides represent the second.

Where do the pollutants come from? Communities generate thousands of tons of municipal sewage daily. Industries, the greatest users of water, utilize more than half of all the water consumed in the United States for raw material, heating and cooling processes, and transporting, sorting, and washing operations. Agriculture, the second largest user, requires millions of gallons of water for irrigation and drainage; for spraying orchards and crops, often with insecticides, fungicides, or herbicides; for removal of animal and other organic wastes; and for manufacturing opera- tions such as meat packing and can- ning.

Chemical Contamination

The continuing proliferation of chemicals, many of them toxic, suggests the dimensions of the problems relating to water pollution. One estimate by the EPA's Office of Toxic Substances indicated that more than 70,000 chemicals are manufactured or processed commercially in the United States. About 1,000 new chemical compounds are added annually. Literally hundreds of these compounds find their ways into the nation's water supply, some in potentially dangerous concentrations.

How directly and to what degree chemical contaminants contribute to America's health bill cannot be gauged with accuracy. But the roles of these contaminants as carcinogens is widely accepted. Federal health officials have estimated that environmental carcinogens, including those in water, account for 55 to 60 percent of all U.S. cancer cases annually. Some estimates run much higher.

Heavy Metals

Attention has focused on the heavy metals. A study by the U.S. Geological Survey reported that small amounts of seven toxic metals were present in many of the nation's lakes and streams, with dangerous concentrations occurring occasionally. The metals are mercury, arsenic, cadmium, chromium, cobalt, lead, and zinc. Aside from being generally poisonous, some of these metals are implicated in specific health problems. Cadmium, as one example, has been linked to hypertension caused by kidney malfunction. Some other substances represent special situations.

Mercury

Because mercury is heavier than water, experts thought for years that it could be dumped into lakes, the oceans, and waterways. In theory, the mercury would lie harmlessly on the bottom. In reality, bacteria can convert some of the metallic part of the element into water-soluble form. The new compound enters the food chain and ends up in fish. When dangerous levels of this form of mercury were found in some waters and in food fish, warnings were issued regarding canned tuna and swordfish. The government later announced that 97 percent of the tuna on the market was safe to eat. But lakes and rivers across the country were closed to commercial and sport fishing.

An extremely toxic substance, mercury can, even in small concentrations, produce blindness, paralysis, and brain damage. The U.S. Food and Drug Administration has established the safe limit of mercury in food at half a part per million—about the equivalent of a thimbleful in an Olympic-sized swimming pool.

PCBs

Among the chief water pollutants today are the *polycholorinated biphenyls* (PCBs), highly toxic chemicals used industrially in carbonless copying paper and as an additive in lubricants, paints, printing inks, coatings, waxes, and many other products. PCBs, which are *biodegradable* (capable of decomposing) only over a period of years, have been found in unusually large quantities in waterways downstream from manufacturing plants. The EPA banned the direct discharge of PCBs into any U.S. waterway in 1977 after tests showed that fish in some rivers, like the Hudson, had levels of PCBs far higher than the permissible levels.

No one knows what the long-term effects of ingesting small quantities of PCBs will be. But the chemical is a suspected carcinogen. PCB's have also caused severe skin and eye irritations and have been implicated in reproductive disorders, kidney damage, and liver ailments. Researchers believe that the millions of pounds of PCBs in the nation's water or in landfills will take many years to dissipate.

Sludge

Sewage treatment plants around the country also face the major health challenge of disposing of the sludge, or solid matter, that is removed from sewage in the treatment process. Sludge contains not only human wastes but the residues of petroleum products, detergents, toxic heavy metals such as cadmium, lead, and zinc, and many other contaminants. Disposal methods range from dumping on land to burning and to composting for use as fertilizer. But environmental experts maintain that the use of sludge as fertilizer constitutes a health hazard; and major food processors will not accept food grown with sludge as fertilizer. In refusing such food, the companies are follow-ing guidelines set by the National Food Processors Association, which has expressed concern for farm workers' health and for the health of the consumer.

The sludge comes from an estimated 6.8 billion gallons of sewage flushed daily into America's sewers. The sewage itself contains microorganisms that can endanger health. You may be risking gastrointestinal upsets if you swim at a beach that is posted with a sign proclaiming "polluted water." Scientists warn that the fish caught in sewage-polluted coastal waters and harbors may not only be cancerous; they may also be carcinogenic. A number of states including Michigan and New York have restricted or banned sales of tainted fish such as naturally grown carp, catfish, and striped bass.

Oil Spills

With the increasing reliance on supertankers to carry industrial and heating oil from abroad, the danger of major water-polluting oil spills in coastal areas has grown substantially. Several of these huge ships have gone aground and broken apart under heavy pounding by sea waves. Their cargoes have spilled into the oceans, where currents usually carry them many miles before they float ashore or sink to the ocean floor. The oil reaching land fouls beaches and kills water birds. Similar accidents on inland waterways have polluted rivers and lakes, killing fish and spoiling recreational areas.

Noise Pollution

"Pollution" refers generally to the various forms of physical pollution by liquids, gases, or solids. Few persons realize that we are all threatened by a pollutant so common that it tends to be overlooked: noise.

Noise assails us nearly everywhere. It fills homes with loud music or the dog's barking or the grinding of the washing machine and the workplace with the chatter of drill presses and the roar of huge engines. Neither city dwellers nor country people can live noise-free today; none of us can escape car and truck horns, motorcycles that belch sound, and the noisy throb of machinery.

Effects of Sound on the Eardrum

Noise is not just annoying; it is potentially dangerous, both physically and mentally. It has been described as "a slow agent of death." A form of energy, sound or noise is caused by anything that vibrates, that moves back and forth. Our ears receive the effects of this vibrating motion from a distance, great or small, via sound waves. These waves are successive series of regions of compressed air and partial vacuums, or areas of high and low air pressure. Sound can also travel through liquids and solids. We *hear* sound because our eardrums are moved back and forth by the changes in air pressure. The eardrum, or *tympanic membrane,* may perceive a sound that moves it only one billionth of a centimeter—the threshold of hearing. If the intensity of sound pressure becomes too great, we experience pain, and the eardrum or the delicate structures inside the ear may be damaged.

The intensity of sounds is often measured in units called *decibels,* or *db.* These units are logarithmic, that

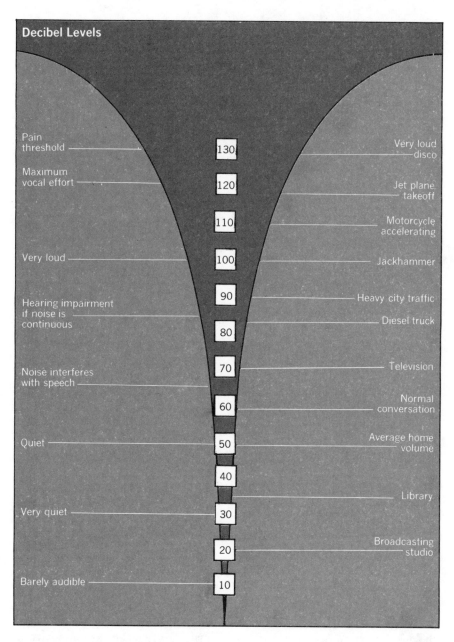

Decibel Levels

Pain threshold —	130 — Very loud disco
Maximum vocal effort —	120 — Jet plane takeoff
	110 — Motorcycle accelerating
Very loud —	100 — Jackhammer
	90 — Heavy city traffic
Hearing impairment if noise is continuous —	80 — Diesel truck
	70 — Television
Noise interferes with speech —	60 — Normal conversation
Quiet —	50 — Average home volume
	40
Very quiet —	30 — Library
	20 — Broadcasting studio
Barely audible —	10

is, 10 db is ten times as powerful as 1 db, 20 db is 100 times as powerful, 30 db is 1,000 times as powerful, and so on. On this scale, 0 db is at the threshold of hearing; rustling leaves, 20 db; a quiet office, about 50 db; conversation, 60 db; heavy traffic, 90 db; a pneumatic jackhammer six feet away, 100 db; a jet aircraft 500 feet overhead, 115 db; a Saturn rocket's takeoff, 180 db.

For most people, the pain threshold is about 120 db; deafening ear damage can result at 150 db. But damage of various kinds can come from much lower exposures. Temporary hearing impairment can result from sounds over the 85 db now found in modern kitchens with all appliances going. If the ears do not get a chance to recover, the impairment will become permanent.

Damage to the Inner Ear

Although very loud noise can damage the eardrum, most physiological damage from noise occurs in the snail-shaped, liquid-filled *cochlea*, or inner ear. Sound transmitted to the cochlea produces waves in the liquid, which in turn move delicate and minute structures called hair cells or *cilia* in that part of the cochlea known as the organ of Corti. The motion of the cilia is transformed into electrical impulses that conduct the sensation of sound to the brain.

The cilia can easily be fatigued by noise, causing a temporary loss of hearing, or a shift in the threshold of hearing. If they are not given a chance to recuperate, they will be permanently damaged, and irreversible hearing loss will result. There are some 23,000 cilia in the average cochlea; different sets of cilia respond to different frequency bands. The cilia responding to sound frequencies of 4,000 to 6,000 cps (cycles per second) are especially vulnerable to damage. The region of 85 to 95 db is generally regarded as the beginning of dangerous sound intensities. In general, the louder the noise, the longer it lasts, the higher it is, and the purer in frequency, the more dangerous it is. Thus, jet engines and powerful sirens are particularly hazardous.

Noise and Stress

The EPA has estimated that some 20 million Americans live or work at noise levels that could cause hearing losses; about 18 million have experienced at least some hearing loss because of noise exposure. But sound, or noise, can lead to physical and psychological problems ranging from irritability to migraine headaches. Linked with many such problems is stress, which has been found to cause high blood pressure, insomnia, ulcers, digestive disorders, alcoholism, anxiety, and many other ills.

Excessive noise has been implicated in such problems as adrenaline flow, elevated heart rates, and blood pressure. All are associated with heart disease. Noise can also affect children in special ways. For example, researchers believe it can retard language development and impair reading ability. Pregnant women exposed to excessive noise may show symptoms of stress and may pass on the harmful effects to their unborn babies. Studies in several countries have shown that the newborns of women living near airport runways experience a higher than normal incidence of birth defects.

Noise-related stress has a definite effect on mental well-being. No one knows exactly how, but noise can produce irritability, tension, and nervous strain. More seriously, British medical authorities have reported a significantly higher incidence of mental illness among people exposed constantly to aircraft noise.

Workplace Noise

Workplace noise presents special problems. Persons working in such industries as construction, mining, steel, lumber, and textiles are almost universally exposed to loud noises. Certain operations in other industries expose workers to high decibel levels. Overexposure takes place when employees work eight hours a day at sites with noise levels exceeding 90 decibels. Such standards, established by the government's Occupational Safety and Health Administration (OSHA), provide also that overexposure occurs where workers are subjected to higher decibel levels for shorter periods.

Workplace noise can lead to problems similar to those produced by overexposure elsewhere. But many workers have little choice as regards the places where they work. For their parts, companies may have limited options insofar as noise control or abatement is concerned. Changing the gears of a machine or building an enclosure around it may not always be feasible.

Some professional musicians find it difficult or impossible to avoid excessive noise on the job. Rock music artists, for example, spend hours at a stretch in enclosed places that magnify sound that is already greatly amplified. Such persons may be at serious risk of incurring hearing losses.

Food Hazards

Contaminants found in water often make their way into food products in the cooking and packaging processes, so that many of the comments on water pollution apply here. Some dilute water pollutants become highly concentrated as they pass up the food chain and end in fish or other foods for man. Mercury was cited earlier as one example. Contamination of food with harmful microorganisms is an everpresent concern wherever standards of cleanliness and sanitation are low.

Additives

Food entails a whole new set of problems because of the thousands of new ingredients that have been added to it, directly and indirectly, in recent years. These substances include many that have been deemed necessary because of the revolution in food technology: the rise of packaged convenience foods of all kinds. Labels on today's convenience foods list preservatives, nutrients, flavors, colors, and processing agents. The trouble with food additives is that we have had little time to learn about their long-term effects on the body. The Food and Drug Administration does set standards in this area; but in the opinion of many experts, these safeguards are inadequate.

What do the additives do and what are they? What kinds of health hazards do they present? The principal kinds are explained below.

Nutrients

Some additives are simply vitamins and minerals that increase the nutritional value of food. Iodine is added to salt as a goiter preventative; vitamins A and D go into fortified milk. The vitamin and mineral additives are generally beneficial.

Preservatives

Preservatives do what the name implies: they protect against spoilage from molds, yeasts, or bacteria, or prevent oxidation. In the first category are such substances as salt, sugar, vinegar, and—among the controversial additives—sodium nitrate, sodium nitrite, and the sulfiting agents. Where some of these substances guard against illnesses like salmonella and *Clostridium botulinum,* or botulism, a deadly form of food poisoning, the controversial types may cause serious illnesses and even cancers. For example, nitrates and nitrites can combine with the amines in protein to become nitrosamines, powerful carcinogens.

The antioxidants include lecithin from soybeans, ascorbic acid (vitamin C), and *butylated hydroxytoluene* (BHT) and *butylated hydroxyanisole* (BHA). The latter two have been studied because they appear to protect against stomach cancer and liver damage.

Flavors

Of the more than 1,500 different flavors used in food, some are natural and some synthetic. Among the natural flavors are cinnamon, vanilla, and citrus oils. The synthetics, some of which, like vanillin, have exactly the same chemical compositions as their originals, include monosodium glutamate (MSG), hydrolyzed vegetable protein, and maltol. MSG in particular has become controversial because it can cause "Chinese restaurant syndrome," with temporary headaches, dizziness, and other unpleasant symptoms.

Colors

As a group, the color additives are the most controversial. But they range from beta carotene, a yellow coloring that is used in carrots and sweet potatoes and is beneficial, to a number of coal tar dyes. The FDA has banned as unsafe more than a dozen of the latter in recent years. Others are readily available and are widely used in cereals, baked goods, ice cream, and beverages.

Processing Agents

Many useful processing agents, including yeast and baking soda, are standard kitchen items. They help to control stability, moisture, texture, and other food qualities and characteristics.

Chemical Residues

Some toxic substances found in food appear in the natural environment. An example: the trace amounts of arsenic in cow's milk. Other poisons are introduced into the environment by humans. These, including fungicides, herbicides, and pesticides, have aroused deep concern among environmentalists and a growing number of private physicians.

American farmers use more than 350 approved agricultural chemicals, including about one billion pounds of insecticides annually. Because of such heavy use, about 52 percent of the average American's diet contains one or more kinds of chemical residues.

Measured often in parts-per-billion, these can collect in human bodies. Permanent damage can result, according to researchers. Among the compounds are not only weed- and bug-killers like parathion but also growth-enhancers like daminozide.

Researchers warn of other problems with contaminated food. The use of antibiotics in livestock feed, for example, promotes the development of bacteria that resist antibiotics. As one result, humans who eat beef or pork that is improperly cooked may acquire infections that resist penicillin or tetracycline.

Irradiated Foods

Consumer groups have urged further study and cautious use of irradiation as a means of preserving many foods. At least 30 countries have approved radiation exposure to retard spoilage and aging; but concerns remain. They focus particularly on the nutritional losses thay may occur if foods are exposed to more than one kind of preservative, on the effects of radiation exposure on workers handling irradiated foods, and on environmental hazards that could emerge in the transport, storage, and handling of radioactive food-processing wastes.

The possible long-term effects of irradiation have led to other concerns. Radiation kills the salmonella microorganism, but may not affect more virulent and dangerous bacteria such as those responsible for botulism and may, over time, strengthen those other organisms. Irradiation might even produce dangerous mutations of some bacteria. Researchers point out further that meat can become contaminated after irradiation, indicating that other preservatives might have to be used.

Other Hazards

Toxic Wastes

Various estimates place the number of toxic-waste disposal sites in the United States at 14,000 to 20,000. Poisonous substances left over from industrial processes are buried or simply dumped at these sites, many of which present serious health hazards. Primarily, according to scientists, the open dumps, landfills, bulk storage containers, and surface impoundments at the thousands of sites spill toxic chemicals into the surrounding soil and through it into groundwater systems. Noxious fumes and even flames burst from some sites at unpredictable moments. The wastes include a huge variety of substances, among them chlorinated solvents, aromatic hydrocarbons, pesticides, trace metals, and PCBs.

The locations of many waste disposal sites remain unknown, often, until a health or environmental problem is detected. Thus the health threats posed by waste dumps may lie dormant for years and may surface only after a container has rusted through or seepage has brought poisonous slush into contact with drinking-water sources.

Waste chemicals can enter the body through skin contact and inhalation as well as ingestion. But the latter is the most common method. Where dosage is substantial, ingestion usually leads to toxic effects on the liver and kidneys. Other parts of the body may be affected as well. Skin contact may produce lesions while inhalation can have direct respiratory effects.

Improved methods of disposing of toxic wastes have combined with public awareness and governmental action to build hopes of reduced waste problems in the future.

Nuclear Radiation

Among the most dangerous of all pollutants is nuclear or "ionizing" radiation. Made up of particles of energy, this radiation can attack the atoms that form the body's cells, causing both short- and long-term damage. Human tissues like skin, bone-marrow, and intestinal cells, all of which reproduce rapidly, feel the impact of radiation most intensely. But different isotopes in ionizing radiation concentrate in different body tissues, sometimes causing cancer or genetic mutations many years after exposure. Of the most common radioactive elements in radiation from a nuclear power plant, barium resembles calcium and therefore concentrates in the bones while iodine 131 concentrates in the thyroid.

Completely invisible, radiation reaches the earth from various natural and manmade sources. Some comes from the sun and outer space; larger amounts are given off by radioactive materials, including waste from nuclear power plants, the fallout from nuclear weapons explosions, and various electronic devices. The numbers of such devices are increasing steadily; among them are lasers, X-ray machines, TV sets, and microwave ovens.

The damage done to the human body as a result of exposure to radiation varies with the intensity of the "dose" and the isotopes involved. A dose of radiation above 1,000 rem, a unit of measurement, is always fatal. Smaller doses, with exposure over an extended period of time, may also be fatal. Victims can protect themselves to a limited degree if given time. For example, they can guard against thyroid cancer by taking potassium iodide. Ingested in pill form, the medication loads the thyroid gland with iodine, thus "blocking" the iodine 131 isotope and preventing its concentration in the thyroid.

In a simple operation physicians can transplant marrow into persons exposed to the barium isotope, and thus reduce the possibility of bone-marrow syndrome. This illness cripples the body's immune system. But donor marrow must match that of the victim, and the relatives of a victim are those most likely to supply marrow that is a genetic match.

Workplace Dangers

Air and noise pollution are, as noted, common in certain industries. The materials and machines used in manufacturing processes are the usual causes of such pollution. Many controls have been mandated by the federal Occupational Safety and Health Administration, but researchers have reported that some industries are experiencing increased health hazards, largely because of the materials they use.

High-tech microelectronics plants are especially threatened. According to scientists, many such plants use toxic chemicals that have been linked to reproductive disorders in both men and women. Among the high-tech hazards usually cited are glycol ethers, widely used as a solvent by manufacturers of printed circuit boards; arsenic, an element in the manufacture of some semiconductor chips; and lead, used in soldering and other operations. Some semiconductor plants are also employing radio-frequency radiation in potentially dangerous amounts to etch and clean silicon wafers.

31

Health Insurance

Health insurance has two basic purposes. It provides for reimbursement to families or individuals for health care costs. It may also guarantee replacement income when a person is unable to work because of sickness or injury. Reimbursement insurance can cover virtually all types of expenses connected with hospital care, medical treatment, and related services. Disability insurance usually calls for periodic payments to make up for lost income.

From another perspective, health insurance offers protection to both groups and individuals. The groups may be company work forces that have *group insurance* as a benefit. Individuals can buy insurance from as many as 1,000 commercial insurance companies offering a huge variety of plans.

Some insurers are general insurance companies. Others are hospital and medical service plans such as Blue Cross and Blue Shield, group medical prepayment plans such as health maintenance organizations (HMOs), and others.

What Health Insurance Is and Does

"Health insurance" means a number of things. It may be called "accident and health insurance" or "disability insurance." Various types of policies have other names. The different descriptions indicate that the policies vary as regards the types of expenses covered. While some policies cover hospital expenses only, others may cover virtually all kinds of medical expenses.

Two Types of Coverage

In general, private health insurance coverage is one of two kinds: *group* and *individual*. Employers, unions, and other kinds of organizations typically provide group insurance as an employee or membership benefit. An individual can buy individual insurance whether or not he or she is covered under a group policy. But a good group policy usually covers all the major health problems or contingencies that a person could face under normal circumstances.

Group insurance has a number of specific advantages over individual coverage, among them the following:

- Because a number of people can be included under a single contract, with consequent savings to the insurer in sales, administrative, and claims costs, the insurer can charge less per individual covered.

- In most cases the company, union, or organization holding the group contract pays part or all of the individual premiums.

- With group insurance the health of the individual insured person is usually not a major factor in determining eligibility. The insurance company is more interested in the average age and overall health status of the group. The health of individuals may become a selection factor, however, where small groups, 10 or fewer persons, are involved.

- Unless an individual leaves a job or gives up a membership, his or her group coverage cannot be canceled. Termination of the group plan itself would, of course, terminate coverage.

Despite such advantages, individual and family policies fulfill at least two fundamental needs. First, they provide coverage for persons who are not members of an insured group. Such policies may also cover those who cannot, for whatever reason, obtain group coverage. Second, the individual or family policy can provide supplementary coverage where a group plan does not meet all basic health insurance needs.

Group and individual plans differ in basic ways. Where a group policy establishes the level of benefits for all group members, the individual policy can more easily be tailored to specific requirements. With the individual policy, too, each person or family is enrolled separately. The cost of individual insurance is usually substantially higher because the insurer considers the age, health status of the insured, and other factors when setting premium rates.

Principles of Health Insurance

Private or commercial health insurance programs function according to some key principles. Primarily, these programs are based on the theory that a relatively small, regular payment, the premium, can protect the insured against what might be a sizable loss.

A companion principle holds that the insured must pay the expenses of operating an insurance system. These expenses include the costs of maintaining offices, investigating claims, and otherwise administering the system as well as paying benefits.

Two other principles underlie the operation of most health insurance programs:

- The *large-loss principle,* which holds that the insured should try to obtain protection only against those costs or losses that he or she could not bear financially. Under this principle the contract may exclude from reimbursement some specific kinds of costs. Most such policies contain a "deductible"

clause specifying that the insured must pay a certain amount of initial costs.

Major medical insurance plans probably exemplify best the large-loss, or large-risk, principle. These policies nearly always provide for a deductible. The higher the deductible, as a rule, the lower the premium.

- The *first-dollar principle,* under which the policy pays the full cost of all covered hospital and medical expenses. Policies of this kind have no deductible clauses.

  Advocates of first-dollar policies stress the need for preventive health care. The policy in theory encourages the insured to see a physician and obtain treatment before a health problem becomes worse or even unmanageable.

Kinds of Insurance Plans

Voluntary or private health insurance plans offer protection against a broad range of hospital and medical expenses. Some policies offer protection against a single illness such as cancer while others insure individuals, families, or groups against nearly all medical contingencies. Some of the many kinds of coverage are as follows:

Hospital

Blue Cross plans and most other commercial plans provide room benefits at a specified rate per day. Usually, they also cover miscellaneous hospital services, including drugs, operating room, and laboratory services up to a given cost level. Some commercial plans and most Blue Cross plans cover all costs in a semiprivate, or shared, room.

Surgical

Typically, health insurance policies cover the costs of surgery according to a schedule that establishes specified amounts for listed procedures. The insurance contract sets a payment of so many dollars for an appendectomy or a tonsillectomy, for example, with that payment going toward coverage of the surgeon's bill. In the case of Blue Shield, certain surgeons perform surgical operations for low-income subscribers for no additional charge.

Regular Medical

This is a form of insurance that provides coverage of physicians' fees in cases that do not involve surgery. The medical care may be provided in the home, in a hospital, or in a physician's office. A regular medical policy may also cover diagnostic X-ray and other laboratory expenses.

Major Medical

As noted, major medical policies usually provide for deductibles. After an insured has reached a specified hospital-medical expense level, the insurer will also pay, for example, 80 percent of all remaining expenses to a set maximum. The maximum may be $1 million or more. Some policies offer unlimited coverage. In some cases the policy sets a maximum, perhaps $5,000, $10,000, or $25,000, for a given illness in a one- or three-year period. Where an insurance company and the insured pay percentages of all costs beyond a deductible, the policy is said to be a form of "coinsurance."

Comprehensive or Comprehensive Major Medical

This kind of health policy combines hospital, major medical, and surgical coverage in one contract. Generally, little or no deductible applies to hospital and surgical charges. But the major medical coverage ordinarily comes with a deductible.

Dental

Basic or comprehensive protection, covering the costs of hospital care, surgery, and physicians' services, may also include dental insurance. A basic plan may establish a set of allowances for each procedure to an annual maximum of, for example, $500 or $1,000. A comprehensive policy would cover, typically, 80 percent of all dental expenses above a specified minimum.

Special Perils

While frowned upon by many insurance experts, "special perils" plans continue to appear. They cover such specific health hazards as cancer, polio, and vision problems.

Auto and Travel

Many insurance companies offer auto and travel policies that cover insured persons in the event of injury or death in an accident. Such policies may pro-vide protection against almost any travel accident in various kinds of vehicles.

Income

Insurance against loss of income gives the insured person a flow of cash if, because of illness or disability, he or she cannot work. A commercial policy that limits coverage to accidental disability usually costs much less than broader coverage, or it provides for greater benefits. Accidental disability payments, usually monthly, may continue for life. Payments for disability resulting from illness are commonly limited to 6, 12, or more months depending on the terms of the contract.

Many policies provide only for *hospital income insurance*. Such insurance pays a stipulated cash payment for every day of hospitalization. Insurance companies offer these policies to individuals only, not to groups.

Basic Protection

Of the various kinds of comprehensive health insurance, the so-called "basic protection" plan ranks among the most common. Basic protection offers coverage for the costs of hospital care and services and physicians' services.

Most basic protection policies specify that hospital room and board benefits will be paid in one of two ways. One kind of policy provides for reimbursement for actual room and board charges up to a set daily maximum. Another kind offers a service type of benefit equaling the hospital's established semiprivate room and board rates. If the insured occupies a private room, he or she pays the additional room charge.

Surgical-Expense Insurance

Basic policies that provide hospital expense coverage generally offer surgical-expense benefits as well. That means coverage may extend to operations and postoperative, inpatient physicians' visits. The policy then becomes a "hospital-and-surgical-expense" or "hospital-surgical" plan.

Surgical-expense insurance normally pays benefits whether illness or accident makes the surgery necessary. Coverage may include benefits for anesthetics. A schedule of surgical procedures and specified maximum benefits for each may be part of such a policy. Physicians' fees may be covered to a "reasonable and customary" level for the particular city or region. In this case the policy would not contain a surgical schedule.

Physician's-Expense Insurance

The counterpart of the surgical-expense policy is the physician's-expense plan. This policy offers benefits to help cover the costs of nonsurgical physicians' services in a hospital, home, or office. The terms of the policy usually provide for maximum payments for specified services. The latter may include diagnostic X-ray and other laboratory expenses.

Policy Provisions

Purchasing health insurance calls for close attention to the provisions of any given policy. Little standardization exists among the hundreds of types of policies, a factor that makes the buyer's task a difficult one. In four areas in particular the buyer should scrutinize closely the "fine print" in an individual, but not a group, policy.

Provisions Relating to Other Policies

Many policies include clauses that limit or prohibit payments where the policyholder has other insurance covering the same loss or expense. In this way insurers protect themselves against overpayments for specific losses. A typical clause of this kind reduces benefits payments to the policy's prorated share of the insured person's actual expenses.

Preexisting Conditions

Most individual health insurance policies exclude preexisting conditions. That means they do not cover at all, or do not cover for a stated period, physical or health problems that existed before the policy became effective. The waiting period that must elapse before coverage for a preexisting condition begins may be 30, 60, or more days.

Cancellation and Renewal

All health policies contain cancellation and renewal provisions. One type, the most favorable to the policyholder, specifies that the insurer cannot cancel or refuse to renew the policy before the insured turns 65. The same clause may state that the premium cannot be increased. Because it provides guaranteed coverage, this kind of policy is usually the most expensive.

Many policies contain a widely used modification of the no-cancel, guaranteed renewal clause. This alternative provides that the company must continue the coverage until the insured reaches 65, but that the premium can be increased for entire groups of insured persons. In a third variation, some policies permit the insurer to cancel or refuse to renew the coverage at any time by giving written notice to the policyholder. This kind

of policy is the least advantageous to the insured.

"Good-Health" Discounts

Increasingly, the disability, hospital, or medical policy provides for discounts for persons in good health. For example, the policy may specify that the applicant be a nonsmoker who exercises three to five times a week and does not have a high-risk job or hobby. Race-car driving would fall in the latter category.

Discounts of 5 to 15 percent have been available to nonsmokers since the 1960s. New discount arrange-

ments broaden the range of qualifying factors and increase the discount levels. The new trend takes as a model the life insurance plan that may offer discounts of up to 50 percent if the applicant observes basic rules of health and safety. These include, in addition to those named, adhering to a nutritious diet, using seat belts while riding in a car, and avoiding excess salt in diet.

Meeting Special Needs

Some health insurance policies are designed to meet special needs. One common kind of coverage protects persons who are above-average risks: persons with poor health histories,

existing problems or illnesses, or chronic disorders of one kind or another. Other types of policies serve other purposes.

Existing Health Problems

Because persons with existing health problems are not average risks, insurance for them may be costly. But an approach to insurance may be made in at least three ways.

1. A policy may exclude entirely the usual benefits for the specified existing condition. The insurance may then provide protection for all or many other conditions. Standard rates or premiums may be charged.

2. Charging a standard rate, the insurer may amend the policy to pro-

vide for a longer waiting period before coverage begins. In such a case standard benefits may be available.

3. The policy may call for a higher than normal premium to compensate for the greater degree of risk. Regular benefits might be available.

Some special health coverages have become relatively common. For example, dental-expense insurance helps pay for normal dental care as well as accidental damage. Insurance companies, prepayment plans, and some state dental associations make such coverage available, usually providing for a deductible and for coinsurance.

Special coverage may, finally, be provided for eye care. Many group policies have such coverage.

Insuring the Unemployed and Divorced

Most Americans have health insurance as a job-related benefit. Coverage terminates, however, if an individual quits his or her job, is laid off, or loses the job for whatever reason.

An employee who is leaving a job should find out how long, if at all, coverage will continue after employment terminates. A normal period would be 30 days. In that period the employee is usually allowed to convert the coverage from group to individual. The conversion option means the employee can remain insured by the same company while retaining, usually, reduced benefits. The premium payments generally increase, sometimes dramatically. Where a group policy permits conversion, the insured has the right to convert regardless of existing health problems. No medical examination is required.

Many group policies provide for conversion from group to individual coverage where a divorced person was dependent for protection on the former spouse's group plan. The person needing health coverage has to apply within the specified period, but cannot be rejected for health reasons.

By the middle 1980s, some 25 states had laws requiring "group continuance." By the terms of these laws a divorced spouse or unemployed person could remain in the group and receive the same benefits as before. The insured had only to assume the group cost formerly contributed by the employer for each insured individual. The effect of the group continuance laws was to make it possible for divorced or unemployed persons to retain group coverage for about half of what an individual policy would cost. With some exceptions, state laws limited group continuance periods to a year or less.

"Medigap" Insurance

An estimated 95 percent of all Americans over 65 are protected by Medicare. But the government program covers only a portion of all possible physician and hospital expenses—less than 50 percent. To help bridge the gap between Medicare and the 100 percent coverage that most persons need and want, private insurance companies have developed "medigap" policies.

What do the medigap policies cover? Their terms vary. Most help insured persons to expand existing Medicare coverages. But few offer even partial protection against hospital and medical costs that Medicare does not cover, or does not cover fully. These areas include: routine physical checkups; most prescription drugs; hearing tests and hearing aids; eye examinations and eyeglasses; most dental care, including dentures; private nursing care; and custodial home nursing care.

Because neither Medicare nor medigap insurance covers these areas thoroughly, many elderly persons remain vulnerable. But some medigap policies, including those offered by Blue Cross/Blue Shield and some associations for the elderly, provide for good hospital and physician coverage.

Congress set minimum standards for medigap insurance in 1980. But the Better Business Bureau has warned that the older person in need of additional insurance should shop carefully. Some groups, the BBB states, offer insurance as a means of building membership rolls. The BBB also advises as follows:

- Older buyers should make sure they have the Medicare medical insurance (Part B) as well as the hospital coverage (Part A).

- Insurance buyers should check the reputation of any potential private insurer with the state insurance department and the local Better Business Bureau. Insurance companies are also rated according to their financial health in *Best's Insurance Reports: Life and Health Insurance,* available in most libraries.

- The practice of switching from one insurance company to another because of premium levels can be hazardous: rates charged by any company can increase.

- As a rule, premiums should not be paid for years in advance. Your needs may change.

Five Innovative Plans

Pressures to cut the costs of medical care have given rise to basic changes in the methods of delivering such care in the United States. No longer do most persons simply call their family physicians and, if the physician so advises, go to a specific hospital. More and more, insurance plans and programs offer both choices and restrictions. Five innovative programs in particular have gained in popularity.

Health Maintenance Organizations (HMOs)

Operating clinic-style facilities, HMOs require that their subscribers pay a set monthly premium. In return the HMO provides full medical care. But members have to select their physicians from a list provided by the HMO. If hospitalization is necessary, the subscriber goes to a hospital selected by the organization.

Charging premiums that may be 10 to 20 percent lower than those for equivalent insurance coverage,

HMOs provide incentives to avoid unnecessary expenses or treatments. HMOs, for example, encourage subscribers to make use of preventive care to stay healthy. Thus most HMOs offer eye and hearing checkups, as well as podiatry and dental services, at little or no cost beyond a monthly fee.

Many subscribers point to the convenience of HMOs as their major attraction. Subscribers not only have the convenience of full medical and hospital services at one facility; they pay no deductibles and have no claim forms to fill out.

HMOs have won federal support. New rules published in 1985 encouraged Medicare recipients to drop out of the government's medical insurance program and to join HMOs. The usual HMO restrictions on choices of physicians and hospitals would apply; applicants would join a central hospital facility, with its own physicians and specialties, and would be directed to specific physicians approved for HMO patients. Those who make the change have to retain the Medicare Part B coverage.

Former Medicare beneficiaries have various ways to report grievances. They can, for example, write to the U.S. Department of Health and Human Services Office of Health Maintenance Organizations, Compliance Division, Room 9-11, Parklawn Building, 5600 Fishers Lane, Rockville, MD 20857.

Preferred Provider Organizations (PPOs)

In the PPO, subscribers receive care at a discount if they go to physicians and hospitals recommended by the insurer. Generally, the insurance company underwriting the PPO allows employees in insured groups to go to a nonparticipating physician. But in such a case the costs of care rise considerably, sometimes to twice those charged by the listed physicians.

Under the PPO arrangement, physicians, hospitals, and insurers work together to keep down overall costs. A PPO hospital provides care for insured persons at reduced rates. In exchange, the hospital enjoys increased utilization of its facilities.

Managed Care

Unlike the HMO and the PPO, a managed care program gives members the freedom to pick the physicians and hospitals they prefer. But severe cost-containment rules apply. The restrictions may include the following:

- Preadmission reviews of hospital stays by panels of physicians and nurses. A panel would have to agree in all cases, except for maternity care and emergencies, that hospitalization and the proposed care are necessary.

- Reviews during hospitalization to ensure that continued inpatient care is necessary.

- Mandatory second opinions before some operations to make certain a particular procedure is necessary.

- As in some newer group plans, surgery is performed on an out-patient basis where possible.

Companies adopting managed care plans may offer HMO and PPO plans as well. An eligible employee in such a firm then has a choice of program.

Hospital Chains

Competition among health care providers has led to still another approach to both cost control and hospital utilization. Some for-profit hospital chains have bought insurance companies to obtain insurance licenses, then provided health insurance programs that required the insured to use the chain's facilities.

A variation on the HMO and PPO systems, the hospital chain approach makes possible insurance costs that are 10 to 15 percent lower than those of traditional plans. Chain officials contend that the lower charges are justified by more efficient hospital operation.

Insurance experts note characteristics of the hospital chains' programs that appear to justify caution on the part of the potential buyer. For example, the policies sold by the chains usually impose limits on lifetime benefits. Unlike the plans of such nonprofit groups as Blue Cross/Blue Shield, the chains' policies provide for the termination of certain benefits at specified ages.

Nursing Home Care

Increasingly, major insurance companies have begun to devise policies that would cover the costs of nursing home care for the elderly. Such specialized plans face a double difficulty. First, the insurance company needs to make a profit off the program of coverage. Second, nursing home costs ranging generally from $15,000 to $50,000 and more per year raise the possibility of enormous claims that could continue for years.

Long-term care insurance marks a start toward a solution. Major insurers have begun to market policies that differ on such points as home health care benefits and the right to renew. But because no actuarial figures are available to show, for example, how many younger policyholders would be needed to offset older beneficiaries, the companies have worked through organizations such as the American Association of Retired Persons (AARP). The memberships of such groups are usually numerous enough to reduce the risks of major claims.

32

Home Care of the Sick

Patients suffering from serious illnesses or from certain communicable diseases should be hospitalized. Home care facilities do not normally include the expensive and delicate medical equipment required for the complete care of these diseases.

If, however, the physician in charge of a case decides that his patient does not need hospitalization and that adequate home nursing care can be provided, the well-being of the patient can be greatly enhanced by his being cared for in the comfortable and familiar surroundings of his own home.

When the decision to treat a patient at home is made, it must be understood that the physician's orders regarding rest, exercise, diet, and medications have to be rigorously adhered to. Nursing responsibilities assigned to the patient and whoever else is tending to the patient's recovery should be carried out as conscientiously as they would be if the patient's care were entrusted to a team of medical professionals in a hospital environment.

The physician in charge of a case should, of course, be notified of any significant changes in the condition of the patient. The physician should be contacted if, for example, the patient complains of severe pain, pain of long duration, or pain that apparently is not directly related to an injury or surgical procedure. The location and characteristics of the pain should be noted, and the physician will want to know whether the pain is affected by changing the position of the patient or if it seems to be related to the intake of food or fluids.

In addition to being informed of such potentially dangerous developments, the physician should get daily or frequent reports on the patient's progress. The easiest and best way to see that this is done is to keep a written record of the following functions, symptoms, and conditions of the patient:

- Morning and evening body temperature, pulse rate, and respiration rate

- Bowel movements—frequency, consistency of stools, presence of blood

- Urination—amount, frequency, presence of burning sensation, color

- Vomiting or nausea

- The amount and kind of solid foods and liquids taken by the patient

- Hours of sleep

- Medications given (should be administered only on the instructions of the physician)

- Patient's general appearance (includes any unusual swelling, skin rash, or skin discoloration)

- General mental and psychological condition of the patient, such as signs of irritability or despondency

Checking the Pulse and Respiration

The pulse and respiration are usually checked in the morning and again in the evening; the physician may recommend other times as well.

Pulse

The home nurse should learn how to measure the pulse rate in beats per minute. A watch with a second hand or a nearby electric clock will help count the passage of time while the pulse beat is counted. The pulse can be felt on the inner side of the wrist, above the thumb; the pulse also can be checked at the temple, the throat, or at the ankle if for some reason the wrist is not conveniently accessible.

The patient should be resting quietly when the pulse is counted; if the patient has been physically active the pulse count probably will be higher than normal, suggesting a possible disorder when none actually exists. Temperature extremes, emotional upsets, and the digesting of a meal also can produce misleading pulse rates.

What is a normal pulse rate? The answer is hard to define in standard or average terms. For an adult male, a pulse rate of about 72 per minute is considered normal. The pulse of an adult woman might range around 80 per minute and still be normal. For children, a normal pulse might be one that is regularly well above 100 per minute. Also, a normal pulse may vary by a few beats per minute in either direction from the average for the individual. The home nurse with a bit of practice can determine whether a patient's pulse is signifi-cantly fast or slow, strong or weak, and report any important changes to the physician.

Respiration

The patient's respiration can be checked while his pulse is taken. By observing the rising and falling of the patient's chest, a close estimate of the rate of respiration can be made. An average for adults would be close to 16 per minute, with a variation of a few inhalations and exhalations in either direction. The rate of respira-tion, like the pulse rate, is higher in children.

Sometimes the respiration rate can be noted without making it obvious to the patient that there is concern about the information; many persons alter their natural breathing rate unconsciously if they know that function is being watched.

Body Temperature

A fever thermometer, available at any drugstore, is specially shaped to help the home nurse read any tiny change in the patient's temperature, such changes being measured in tenths of a degree. Instead of being round in cross-section like an ordinary thermometer, a fever thermometer is flat on one side and ridge-shaped on the other. The inner surface of the flat side is coated with a reflective material and the ridge-shaped side actually is a magnifying lens. Thus, to read a fever thermometer quickly and properly, one looks at the lens (ridged) side.

How To Take the Temperature

The usual ways of taking temperature are by mouth (oral) or by the rectum (rectal), and fever thermometers are specialized for these uses. The rectal thermometer has a more rounded bulb to protect the sensitive tissues in the anus. Normal body temperature taken orally is 98.6° F. or 37° C. for most people, but slight variations do occur in the normal range. When the temperature is taken rectally, a normal reading is about 1° F. higher—99.6° F. or about 37.5° C.—because rectal veins in the area elevate the temperature slightly.

Before a patient's temperature is taken, the thermometer should be carefully cleaned with soap and water, then wiped dry, or sterilized in alcohol or similar disinfectant. The thermometer should then be grasped firmly at the shaft and shaken briskly, bulb end downward to force the mercury down to a level of 95° F. or lower—or 35°

C. or lower if the thermometer is calibrated according to the Celsius temperature scale. See the chart *Body Temperature in Degrees* for comparative values of the Fahrenheit and Celsius scales.

If the temperature is taken orally, the thermometer should be moistened in clean fresh water and placed well under the tongue on one side. If the temperature is taken rectally, the thermometer should be dipped first in petroleum jelly and then inserted about one inch into the opening of the rectum. If an oral thermometer is used in the rectum, special care should be taken to make sure that the lubrication is adequate and that it is inserted gently to avoid irritating rectal tissues. Whichever method is used, the thermometer should be left in place for at least three minutes in

Body Temperature in Degrees		
Fahrenheit		**Celsius**
105.5		40.8
105		40.6
104.5		40.3
104		40
103.5		39.7
103		39.4
102.5		39.2
102		38.9
101.5		38.6
101		38.3
100.5		38.1
100		37.8
99.5		37.5
99		37.2
98.6	Normal	37.0
97.8	Range	36.6

order to get an accurate reading.

If circumstances preclude an oral or rectal temperature check, the patient's temperature may be taken under the arm; a normal reading in that area is about 97.6° F. or 36.5° C.

Above-Normal Temperature

If the patient's temperature hovers around one degree above his normal reading, the home nurse should note the fact and watch for other signs of a fever that would indicate the presence of an infection or some other bodily disorder. A mild fever immediately after surgery or during the course of an infectious disease may not be cause for alarm. Also, the normal body temperature of a mature woman may vary with hormonal changes during her menstrual cycle. But when oral temperatures rise above 100° F. the change should be regarded as a warning signal. A rise of as much as three degrees above normal, Fahrenheit, for a period of several hours or more, could be critical, and a physician should be notified immediately.

Sleep

Another item to be checked each day for the at-home medical records is the patient's sleeping habits. While there is no standard number of hours of sleep per day preferred for healthy individuals, a regular pattern of sleep is very important during recovery from disease or injury, and an obvious change from such a pattern can suggest tension, discomfort, or other problems. Typical daily sleep periods for most adults range from 7 to 9 hours, while children and infants may sleep as much as 12 to 20 hours per day and be considered normal; sleep in the form of naps should be included in total amounts per day.

Making the Patient Comfortable

A good deal of the patient's time at home will be devoted to sleep or rest, most or all of it in bed. The bed should give firm support to the body; if the mattress does not offer such support, place a thick sheet of plywood between the springs and mattress. Pillows can be placed under the head and shoulders of the patient to raise those parts of the body from time to time. When the patient is lying on his back, a small pillow can be slipped under the knees to provide support and comfort. A small pillow can also be placed under the small of the back if necessary. Additional pillows may be placed as needed between the ankles or under one foot or both feet.

If the pressure of bed clothing on the feet causes discomfort, a bridge made from a grocery carton or similar box can be placed over the feet but beneath the blankets. To help maintain muscle tone and circulation in the feet and legs, a firm barrier can be placed as needed at the foot of the bed so the patient can stretch his legs and push against the barrier while lying on his back.

Changing Position

Helping the patient change position in bed is an important home-nursing technique. Unless a definite effort is made to help the patient change positions at regular intervals, the sick person may tend to curl up into a sort of fetal position, with the hips and knees flexed and the spine curved. While this position may be preferred by the patient in order to increase body warmth or to relieve pain, the practice of staying in one position for longer periods of time can lead to loss of muscle tone and even deformities.

Moving or positioning the patient in bed should, of course, be done according to directions outlined by the doctor for the specific medical problem involved. Body movements should not aggravate any injury or other disorder by placing undue strain or stress on a body part or organ system that is in the healing stage. At the same time, the patient should be stimulated and encouraged to change positions frequently and to use as much of his own strength as possible.

If the patient is likely to need a very long period of bed rest, and the family can afford the modest expense, it may be wise to purchase or rent a hospital-type bed. The basic hospital bed is higher from the floor than ordinary beds, making the tasks of changing bed linens, taking temperatures, etc., easier for the home nurse. More sophisticated hospital beds have manual or electrical controls to raise the head and foot of the bed.

Helping the Patient Sit Up

The patient can be helped to a sitting position in bed by placing one arm, palm upward, under the patient's shoulder while the patient extends an arm around the nurse's back or shoulders. The nurse also may slip both hands, palms facing upward, under the patient's pillow, raising it along with the patient's head and shoulders. The same procedures can be used to help move a patient from one side of the bed to the other if the patient is unable to move himself.

When the patient has been raised to a sitting position, he should try to brace his arms behind him on the bed surface with elbows straightened. If the patient feels dizzy or faint as a result of the effort, he can be lowered to the back rest position again by simply reversing the procedure.

When the patient is able to support himself in a sitting position, he should be encouraged to dangle his legs over the side of the bed, and—when his strength permits—to move to a chair beside the bed and rest for a while in a seated position.

Bathing the Patient

A patient who is unable to leave the bed will require special help in bathing. When bath time comes, the nurse will need a large basin of warm water, soap, a washcloth, and several towels, large and small. A cotton blanket also should be used to replace the regular blanket during bathing, and pillows should be removed from the bed unless they are necessary at the time.

One large towel should be placed under the patient's head and another should be placed on top of the bath blanket, with part of the towel folded under the bath blanket. This preliminary procedure should help protect the bed area from moisture that may be spilled during the bathing procedure.

The bath should begin at the area of the eyes, using only clear water and brushing outward from the eyes. Soapy water can be applied to the rest of the face, as needed, with rinsing afterward. After the face, bathing and rinsing are continued over the chest and abdomen, the arms and hands, the legs and feet, and the back of the body from the neck downward to the buttocks. The external genitalia are washed last.

During the washing procedure, the nurse uses firm strokes to aid circulation and checks for signs of pressure areas or bed sores. Skin lotions or body powders may be applied, and a back rub given, after washing. The teeth may be brushed and the patient may want to use a mouthwash. After the personal hygiene routine is completed, a fresh pair of pajamas can be put on. If bed linen needs to be changed, the bathing period provides a good opportunity for that chore.

Changing the Bed Linen

Changing the bed linen while the patient is in bed can be a challenge for any home nurse. However, there are a few shortcuts that make the task much easier. First, remove all pillows, or all but one, as well as the top spread if one is used. Loosen the rest of the bedding materials on all sides and begin removing the sheets from the head of the bed, top sheet first. By letting the patient hold the top edge of the blanket, or by tucking the top edges under his shoulder, the blanket can remain in place while the top sheet is pulled down, under the blanket, to the foot of the bed. If the top sheet is to be used as the next bottom sheet, it can be folded and placed on the side with the top spread.

Next, the patient must be moved to one side of the bed and the bottom sheet gathered in a flat roll close to the patient. Then the clean bottom sheet is unfolded on the mattress cover and the edges, top, and bottom,

Changing Patients Bed

New sheet   Old sheet   New sheet   Old sheet

tucked under the mattress. The rest of the clean sheet is spread over the empty side of the bed and pushed in a flat roll under the soiled sheet next to the patient's back.

The next step is to roll the patient from one side of the bed onto the clean sheet that has been spread on the other side. The soiled bottom sheets can be pulled out easily and the new bottom sheet spread and tucked in on the other side.

The new top sheet can be pulled up under the blanket, which has been used to cover the patient throughout the change of bed linens. Finally, the top spread and pillows can be replaced, after the pillow cases have been changed. A special effort should be made, meanwhile, to keep the mattress cover and bottom sheet of the patient's bed as flat and smooth as possible and to allow room for the feet to move while the sheets are firmly tucked in at the foot of the bed.

The home nurse should handle the soiled linens carefully if the patient is being treated for an infectious disease; they should never be held close to the face.

Bowel Movements and Urination

If the patient is expected to remain bedridden for a long period of time, the home nurse should acquire a bedpan and perhaps a urinal from a drugstore. A sheet of oilcloth, rubber, or plastic material should also be provided to protect the bed during bowel movements and urination.

If the patient is unable to sit up on a bedpan because of weakness, his body can be propped up with pillows. If he is capable of getting out of bed but is unable to walk to the bathroom, a commode can be placed near the bed and the patient can be helped from the bed to the commode and back. Another alternative is to use a wheelchair or any chair with casters to move the patient between the bedroom and bathroom.

Administering an Enema

Occasionally, a physician may recommend an enema to help the patient empty his bowels or to stimulate the peristaltic action associated with normal functioning of the intestinal tract.

Since enemas are seldom an emergency aspect of home nursing, there usually is time to purchase disposable enema units from a drugstore. The disposable enema contains about four or five ounces of prepared solution packaged in a plastic bag with a lubricated nozzle for injecting the fluid into the patient's rectum. The entire package can be thrown away after it has been used, thus eliminating the need to clean and store equipment. The alternative is to use a traditional enema bag filled with plain warm water or a prescribed formulation.

An enema is best administered while the patient is lying on his side with his knees drawn up toward his chest. When using the disposable enema unit, the home nurse simply squeezes the solution through the lubricated nozzle that has been inserted into the rectum. When using an enema bag, the home nurse should lubricate the nozzle before insertion.

After insertion of the nozzle, the enema bag should be held or suspended above the patient so that, upon the opening of the valve that controls the flow of the enema, the liquid will flow easily into the patient's rectum.

Feeding the Patient

It may be necessary at times for the home nurse to feed a patient unable to feed himself. An effort should be made to serve meals to the patient in an attractive and, when possible, colorful manner. The bedding should be protected with towels or plastic sheeting and the patient made as comfortable as possible with his head raised.

Liquids should be offered in a spoon filled about two-thirds full with any drops on the bottom of the spoon carefully wiped off. The spoon should be held so that the area between the tip and the side touch the patient's lower lip. Then the spoon is tilted toward the tip so the liquid will run into the patient's mouth. The process takes time, and much patience is required of the nurse. The patient may be slow to swallow and in no hurry to finish the meal.

If the patient can take liquids through a glass tube or plastic straw, the home nurse should see to it that the end of the tube inserted in the container of liquid is always below the surface of the fluid so that the patient will swallow as little air as possible.

A patient who can drink liquids from a spoon or tube may be able to drink from a cup. In making the step from tube or spoon to cup, the home nurse can help the patient by holding the cup by its handle and letting the patient guide the cup to his lips with his own hands.

The nurse should always make sure the patient is fully alert before trying to put food or liquid into his mouth; a semiconscious person may not be able to swallow. The nurse also should test the temperature of the food; cold foods should be served cold and warm foods should be served warm. But foods should never be too hot or too cold for the patient. Finally, the dishes, tubes, or other devices used to feed the patient should be carefully cleaned before storing them.

Ice Bags and Hot-Water Bottles

Ice bags and hot-water bottles frequently are used in home nursing to relieve pain and discomfort. The temperature of the water in a hot-water bottle or bag should be tested before it is placed near a patient's body. The maximum temperature of the water should be about 130° F., and preferably a few degrees cooler. The hot-water container should never be placed directly against the skin of a patient; it must be covered with soft material, such as a towel, to protect the patient against burns. A patient who is receiving pain-killing medications could suffer serious tissue damage from a hot-water bottle without feeling severe pain.

When ice is the preferred method of relieving pain, it can be applied in a rubber or plastic bag sealed to prevent leakage and covered with a soft cloth. Cold applications to very young and old persons should be handled cautiously and with medical consultation, particularly if ice packs are to be applied to large body areas for long periods of time; individuals at both age extremes can lack the normal physiological mechanisms for coping with the effects of cold temperatures.

Steam Inhalators

If the at-home patient suffers from a respiratory ailment that is relieved by steam inhalation, there are several devices to provide the relief he needs. One is the commercial electric inhalator that boils water to which a few drops of a volatile medication are added to provide a pleasantly moist and warm breathing environment. If a commercial inhalator is not available, a similar apparatus can be made by fashioning a cone from a sheet of newspaper and placing the wide end of the cone over the top and spout of a teapot containing freshly boiled water. The narrow end of the cone will direct the hot water vapor toward the face of the patient. If a medication is to be added, it can be applied to a ball of cotton placed in the cone; the steam or water vapor will pick up the medication as it passes through the cone.

If medicated vapor is intended for a small child or infant, the end of the cone can be directed into a canopy or tent made of blankets placed over a crib or the head of a bed. This arrangement should produce an effective respiratory environment for the child while keeping his body safely separated from the hot teakettle.

Still another method of providing steam inhalation for a patient requires only an old-fashioned washstand pitcher and bowl plus a grocery bag. An opening is cut in one corner of the bottom of the bag which is placed upside down over the pitcher filled with hot steaming water and, if needed, a medication. The patient simply breathes the hot moist air seeping through an opening in the bag. The pitcher of steaming water is placed in a bowl or basin as a safety precaution.

Improvising Sickroom Devices

With a bit of imagination, many sickroom devices can be contrived from items already around the house. A criblike bed railing can be arranged, for example, by lining up a series of ordinary kitchen chairs beside a bed; if necessary, they can be tied together to prevent a patient from falling out of bed. The bed itself can be raised to the level of a hospital bed by placing the bed legs on blocks built from scrap lumber. Cardboard boxes can be shaped with scissors and tape into bed rests, foot supports, bed tables, or other helpful bedside aids.

Plastic bags from the kitchen can be used to collect tissues and other materials that must be removed regularly from the sickroom. Smaller plastic bags may be attached to the side of the bed to hold comb, hairbrush, and other personal items.

Keeping Health Records

The family that keeps good records of past injuries and illnesses, as well as immunization information and notes on reactions to medications, has a head start in organizing the home care of a member who suddenly requires nursing. The file of family health records should include information about temperatures and pulse rates taken during periods of good health; such data can serve as benchmark readings for evaluating periods of illness. Also, if each member of the family can practice taking temperatures and counting pulse and respiration rates during periods of good health, the family will be better able to handle home nursing routines when the need arises.

Home Care Equipment Checklist

Following is a convenient checklist of basic supplies needed for home care of the sick:

1. Disinfectants for soaking clothing and utensils used by the sick. Not all disinfectants are equally effective for every purpose. For clothing and food utensils, corrosive or poisonous disinfectants are to be avoided. Antiseptics do not kill bacteria; they only retard their growth. Among the common disinfectants that can be used in the home are:

- Alcohol, 75 percent by weight, used for disinfecting instruments and cleaning the skin

- Lysol, for decontaminating clothing and utensils

- Soap with an antibacterial agent for scrubbing the hands

- Carbolic acid (phenol) for disinfecting instruments and utensils (it is corrosive, poisonous, and very effective if used in 5 percent solution)

- Cresol in 2.5 percent solution for disinfecting sputum and feces (less poisonous than phenol and can be obtained as an alkali solution in soap)

- Boric acid, a weak antiseptic eyewash

- Detergent creams, used to reduce skin bacteria

2. Disposable rubber gloves, to be used when handling patients with open wounds or contagious diseases, as well as for cleaning feces.

3. Paper napkins and tissues for cleaning nasal and oral discharges.

4. Rectal and oral thermometers. The former is used primarily for infants, while the latter is used for adults and older children. Thermometers should always be thoroughly disinfected after use by soaking in iso-propyl alcohol, and they should be washed prior to reuse.

5. Eating and drinking utensils to be used only by the patient. Disposable utensils are preferable.

6. Urinal, bedpan, and sputum cup for patients who cannot go to the toilet. After use, they should be thoroughly disinfected with cresol and washed with liquid soap containing an antibacterial agent.

7. Personal toilet requisites: face cloths and towels, toilet soap, washbasin, toothbrush and toothpaste, comb, hairbrush, razor, and a water pitcher (if running water is not accessible to the patient).

8. Measuring glass graduated in teaspoon and tablespoon levels for liquid medication.

9. Plastic waste-disposal bags that can be closed and tied.

33

Health Care Delivery

A Changing Service

Unending change has characterized American health care in recent decades. The general practitioner in private practice, once the institutionalized symbol of medical care in the United States, has largely given way to specialists of many kinds. Where the general practitioner once sent a handwritten bill for services to the family home, he or she may now send a computerized invoice to an insurance company or a government agency. The "house call" has virtually disappeared.

Technology has taken over. Hospitals and other health care institutions may pay sums in seven figures for equipment that can save lives but that also demands to be used. A "technological imperative" requires that the new approach or instrument or drug at least be tried—experimented with, proven useful or useless, and made available to those who need it. In diagnosis and therapy in particular, physicians and other professionals are continually seeking the new and better.

Some seven million people work in the American health care system. Half a million of those are physicians. The facilities in which the system's personnel work range from rural clinics to high-technology urban medical centers. On balance, the consumer dealing with this system has many choices. Understanding those choices may make the difference between a beneficial experience and a frustrating search for help.

Health care reaches the American public at three broadly defined levels. The three are primary, secondary, and tertiary care.

Primary Care

Essentially, *primary care* refers to "first contact" care as provided in physicians' offices or hospitals. Such care may also be provided in emergency rooms and outpatient clinics. The individual can obtain primary care without referral by a physician, but referrals from this level of care are generally necessary to ensure that the patient will receive treatment at the next higher level. Among the types of services provided at the primary care level are health maintenance for infants and children, screening for infectious and communicable diseases, and treatment for minor injuries.

Secondary Care

At the *secondary care* level the patient usually comes under the care of a specialist, often in a community hospital or other, similar setting. Secondary level specialties include such well-known areas of medicine as obstetrics and gynecology, dermatology, otolaryngology, and cardiology. While physicians often refer their patients for secondary level care, many persons "refer themselves."

Tertiary Care

At the tertiary care level, the patient receives highly specialized, high-technology care and treatment. Complex programs and unusual procedures, among them open heart surgery, heart or kidney transplantation, and neurological surgery, are provided by physicians with extensive training and the advantages of sophisticated equipment for diagnosis and treatment. Often, care at this level is obtainable only if the patient enters a hospital with specialized facilities. Of the various tertiary care institutions, three key ones are hospitals specializing in a certain disease or a group of diseases, hospitals associated with medical schools, and large regional referral centers. Many such institutions would be expected to have diagnostic equipment for such procedures as cardiac catheterization, nuclear magnetic resonance testing, and CT scanning.

Importantly, the three levels of care overlap. The distinctions among them are not always clearly drawn or defined. For the patient, the most important factor may be the need for referrals at some levels and not at others.

Health Care Delivery Formats

The average American visits a physician five times a year. That statistic appears in a U.S. Public Health Service survey that also defines a visit as an encounter with a physician or other health professional under a physician's direction or supervision. The "encounter" can take place in the physician's office, in the patient's home, by telephone, or in some other ambulatory care setting. The physician initiates about half of the encounters, usually as part of follow-up care.

Office and Clinic Care

In the main, the patient sees his or her physician in an office or at a site reserved for group practice; in a hospital outpatient department; in an ambulatory surgical center; or in a free-standing surgical center.

Office-Based Practice

Most physicians practice on their own; even so, the solo practice is declining as a way of medical life. The solo practitioner survives in isolated or rural areas, but hardly at all elsewhere. For the physician, solo practice is both simpler because of the independence and freedom it guarantees and more complex because the service responsibility may continue 24 hours a day, seven days a week. For the patient, the main advantage of solo practice is both the closer relationship that can develop and less fragmented care.

Partnerships

Very common today is the partnership, an agreement between two or more physicians under which the participants share office space, staff, and equipment. The physicians retain their independence in the sense that they have their own practices, but they usually share patient responsibilities under given circumstances. A physician who has to be out of contact with the office may, for example, give a patient another partner's number so as to have continuous backup. Spreading the care responsibilities and reducing the workload, each physician may also have more time for each patient.

The patient may find major advantages in the partnership. He or she can become acquainted with the physician's partner and in this way obtain personalized care at all times. Backup support may be especially important in obstetrics, where deliveries may occur without warning, and in cardiology, where emergencies are equally unscheduled.

Groups

Where three or more physicians associate in an arrangement that is normally less formal than a partnership, it is termed a *group*. The physicians belonging to the group may practice in a single specialty or in diverse fields of medicine. An example of the latter would be a group of three doctors offering internist, obstetrics-gynecological, and pediatric services. In other ways the group shares the advantages and disadvantages of the typical partnership. Like the partnership, the group has one particular advantage, however: other physicians are available for consultation and education. The group format may also make possible relatively sophisticated laboratory and other facilities.

Health Maintenance Organizations

The health maintenance organization (HMO) ranks as a special kind of group practice, one that involves a fixed monthly or annual fee system rather than a fee-for-service arrangement. The fixed fee ensures that the HMO member will receive, at no additional charge, all necessary health services, including hospitalization and the care of specialists. Preventive medicine at no extra cost to the member is a feature of the HMO that has ensured reduced usage of hospital facilities.

Preferred Provider Organizations

Like the HMO, the preferred provider organization (PPO) is at least partly a response to rising health-care costs. Forming a PPO, a group of physicians contracts individually with an insurance company or employer to provide health services for fees that are usually lower than those prevailing in the community or area. The PPO does charge on a fee-for-service basis, but employees making use of the organization's medical services save money because they avoid the copayments of conventional insurance plans and the standard deductibles. Physicians belonging to the PPO have a stable pool of employed members whose health problems may be extremely diverse. For the employer or insurance company, a particular advantage is the ability to bargain for lower fees.

Three Alternative Systems

Obviously, office and clinic care takes many forms. Three alternatives that provide relatively minor, low-level services are the hospital outpatient department, the ambulatory surgical center, and the freestanding emergency center. Each plays a particular role in the health care delivery network.

Hospital Outpatient Departments

Outpatient departments once offered free services as a means of training medical students and residents or because physicians volunteered their services for such departments. Today, outpatient departments charge for their services while delivering health care that varies broadly as regards quality. One hospital in three has an outpatient department or a clinic for ambulatory care while nine of ten community hospitals offer outpatient care in their emergency departments.

Ambulatory Surgical Centers

Sometimes called surgicenters, the ambulatory surgical center may be attached to a hospital or be completely independent. In either case, the surgicenter may be an effective alternative in the traditional situation where a patient needs an abortion, a dilatation and curettage (D & C), hernia repair, or tissue biopsy. Because they perform lower-risk procedures, ambulatory surgical centers can keep costs down. Local anesthesia is the norm, and usually the patient goes home on the day of the operation.

Freestanding Emergency Centers

Sometimes called *urgicenters,* freestanding emergency centers resemble hospital emergency departments. But private, for-profit groups usually run them. Open from 12 to 24 hours daily, they operate on a drop-in basis, meeting a definite need where a hospital emergency room is far away or when all physicians' offices have shut down for the day. Typically, emergency centers treat sprains and bruises, cuts that require stiches, and upper respiratory infections. Charges for such services usually range from visits to physicians' offices on the low side to hospital emergency rooms on the high side.

Community Health Care Facilities

Providing more evidence of the complexity of the United States' health care delivery complex, community health facilities fill a void in health services at a very basic level. At least five different modes of providing health care need to be considered as community facilities.

School and College Health Programs

Once concerned primarily with the control of communicable diseases and screenings for dental, vision, and hearing problems, school and college health programs have taken on new functions. At the elementary and high-school levels, they may help with health and sex education programs, keep vaccination records, and consult with parents. Colleges and universities generally provide infirmary services, meaning inpatient care for acute illness. At larger schools, programs may deal with contraception and pregnancy problems, substance abuse, and neuroses.

Industrial Health Programs

Treatment of work-related injuries and minor illnesses remains a key function of industrial health programs. The programs also continue to give minor physical exams and to provide general medical and dental care. But they have expanded their services in recognition of the value of preventive medicine. Newer or more modern programs offer comprehensive work-site education and screening programs, alcohol abuse counseling, stop-smoking clinics, and aerobic fitness classes.

Health Screening

Provided by local health departments and voluntary health agencies (see Chapter 36), health screening varies from community to community as regards both availability and reliability. Depending on community funding, a local health department may or may not provide tests that screen for infectious or parasitic diseases, including sexually transmitted diseases (see Chapter 17), and chronic disorders such as high blood pressure, sickle cell anemia, or diabetes. Many health departments make referrals to follow-up medical care.

Neighborhood and Primary Health-Care Centers

Neighborhood and primary health-care centers were established first in the 1960s to provide ambulatory care in underserved communities, both rural and urban. Staffed often by U.S. Public Health Service medical personnel or by nurse practitioners, the centers either limited their services according to income requirements or served specific communities. Because of cuts in federal spending, experts note, many such centers have been or are being phased out.

Women, Infant, and Child Care

Also federally funded, the women, infant, and child care program emphasizes provision of well-baby care, nutritious food, and nutrition education for pregnant women, infants, and children under three. Estimates indicate that the program saves three dollars for every dollar spent. But federal budget cuts have begun seriously to scale back the program.

Disease Prevention and Control

County or city health departments usually establish disease prevention and control programs to help control the spread of communicable diseases. Methods used include immunization, screening, and follow-up. Typical concerns include immunization for childhood diseases like diphtheria, measles, and polio; tuberculosis and sexually transmitted diseases; and influenza immunization for older persons.

Hospitals

Viewed a century ago as a death-house, the hospital has a new image in the 1980s. With an entirely revised role built on its ability to provide comforts and even amenities, the hospital has added a "hotel" function to its fundamental "healing" function. But the hotel role does not affect the hospital's main medical purpose: to provide, within budgetary and other limits, sophisticated, technologically up-to-date care. The hospital has become the place to go for diagnostic and therapeutic care that a physician's office cannot provide.

A basic method of classifying hospitals is by length of the patient's stay. Viewed this way, hospitals fall into two groups, long-term or extended-care institutions and short-term hospitals. The former will be discussed later; the second group includes community, teaching, and public hospitals.

Community Hospitals

Most Americans receive medical care in community hospitals. Usually quite small, with 50 to 500 beds, this kind of hospital generally provides good to excellent secondary-level care. Traditionally, community hospitals were nonprofit corporations that depended heavily on community support. Today, the community hospital is increasingly likely to be proprietary. That means it is run for profit by investor-owned groups or corporations.

The costs of medical care at a proprietary community hospital may not be significantly different from those charged by a voluntary or nonprofit hospital.

Teaching Hospitals

Ranging in size from a few hundred to a few thousand beds, teaching hospitals universally offer training for undergraduate medical students, postgraduate students, or fellows. Also, nearly all have ties to major medical schools. A state government may own a teaching hospital that is used by state medical schools; others are owned by the associated university or by a nonprofit corporation. Teaching hospitals provide care at all three levels.

Public Hospitals

Public hospitals include not only county hospitals but others supported by public funds, among them public health service hospitals, Veterans Administration (VA) hospitals, and municipal short-term-stay hospitals. Many such institutions that are owned by federal, state, or city governments are teaching hospitals, and many also have associated rehabilitation units and nursing homes.

The Elderly: Home Care

Surprisingly, most elderly persons live at home and receive care from relatives and others who may visit the home to help out. Younger family members may need home care because of illness or injury, but typically the disabled or ill older person is the one receiving such care. A number of community resources are available to make home care—or self-care for those living alone—easier. These resources include home health workers, such services as Meals-on-Wheels, and various day-care programs.

Invaluable aids for those responsible for home care for an aging relative are unskilled companions and temporary help. With this kind of assistance, the elderly person may be able to enjoy continuity of care and independence while maintaining ties with family, home, and community.

Home Health Services

Some 2,500 home health agencies operate under the general direction of physicians to provide two kinds of services: skilled and supportive. Of the many types of home health service providers, the best known are private, either profit-making or non-profit; public health agencies such as neighborhood health centers; hospital-based services; and local or county health department or community and church programs. The nationwide Visiting Nurses Association is perhaps the most familiar.

Different communities and areas enjoy different levels and types of home health services. But most such agencies provide care to anyone who requests it. Fees vary, and may be paid by the individual or the family accepting the care. In other cases the government or individual insurance plans may reimburse the family, partially or totally, for the fees charged. Hospital social workers or discharge-planners, the Area Agency on Aging, the local office of the Social Security Administration, day-care centers, and churches and synagogues normally provide information on home health services.

Voluntary Health Agencies

Many voluntary health agencies provide aid and support to the disabled or sick elderly person (see Chapter 36). Such groups and organizations as the American Cancer Society and the Easter Seal Society may even offer "friendly visitor" services in specific communities. Most of the groups see education of the public as functional to their roles. Thus they may provide films, lecturers, books and pamphlets, and other materials of interest to groups and organizations of many kinds. Many such agencies have specialized equipment for those who need it as well as listings of community resources.

Drugstores and Medical Supply Houses

Two other basic sources of specialized equipment and sickroom supplies, the medically oriented drugstore and the medical supply house, play important roles. In many cases the family discharging home care responsibilities can obtain wheelchairs, walkers, portable oxygen equipment, and hospital beds from one source or the other. Often, the supplier will rent or sell the specialized equipment; the choice may be the family's to make.

Community Facilities for the Aged

An entire new category of health care facilities has come into being in recent years in response to the needs of the elderly. These community facilities are designed specifically for those elderly persons living at home who are not housebound.

Adult Day Care

A broad variety of community-based centers schedule adult day-care programs for the elderly. To some extent the programs provide an alternative to institutionalization. In each case the programs are tailored to meet specific needs. Each type has a basic therapeutic objective.

Day Hospitals

Generally located at an extended-care facility or hospital, the day hospital provides medical care and supervision for persons recovering from acute illnesses. A physician's referral is normally required; fees closely parallel those charged for other hospital services. The day hospital that treats primarily patients discharged from an institution is sometimes called an aftercare clinic.

Medical Day Care

Where chronically ill or disabled persons do not require frequent or intensive medical intervention, the medical day care service may be the solution. Located usually in a long-term care institution or freestanding center, such a care service may include nursing and other supports. A physician's referral is required, and rehabilitation and maintenance are primary therapeutic goals. Reimbursement is by third-party (insurance company) payments on a sliding scale. Medicaid pays for medical day care in some states.

Mental Health Day Care

Offering a supervised environment along with mental health services to adults with organic or functional mental illness, the mental health day care service is usually located in a psychiatric institution or freestanding center. Referral by a psychiatrist is required. Three basic therapeutic goals are supervision, assistance with coping skills, and safety for the patient. Reimbursement is by third-party payment.

Social Adult Day Care

Title XX of the Social Security Act provides for funding of many social adult day care facilities, all of which are geared to the needs of adults who have difficulty functioning independently. Both families and health facilities can make referrals, but examination by a physician is normally required before admission. Third-party reimbursement is the norm. Program objectives and services vary widely, and are usually formulated by the funding source and the sponsoring organization. Program participants may attend part-days or full days five days a week; the facility may provide a midday meal and transportation within a specified area.

Nutrition Services

Nutrition ranks as a critical need for both homebound and more independent elderly persons. Meals-on-Wheels, a community service offered under voluntary auspices but funded partly by public funds, caters to the homebound. For a reasonable charge the service provides at least one hot meal daily for persons 60 and older. For the elderly attending senior centers, the Area Agency on Aging provides both adequate nutrition and a chance to socialize. Agency personnel can keep in touch with clients' physical and social situations, giving the program an important outreach and prevention dimension.

Extended-Care, Long-Term Care, Nursing Homes

Closely related, the extended-care facility, long-term care facility, and nursing home nonetheless meet different needs. A relatively recent innovation, the extended-care facility provides a service that falls between that given in an acute-care hospital and that provided in a skilled nursing facility or nursing home.

Extended-Care Facility

Despite its name, the extended-care facility provides short-term inpatient care. This type of facility is designed mainly to aid patients who have been hospitalized but no longer need the full complement of hospital services. Such patients still require professional nursing and medical supervision. Typically attached to a hospital, the extended-care facility may also serve those who are not acutely ill but who require skilled care.

Because most extended-care facilities are physically attached to hospitals, patients often simply move from one hospital wing to another. Some nursing homes also meet the standards set for qualification as extended-care facilities by the Joint Commission on the Accreditation of Hospitals (JCAH). For the most part, extended-care facilities charge much less than the typical hospital.

Long-Term Care Facilities

Patients with chronic conditions that cannot be treated effectively in a general hospital generally qualify for care in a long-term care facility. Such conditions range from tuberculosis to mental retardation. The facilities also include chronic disease hospitals, rehabilitation hospitals, and psychiatric hospitals for both children and adults.

Nursing Homes

Also falling in the category of long-term care facilities, nursing homes comprise a special group of facilities of different kinds. They offer services ranging from sheltered living arrangements to around-the-clock nursing care. All nursing homes rank as residential facilities.

The approximately 18,000 nursing homes in the United States have between 1.3 and 1.5 million beds. Three-quarters of these nursing homes are proprietary, or for-profit, institutions that house about two-thirds of all the beds. Nonprofit organizations operate 15 percent of all the nation's nursing homes and make available about 20 percent of the beds. The government operates the remaining homes.

Nursing homes accommodate persons of all ages. A few younger residents have serious congenital illnesses or disorders, or have been recently discharged from a hospital. Others are recovering from recent surgery. But most patients are the chronically ill elderly. Typically, a nursing home resident is a woman in her 80s, single or widowed. Afflicted with three or more serious chronic illnesses, she has very likely exhausted all her assets except her monthly Social Security payments.

Residential-Care Facilities

Standing at the lowest level of nursing home care, the residential-care facility is usually appropriate for the person who can no longer live alone and manage household chores. This "typical" resident does not need extensive medical attention but does require sheltered living, prepared meals, and some medical monitoring. The latter may include supervision of medications and tracking of signs and symptoms.

Intermediate-Care Facilities

The intermediate-care facility supplements typical RCF services with regular, but not round-the-clock, nursing care for residents who are unable to survive on their own. The intermediate-care facility may also make provision for social and recreational activities. Programs of physical therapy and rehabilitation, occupational therapy, speech therapy, and social work services may also be offered.

Skilled Nursing Facilities

With staffs of registered nurses, licensed practical nurses, and nurses' aides, skilled nursing facilities can provide 24-hour care. They are, thus, appropriate for persons in need of intensive nursing care and rehabilitation. Like intermediate-care facilities, skilled nursing facilities are state-certified for the most part, a factor that makes them eligible for public funds as payment for services. Lack of certification may mean that an ICF or SNF has serious deficiencies.

Hospices

Described sometimes as more a philosophy than a type of physical facility, the hospice is a form of care for the terminally ill. The family and the patient merit equal consideration in the typical hospice; the purpose is to minimize the twin fears associated with dying, fear of isolation and fear of pain. Typical palliative care involves the careful control of pain and the management of other symptoms of terminal disease or illness.

A growing number of communities have hospice facilities. But no pattern appears in the types of institutions— or sections of institutions—devoted to the care of the terminally ill. A hospice may be a wing in a hospital or simply a group of hospital beds that can be made available as needed. A hospice may also be a separate building or institution. While families provide much of the care as long as patients are at home, a team including a physician, nurses, counselors, home health aides and others may be continually on call. The team provides continuity between home and hospice when patients must be institutionalized. At all times, the individual patient's comfort is a prime consideration.

Patients enter hospice programs at their own requests. A physician's referral, indicating that the prognosis is no more than six months, may also be required.

34

Voluntary Health Agencies

Major Agencies

The establishment of more than 100 voluntary health agencies since the beginning of this century has been a major factor in the growth of health services to the American public. These agencies, whose activities are made possible by donations of time and money from the public, occasionally augmented by government grants for special projects, have the following objectives: spreading information about various diseases to the professional and lay public; sponsoring research; promoting legislation; and operating referral services on the community level to patients in need of diagnosis, treatment, and financial aid.

Some of these agencies, such as the American Diabetes Association or the Arthritis Foundation, focus on a particular disease; others deal with problems arising from related disorders, such as the National Association for Mental Health and the American Heart Association. Still others, such as Planned Parenthood and the American Social Health Association, have programs vital not only to individuals, but to society as a whole.

To coordinate the activities of these many groups, to promote better health facilities, and to establish standards for the organization and conduct of these agencies, the National Health Council was founded in 1920. Its membership includes government, professional, and community associations, as well as the 21 voluntary health agencies described below, which command a total budget of almost $1.5 billion and involve the services of almost 12 million volunteers.

All of these organizations function on the national, state, and community level. Information and literature may be obtained through local chapters or by writing to the national office of the organization. Volunteers may offer their services in a variety of ways: as office workers, fund raisers, speakers, and community coordinators.

On the following pages, voluntary health agencies are discussed under the subjects with which they are concerned; the subjects are arranged alphabetically. Following these agencies is a brief discussion of other voluntary health agencies. Because of limitations of space, however, many worthwhile organizations have had to be omitted.

Accident Prevention

The National Safety Council, 444 North Michigan Avenue, Chicago, Illinois 60611, was founded in 1913 to improve factory safety but soon broadened its activities to preventing every type of accident. The Council is now composed of groups and individuals from every part of the population: business, industry, government, education, religion, labor, and law. Its main efforts are devoted to building strong support for official safety programs at the national, state, and community levels in specific areas, such as traffic, labor, and home.

The Council believes that practically all accidents can be prevented with the application of the right safeguards. These safeguards include public education and awareness of danger, enforcement of safety laws and regulations, and improved design standards for machines, farm equipment, and motor vehicles.

It maintains the world's largest library of accident prevention materials, distributes a wide variety of safety literature, and issues awards for outstanding safety achievements.

It also serves as a national and international clearing house of information about the causes of accidents and how they can be prevented.

In addition to campaigning for increased safety legislation on the national and state level, the Council's current programs include a defensive driving course, which provides effective adult driver training on a mass scale; a safety training institute; environmental and occupational health and "Right-to-Know" educational materials; and several approaches to the alcohol and driving problem.

Its publication, *Family Safety and Health,* has record circulation of more than two million readers, and its manual called *Fundamentals of Industrial Hygiene* provides more than 1,000 pages of material essential to the safety of factory workers.

The Council in recent years has expanded its safety promotion work to include both on- and off-the-job safety for workers and their families, as well as 24-hour-a-day safety for all persons in all activities.

Alcoholism

The National Council on Alcoholism and Drug Dependence, 12 W. 21st Street, New York, New York 10010, is the only national voluntary health agency founded to combat alcoholism as a disease by an extensive program on the professional and community level. The Council is completely independent of Alcoholics Anonymous, although the two organizations cooperate fully.

In nearly 200 cities where the Council has affiliates, alcoholism information centers have been established that provide referral services for alcoholics and drug addicts and their families as well as educational materials for all segments of the community, including physicians and nurses, the clergy, the courts, social workers, and welfare agencies. Local affiliates also help to develop labor-management programs that provide help for employees who suffer from the disease.

The Council also sponsors research, professional training, and legislative action. Its publications department distributes a variety of fact sheets, pamphlets, posters, and videos. For a listing of publications or information on the Council's programs, write the national headquarters or contact the nearest local affiliate.

Arthritis

The Arthritis Foundation, 1314 Spring Street N.W., Atlanta, Georgia 30309, was established to help arthritis sufferers and their physicians through programs of research, patient services, public health information, and education on the professional and popular level. Its long-term goal is to find the cause, prevention, and cure for the nation's number one crippling disease.

The Foundation operates local chapters throughout the United States whose chief concern is the patient who has or might have arthritis. These chapters are centers for information about the disease itself and also serve as referral centers for treatment facilities. In addition, they distribute literature and sponsor forums on the latest developments in research and patient care.

Some chapters support arthritis clinics and home care programs; most conduct patient self-help programs such as discussion groups and exercise classes. Parent groups are often maintained for parents of children with arthritis.

Two special groups work within the Foundation: the Arthritis Health Professions Association which devotes itself to continuing education for health professionals caring for arthritis patients and the American Juvenile Arthritis Organization for those with a special interest in arthritis in children. A major part of the Foundation's work at the national level is providing funds for fellowships to young physicians and scientists so that they may continue their work in arthritis research and in funding through annual grants research at major institutions throughout the United States.

Cancer

The American Cancer Society, 1599 Clifton Rd. N.E., Atlanta, Georgia 30329, was established in 1913 by a small group of physicians and volunteer workers to inform the public about the possibility of saving lives through the early diagnosis and treatment of cancer. The Society now has 57 regional groups, one in each state plus one in the District of Columbia and six other metropolitan areas, devoted to the control and eradication of cancer. In addition to the physicians, research scientists, and other professional workers engaged in the Society's activities, more than two million volunteers are connected with its many programs.

The American Cancer Society conducts widespread campaigns to educate the public in the importance of annual medical checkups so that cancerous symptoms can be detected while they are still curable. Such checkups should include an examination of the rectum and colon and, for women, examination of the breasts and a Pap test for the detection of uterine cancer.

In another of its campaigns, the Society emphasizes the link between cigarette smoking and lung cancer. It also sponsors an extensive program to persuade teenagers not to start smoking. During its annual April Crusade against Cancer, the Society distributes approximately 40 million copies of a leaflet containing lifesaving information on early detection of cancer.

On the professional level, the major objective of the Society is to make every physician's office a cancer-detection center. To achieve this goal, it publishes a variety of literature, offers refresher courses, sponsors seminars, and cooperates closely with local and state medical societies and health departments on the diagnosis and treatment of cancer. It also arranges national and international conferences for the exchange of information on the newest cancer-fighting techniques, and finances a million-dollar-a-year clinical fellowship program for young physicians.

Among its special services to patients are sponsorship of the International Association of Laryngectomies, for people who have lost their voices to cancer; and Reach to Recovery, a program for women who have had treatment for breast cancer and who need support and guidance to return to normal living. On the community level, the American Cancer Society operates a counseling service for cancer patients and their families, referring them to the proper medical facilities and social agencies for treatment and care. Through its "loan closets," it provides sickroom necessities, hospital beds, medical dressings, and so on.

Some local divisions offer home care programs through the services of the Visiting Nurse Association or a similar agency. Although the Society does not operate medical facilities, treat patients, or pay physicians' fees, some of the chapters support cancer detection programs and professionally supervised rehabilitation services.

Cerebral Palsy

The United Cerebral Palsy Associations, 7 Penn Plaza, Suite 804, New York, New York 10001, founded in 1948 by a small group of concerned parents, now has 203 affiliates across the country where those who have the condition may obtain treatment referral, therapy, and education. The Associations also play an important role in vocational training, job placement programs, housing, and recreational services.

The Research and Educational Foundation of this organization supports studies investigating possible causes of cerebral palsy. The Foundation also gives grants to universities and medical schools for research into the causes and prevention of cerebral palsy and new methods of therapy, for training medical and other professional personnel in the management of this condition.

Cystic Fibrosis

The Cystic Fibrosis Foundation, 6931 Arlington Road, No. 200, Bethesda, Maryland 20814, was organized in 1955 by a group of concerned parents whose children were born with this lung disease. The Foundation now concerns itself with all serious lung ailments of children regardless of their medical names, and it engages in a broad program of research, medical education, public information, and the sponsorship of diagnostic and treatment centers.

The Foundation's 58 local chapters offer advice and information to parents of children with severe lung disease, and have direct connections with the more than 120 Cystic Fibrosis Centers throughout the country. They refer patients to sources of financial aid, make arrangements for the purchase of drugs at a discount, and lend home treatment equipment to families who cannot afford to buy it.

The national organization makes grants for research activities, conducts professional conferences, and publishes literature for physicians and the general public on various aspects of childhood lung diseases.

Diabetes

The American Diabetes Association, National Service Center, P.O. Box 25757, 1660 Duke Street, Alexandria, Virginia 22314, was established as a professional society in 1940. In recent years it has enlarged its scope so that it currently has 800 affiliated local chapters throughout the country that promote the creation of better understanding of diabetes among patients and their families; the exchange of knowledge among physicians and other scientists; the spreading of accurate information to the general public about early recognition and supervision of the disease; and the sponsorship of basic research.

Since 1948, the American Diabetes Association has conducted an annual Diabetes Detection Drive supported by widespread publicity in all news media. During this drive, approximately three million testing kits are provided to state and county medical societies to facilitate the early detection and prompt treatment of the disorder. This annual activity hopes to find the estimated 1,600,000 people who are unaware that they have diabetes.

Among the Association's publications of special interest to diabetics and their families are the *Diabetes Forecast,* a national magazine that presents news items on research and treatment; *Meal Planning with Exchange Lists,* prepared with the cooperation of the American Dietetic Association and the U.S. Public Health Services; and *A Cookbook for Diabetics,* which contains attractive recipes for meals that can be served to diabetics.

Other activities of the Association include encouraging the employment of diabetics and providing special groups such as teachers, police, and social agencies with information on the condition. It also established a classification of the disease according to its severity. Guidelines on emergency medical care and the scientific journal *Diabetes* are available to physicians.

Drug Abuse

The American Social Health Association, which was organized originally to combat the spread of venereal disease, expanded its program in 1960 to include drug abuse education. For information about its activities in this field, see below under "Sexually Transmitted Diseases."

Eye Diseases

The National Society to Prevent Blindness, 79 Madison Avenue, New York, New York 10016, was founded in 1908 to reduce the number of cases of infants born with impaired sight. In subsequent years, it merged with the

American Association for the Conservation of Vision and the Ophthalmological Foundation. The Society is now concerned with investigating all causes of blindness and supports measures and community services that will eliminate them. It also distributes information on the proper care and use of the eyes.

The organization's first and most significant victory was the adoption of laws by almost all states requiring that silver nitrate solution be routinely dropped into the eyes of all newborn babies to counteract the possibility of congenital blindness. This resulted in a dramatic drop in the number of children suffering from eye impairment dating from birth.

For almost half a century, the Society has actively campaigned to reduce the number of people suffering from glaucoma, one of the leading causes of blindness in the United States. It has also conducted a national program to educate the elderly in the ease, safety, and advantages of surgery for cataracts, the leading cause of blindness among the aged.

Since 1926, the Society has been conducting preschool vision screening programs administered by teams that travel from big cities to isolated rural communities. Current activities also include research into the cause, treatment, and prevention of eye diseases leading to blindness; assembling data and publishing reports; cooperating with community agencies to improve eye health; promoting conditions in schools and industry to safeguard vision; and advocating eye examinations in early childhood so that disorders can be properly and promptly corrected.

Family Planning

Planned Parenthood Federation of America, 810 Seventh Avenue, New York, New York 10019, is the nation's oldest and largest voluntary family planning organization. Tracing its origins to 1916, when Margaret Sanger founded the first U.S. birth control clinic in Brooklyn, New York, Planned Parenthood maintains that every individual has the fundamental right to choose when or whether to have a child.

Planned Parenthood has five key goals:

- To increase the availability and accessibility of high-quality and affordable reproductive health care services and information, especially for underserved groups

- To reduce adolescent pregnancy and unwanted births to teens

- To meet the challenge of changes in health care delivery systems and maintain high-quality, efficiently run, and creative Planned Parenthood programs

- To further Planned Parenthood's role in the provision of education of human sexuality, reproduction, and population, and on the bioethical and legal implications of reproductive technology

- To increase access to safe and effective methods of voluntary fertility regulation for individuals in developing countries

Each year, more than three million individuals in 49 states and the District of Columbia obtain medical, educational, and counseling services through more than 900 clinics operated by Planned Parenthood's 171 affiliates. The organization is active in more than 100 developing countries throughout the world. In addition, Planned Parenthood conducts clinical research, provides professional training of health and education personnel, and serves as a resource to health agencies, government agencies at the state and federal levels, legislators and other policy makers, and the media.

Heart Disease

The American Heart Association, 7320 Greenville Avenue, Dallas, Texas 75231, was founded in 1924 as a professional organization of cardiologists. It was reorganized in 1948 as a national voluntary health agency to promote a program of education, research, and community service in the interests of reducing premature death and disability caused by diseases of the heart and blood vessels. The complex of heart disorders, including atherosclerosis, stroke, high blood pressure, kidney diseases, rheumatic fever, and congenital heart disturbances, is by far the leading cause of death in the United States.

Since its first Annual Heart Fund Campaign in 1949, the Association has contributed more than $150 million to research and has been a major factor in the reduction of cardiovascular mortality statistics. It has spent more than $2 million since 1959 studying human heart transplantation procedures, and has contributed to the development of an artificial heart, plastic heart valves, and synthetic arteries.

Public and professional education programs designed to reduce the risk of heart attack through avoidance of cigarette smoking, obesity, and foods high in cholesterol are conducted on a nationwide and community level by the Association's affiliates throughout the country. The local chapters are also engaged in service programs for rheumatic fever prevention, stroke rehabilitation, school health, cardiopulmonary resuscitation, and industrial health. In addition, they conduct information and referral services for patients and their families.

The American Heart Association publishes many technical and professional journals as well as material designed for the general public.

Hemophilia

The National Hemophilia Foundation, 110 Green Street, Room 406, New York, New York 10012, was established in 1948 to serve the needs of hemophiliacs and their families by ensuring the availability of treatment and rehabilitation facilities. It is estimated that there are as many as 100,000 males suffering from what is popularly known as "bleeder's disease," an inherited condition passed from mothers to sons.

The long-term goal of the Foundation is to develop a national program of research and clinical study that will provide new information about early diagnosis and effective treatment of the disorder as well as trained professional personnel to administer patient care.

The development in recent years of blood-clotting concentrates is the most important advance to date in the treatment of the disease. This development, supported in part by the Foundation's 48 chapters, makes it possible for patients to have elective surgery and dental work, and to eliminate much of the pain, crippling, and hospitalization of those suffering from hemophilia.

The need for blood supplies from which to extract the clotting factor caused the Foundation to embark on an extensive campaign for blood donations. For this purpose, it has been working closely since 1968 with the American Red Cross and the American Association of Blood Banks. It also maintains close ties with various laboratories and research groups in the development of more powerful concentrates that can be manufactured and sold at the lowest possible cost.

The organization's activities include a national network of facilities with blood banks, clinics, and treatment centers as well as referral services. It has also established a Behavioral Science Department to explore the nonmedical aspects of hemophiliacs' problems, such as education, vocational guidance, and psychological needs.

Kidney Disease

The National Kidney Foundation, 30 E. 33rd Street, Suite 1100, New York, New York 10016, formerly the National Kidney Disease Foundation, was founded in 1950 by a group of parents whose children had a disease with no cure—nephrosis. The ultimate goal was the total eradication of all diseases of the kidney and urinary tract. Today, although there remains no cure for nephrosis, the disease is almost totally treatable. In the past two decades the National Kidney Foundation and its 49 affiliates nationwide have supported more than $20 million in research to find the answers to kidney and urinary tract related diseases.

The National Kidney Foundation and its affiliates sponsor a wide variety of programs in treatment, service, education, and prevention that are designed to aid the patient in the community. Examples of some affiliate programs include: information and referral programs for patients and their families, drug banks, support groups, summer camp programs for children on dialysis and transplantations, transportation services, counseling and screening, and direct financial assistance to needy patients.

The National Kidney Foundation seeks continually to increase the number of organs available for transplantation through its nationwide Organ Donor Program. To date, more than 50 million donor cards have been distributed by the Foundation and its affiliates. Distribution of public and professional educational materials continues to heighten public awareness of organ donation and the "Gift of Life" it can provide to thousands of people waiting for a kidney transplant.

Mental Health

The National Mental Health Association, 1021 Prince Street, Alexandria, Virginia 22314-2971, was founded in 1909 to work toward the improved care and treatment of people with mental illnesses, the promotion of mental health, and the prevention of mental disorders. The original National Committee for Mental Hygiene merged with the National Mental Health Foundation and the Psychiatric Foundation in 1950 to create the organization as it now stands.

The association implements its service programs through its 650 affiliates (local chapters and larger state divisions) across the country. These mental health associations tailor their efforts to the needs of their communities.

The National Mental Health Association is composed of one million volunteers and supporters who have a keen interest in mental health. They include family members whose loved ones have been affected by mental illnesses, current or former consumers, mental health professionals, and lay citizens.

Recent and ongoing activities include:

- Coordinated a national coalition to address the needs of people with mental illnesses who are homeless.

- Serves as a prime source of referral and educational information on mental illnesses and mental health issues through the NMHA Mental Health Information Center.

- Assists local and state MHA affiliates in serving communities through patient and family support groups, housing programs, suicide-prevention hotlines, and school mental health education programs.

- Helped extend the civil rights protection of the 8th and 14th Amendments to the U.S. Constitution to the mentally disabled by representing persons with severe mental illnesses before the Supreme Court.

- Specified a "state-of-the-art" program to prevent severe mental and emotional disabilities in a landmark 1986 report by its National Commission on the Prevention of Mental-Emotional Disabilities.

- Serves as the public-interest policy voice for mental health issues in the Congress and state legislatures.

Multiple Sclerosis

The National Multiple Sclerosis Society, 205 East 42nd Street, New York, New York 10017, was founded in 1946 with the primary goal of supporting research on this chronic neurological disease whose cause and cure are unknown. Some 250,000 Americans are estimated to have multiple sclerosis (MS).

Research aimed at finding the cause and methods of arresting MS is being conducted worldwide. From the beginning the Society has made every effort to increase professional and public awareness of the symptoms of MS and the best ways of treating them. This is done through a network of 143 chapters and branches and some 470,000 active members. The chapters, which are either affiliated with or support MS clinics around the country, provide home and hospital visits, recreational programs, referrals for medical care, job counseling, and other services. The chapters also arrange educational programs for physicians and social workers as well as for patients and their families. The society sponsors public education awards in magazine, radio, and television writing and conducts Project Rembrandt, a biennial competition for artists with MS.

The national office distributes publications for physicians and the interested public, including guides for the development of patient services and a quarterly magazine, *Inside MS*. Films, slide presentations, videocassettes and audiocassettes are available for purchase or loan.

Physical Disabilities

The National Easter Seal Society, 70 East Lake Street, Chicago, Illinois 60601, has grown from its pioneering origins in 1919 to a national organization that serves more than one million disabled people of all ages. Among its network of facilities are comprehensive rehabilitation centers, treatment and diagnostic centers, and vocational training workshops, residential camps, special education programs, and transportation services in many different parts of the country.

Because many disabled children and adults in rural areas and small communities are unaware of the services available to them, the Society gives top priority to publicizing its information, referral, and follow-up activities. In recent years, it has also established mobile treatment units in hospitals and nursing homes in rural areas.

Other innovative activities include screening and testing programs to detect hearing loss in newborns and learning disabilities in preschool children, and providing treatment and referral for those who are disabled by respiratory diseases.

The Society collaborates with federal and professional agencies in all programs designed to eliminate architectural barriers to the disabled, and was instrumental in the enactment of legislation making it mandatory that all buildings constructed with government funds be fully and easily accessible to the disabled. It also initiates and supports significant studies in rehabilitation procedures as well as scientific research in bone transplant techniques.

Extensive literature is distributed to professionals, the public, parents, and employers. It also assembles special educational packets for parents of the disabled.

Sexually Transmitted Diseases

The American Social Health Association, P.O. Box 13827, Research Triangle Park, North Carolina 27709, was organized in 1912 to promote the control of venereal disease and to combat prostitution. In the mid-1980s the Association faced new challenges in the field of sexually transmitted diseases (STDs) while also developing new strategies to augment and complement existing AIDS information programs, promote attention to chlamydia, the most widespread STD in the United States, exert influence in Congress for additional federal funding for STD prevention and control programs, and place STD information in the hands of high-school students.

The Association is in close touch with government agencies such as the Public Health Service, the National Institutes of Health, and the various branches of the armed forces. Through these channels, it promotes its program for STD education in the schools and for research toward the discovery of an immunizing vaccine against syphilis and gonorrhea.

It is the major national voluntary repository for information and consultation on STDs, and maintains the world's most comprehensive collection of source workshops, residential camps, special education programs, and materials on STDs. It constantly helps communities in diagnosing their problems and produces a number of publications for teachers, guidance counselors, and youth workers.

The Association stresses the importance of introducing family life education into the curriculum of elementary and secondary schools and of establishing training programs on this subject in teachers' colleges. These efforts have resulted in the inclusion of family life education in an increasing number of school systems throughout the United States.

Tuberculosis and Respiratory Diseases

The American Lung Association, 1740 Broadway, New York, New York 10019, is the direct descendant of the first voluntary health organization to be formed in the United States. In 1904, when the National Association for the Study and Prevention of Tuberculosis was organized, this disease was the country's leading cause of death. Since 1973, with the sharp increase in the problems relating to smoking and air pollution, the association has been known by its present name, which was adopted to reflect the broader scope of its activities.

It now concerns itself not only with the elimination of tuberculosis but with chronic and disabling conditions, such as emphysema, and with acute diseases of the respiratory system, such as influenza. Through its affiliates and nationwide state organizations, it is actively engaged in campaigns against smoking and air pollution.

The early endeavor of the association to have tuberculosis included among the reportable diseases was accomplished state by state, and since the 1920s all states have required that every case in the country be brought to the attention of local health officials.

Public awareness of better care and the development of effective drugs have dramatically reduced the number of TB patients, but the association continues to concern itself with the fact that provisional data indicate that there are still about 22,000 new cases each year.

Through its local affiliates, the American Lung Association initiates special campaigns to combat smoking and air pollution, using radio and television announcements, car stickers, posters, and pamphlets, as well as films and exhibits. Educational materials on respiratory diseases are regularly distributed by the national office to local associations for physicians, patients, and the general public. Funds raised by the annual Christmas Seal drive also support research and medical education fellowships.

Other Voluntary Health Agencies

In addition to those voluntary health agencies that are members of the National Health Council, many other organizations function on a national scale and offer specialized services as well as literature and guidance to professionals, patients, parents, and concerned families. The following is a partial list.

Alcoholics Anonymous World Services, Box 459, Grand Central Station, New York, New York 10163, is a fellowship of men and women who share their experiences and give each other support in overcoming the problem of alcoholism. Chapters exist throughout the country and offer referral services, literature, and information about special hospital programs.

Al-Anon Family Group Headquarters, Inc., P.O. Box 862 Midtown Station, New York, New York 10016, is not affiliated with Alcoholics Anonymous, but cooperates closely with it. Al-Anon, which includes Alateen for younger members, is a primary community resource and self-help fellowship for the families and friends of alcoholics. Members share their experiences, strength, and hope at regularly held meetings, and learn to cope with the effects of being close to an alcoholic. Headquarters registers, services, and provides literature to 25,000 groups worldwide, of which 18,000 are in the United States.

Asthma and Allergy Foundation of America, 1835 K Street, N.W., Suite P-900, Washington, D.C. 20006, was established to help solve all health problems related to allergic diseases by sponsoring research and treatment facilities. It also grants scholarships to medical students specializing in the study of allergy.

Alzheimer's Association, 70 E. Lake Street, Suite 600, Chicago, Illinois 60601, was founded in 1980 to heighten public awareness of this degenerative brain disorder, provide support for patients and their families, aid research efforts, advocate for legislation that responds to the needs of Alzheimer's disease patients and their family members, and commemorate National Alzheimer's Disease Awareness Month each November. The network includes more than 140 chapters and affiliates across the country representing over 1,000 Family Support Groups. To obtain the most up-to-date information on Alzheimer's disease legislation and research, and for referral to local chapters, call the Association's toll-free information and referral number, 800-621-0379 (in Illinois only, 800-572-6037) or write to the Association.

The *American Foundation for AIDS Research* (AmFAR), 5900 Wilshire Blvd., 2nd Floor, East Satellite, Los Angeles, California 90036, was created in 1985 as a result of the unification of two not-for-profit public foundations: the AIDS Medical Foundation (AMF), and the National AIDS Research Foundation (NARF). AmFar is an independent, national organization whose directors, committee members, and staff are professionals in the field of AIDS.

The Foundation has two main missions. First, it supports and facilitates research projects to achieve an understanding of the pathogenesis of AIDS, its prevention through the use of a vaccine, and its treatment. Second, the Foundation serves as a clearinghouse for accurate and up-to-date information on AIDS.

The C.D.C. National AIDS Hotline, (800) 342-2437 is operated by the Federal Centers for Disease Control and provides confidential and anonymous information and referrals to local health organizations, counselors, and support groups. *The C.D.C. National AIDS Clearinghouse,* P.O. Box 6003, Rockville, MD 20849, provides free educational materials on HIV and AIDS.

American Foundation for the Blind, 15 West 16th Street, New York, New York 10011, is a national nonprofit organization working with local and national services to improve the quality of life for all blind and visually impaired persons. It stocks consumer products and publications and has recorded and produced millions of talking book recordings for the Library of Congress. Through its staff of national consultants and its six regional offices, the Foundation maintains a direct liaison with state, regional, and local agencies.

The *Association for Voluntary Surgical Contraception,* 122 East 42nd Street, New York, New York 10168, was founded in 1937 to promote the right of each individual to choose sterilization as a method of birth control. A nonprofit membership organization, the AVSC has increasingly collaborated with governmental and private sector providers to ensure effective access to sterilization facilities. The Association also sponsors training, education, and program support for

sterilization and family planning counselors and others; prepares annual estimates of male and female voluntary sterilizations in the United States; issues a quarterly newsletter, the *AVSC News,* and other publications, and initiates and monitors research into medical, legal, psychological, ethical, and public health aspects of voluntary sterilization.

The Epilepsy Foundation of America, 4351 Garden City Drive, Landover, Maryland 20785, is the result of a merger in 1967 of two similar organizations. At present, the Foundation has 85 local affiliates that provide information, referral services, and counseling. It conducts a research grant program for medical and psychosocial investigation and distributes a wide variety of literature on request to physicians, teachers, employers, and the interested public on such subjects as anticonvulsant drugs, insurance, driving laws, and emergency treatment. The national office also maintains an extensive research library.

The Leukemia Society of America, 733 Third Avenue, New York, New York 10017, was organized in 1949 and now has 57 chapters. It supports research in the causes, control, and eventual eradication of the disease. The society has a continuing program of education through special publications directed to physicians, nurses, and the public. Through its local affiliates, it conducts patient-aid services that provide counseling, transportation, and—to those who need financial assistance—drugs, blood transfusions, and laboratory facilities.

The Muscular Dystrophy Association, Inc., 810 Seventh Avenue, New York, New York 10019, has as a primary goal the scientific conquest of muscular dystrophy and related neuromuscular diseases. The Association supports scientific investigators worldwide. In addition, through its 170 chapter affiliates nationwide, MDA provides a comprehensive patient and community services program to individuals diagnosed with any one of 40 neuromuscular disorders. The Association maintains a network of some 240 MDA clinics coast to coast to provide diagnostic services and therapeutic and rehabilitative follow-up care as well as genetic, vocational, and social service counseling to patients and their families. MDA also sponsors a summer camping program for youngsters aged 6 to 21 as well as adult outings, with activities geared to the special needs of those with neuromuscular diseases.

The Association for Retarded Citizens of the United States, P.O. Box 6109, Arlington, Texas 76006, established in 1950, is the nation's largest voluntary organization specifically devoted to promoting the welfare of children and adults with mental retardation. It is estimated that there are six million such persons in the United States. Through its 1,500 affiliates the association conducts and supports research, sponsors employment programs, advocates for progressive public policy, and works for better community services. Counseling and referral services, as well as extensive literature for professionals and concerned families, are available on request.

The March of Dimes Birth Defects Foundation, 1275 Mamaroneck Avenue, White Plains, New York 10605, was founded in 1938 to combat infantile paralysis (polio). In the 30 years since the conquest of polio, through the development of the Salk and Sabin polio vaccines, the March of Dimes has dedicated itself to the prevention of birth defects, the nation's number one child health problem. It does this through programs of birth defects research and medical service and education that provide new knowledge and understanding of birth defects and their prevention. More than a quarter-million babies are born with one or more of the 3,000 known birth defects each year. The Foundation also has established the Salk Institute in La Jolla, California, directed by Dr. Jonas Salk, for the purpose of carrying on basic research in life processes to discover what causes birth defects and other diseases.

Special Health Services and Agencies

Many factors have contributed to the growth of the American system of health services. Specialists in various medical specialties have tried to meet needs for new types of health care. Medical care has become so effective that individual life expectancy has increased enormously; as one result, the number of Americans aged 65 and older tripled in the three-quarters of a century between 1900 and 1975. As the population of the United States has grown older, in percentage terms, the problems of the aged have received more attention. New methods and devices have been developed for the care and assistance of the ill or disabled of any age.

Special health services and agencies help to fill such needs. Many older persons have utilized the services of trained individuals who make survival possible—sometimes at home—or slow down the rate of deterioration. Other institutions and agencies perform simple maintenance tasks for the aged or the seriously ill

or handicapped, or help with rehabilitation. Social service agencies and groups with health roles, for example, provide adult day care, homemaker assistance, and home health services that may include the following:

- Part-time or occasional nursing care, often under the supervision of a registered nurse

- Physical, occupational, or speech therapy

- Medical social services that help the patient and his or her family to adjust to the social and emotional conditions accompanying illness or disability of any kind

- Assistance from a home health aide, including help with such tasks as bathing and going to the bathroom, taking medications, exercising, and getting into and out of bed

- Under some circumstances, medical attention from interns or residents in training